Non-Epileptic Childhood Paroxysmal Disorders

Non-Epileptic Childhood Paroxysmal Disorders

FRANCIS J. DiMARIO, Jr., MD

Professor of Pediatrics and Neurology
The University of Connecticut, School of Medicine
Academic Chief of Pediatric Neurology
Associate Chair for Academic Affairs, Department of Pediatrics
Connecticut Children's Medical Center
Hartford, Connecticut

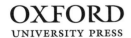

OXFORD
UNIVERSITY PRESS

2009

OXFORD

UNIVERSITY PRESS

Oxford University Press, Inc., publishes works that further
Oxford University's objective of excellence
in research, scholarship, and education.

Oxford   New York
Auckland   Cape Town   Dar es Salaam   Hong Kong   Karachi
Kuala Lumpur   Madrid   Melbourne   Mexico City   Nairobi
New Delhi   Shanghai   Taipei   Toronto

With offices in
Argentina   Austria   Brazil   Chile   Czech Republic   France   Greece
Guatemala   Hungary   Italy   Japan   Poland   Portugal   Singapore
South Korea   Switzerland   Thailand   Turkey   Ukraine   Vietnam

Published by Oxford University Press, Inc.
198 Madison Avenue, New York, 10016

www.oup.com

The science of medicine is a rapidly changing field. As new research and clinical experience broaden our
knowledge, changes in treatment and drug therapy occur. The author and publisher of this work have checked
with sources believed to be reliable in their efforts to provide information that is accurate and complete, and in
accordance with the standards accepted at the time of publication. However, in light of the possibility of human
error or changes in the practice of medicine, neither the author, nor the publisher, nor any other party who has
been involved in the preparation or publication of this work warrants that the information contained herein is
in every respect accurate or complete. Readers are encouraged to confirm the information contained herein
with other reliable sources and are strongly advised to check the product information sheet provided by the
pharmaceutical company for each drug they plan to administer.

Library of Congress Cataloging-in-Publication Data
DiMario, Francis J.
   Non-epileptic childhood paroxysmal disorders / Francis J. DiMario, Jr.
      p.   ;   cm.
   Includes bibliographical references and index.
   ISBN 978-0-19-533537-8
   1. Epilepsy in children—Diagnosis.   2. Nervous system—Diseases—Diagnosis.   3. Children—Diseases—
Diagnosis.   4. Diagnosis, Differential.   5. Neurologic manifestations of general diseases.   I. Title.
[DNLM: 1. Neurobehavioral Manifestations.   2. Child.   3. Factitious Disorders.   4. Migraine
Disorders.   5. Movement Disorders.   6. Sleep Disorders.   7. Somatoform Disorders.
WL 340 D5815n 2009]
RJ496.E6D52 2009
618.92'853—dc22

                                                                                          2008036665

1   3   5   7   9   8   6   4   2
Printed in the United States of America
on acid-free paper

To Sandy, Trevor, and Tyler, may I rise to your expectations, immensely grateful for your being.

Acknowledgments

It has been a long and arduous journey through the final notations on these pages. It began not merely at the moment when this manuscript had its genesis but rather when a childhood desire became a life passion, one that continues to fulfill and enrich. This was a journey joyously taken.

Inspiration emanates from many sources, some unexpected, others consistently depended upon. My entire family has always been a source of dependable and unquestioning encouragement. My parents, Betty and Frank, fostered the curiosity to ask, the determination to try, the humility to accept, and the gratitude to be thankful for all that one has. My wife, Sandy, whom I suspect was cut from a similar stock, has been tolerant of my faults, understanding of my absences, unendingly supportive, and loving beyond all measure. I can only thank you with all my heart and promise to tell you that more often. My children, Trevor and Tyler, have also endured the journey and have been a source of continued pride. Hopefully, they will embark upon their own journeys with an appreciation of that which is truly important in life.

I would like to thank a few others in my past with whom I have had the privilege to work and learn from, even if only tacitly, over my career thus far. I am deeply indebted to Drs. Marcelina Mian and William Rowley, who extended an opportunity and fostered great hope and encouragement; Dr. RJ McKay, the pediatrician's pediatrician, who taught by example; Dr. Paul Young, a pediatrician who embodied what a mentor should be; Dr. ES Emery, a wonderful role model, who shared his talents and dedication to children with enthusiasm; Dr. Peter Berman, an astute clinician and unassuming man to whom I shall always be grateful for offering me the chance of a lifetime, Drs. Arthur Asbury and Gunter Hasse, whose immense funds of knowledge were eclipsed only by their humility and bedside manner; and to Dr. JBP Stephenson, who continues to instill intellectual curiosity with an insistence to always ask questions and seek their answers.

I shall always hold a special fondness for my Connecticut colleagues, with whom I have worked and shared but from whom I have received much more in kind: Dr. Les Wolfson, for always offering support; Dr. Lou Reik, for his pithy interrogatory; Dr. Jim Donaldson, who reminded me that at its core neurology is a wonderful story; Dr. Bob Greenstein, a good friend and sage advisor; Dr. Barry Russman, whose optimism and outlook on life deserve envy; Dr. Bob Cerciello, whose work ethic and dedication I admire and can only attempt to emulate; Dr. Ed Zalneraitis, an esteemed educator, scholar, and healer, a true triple threat; Dr. Phil Brunquell, who personifies conscientious and compassionate care; Dr. Carol Leicher, who exemplifies perseverance and dependability; and Jamie Cubanski and Deb Johnson, two wonderful nurses who have provided immense personal support, an enthusiastic and cheerful presence, and a calm reassuring voice for all my patients.

Finally, I would be remiss if I did not thank the countless children and families for whom I have had the privilege to serve over the years; these children have been the sources of true inspiration, fulfillment, and the journey's motivation.

I would like to extend my appreciation to the medical library staffs at the Lyman Maynard Stowe medical library of the University of Connecticut and the Hartford Hospital medical library that assisted in the acquisition of countless references.

Preface

This is a book written for those of us who evaluate the many quirks and behaviors encountered in the lives of developing children. The number of important pathologic conditions that befall this age group is staggering. However, equally staggering is the number of episodic and often benign or developmentally programmed paroxysmal events encountered in this population. The nature of these episodic events in many circumstances leads to their erroneous identification as epileptic in nature. It is my hope that this book will serve as a compendium of those episodically manifest entities often uniquely observed in childhood.

The book is organized with some foundations in terminology and an in-depth analysis of the epidemiology of many of these disorders. As best possible, epidemiologic data are compiled with incidence and prevalence figures provided for comparisons. Discussion on the deductive approach to their clinical assessment is provided along with emphasis on the diagnostic clues contained within the descriptive and observational information provided during clinical evaluation. A categorization of the differential features and ages of presentation are provided as a means to help direct logical diagnostic considerations. Subsequent chapters are organized by major topic: Syncopes, Sleep Phenomena, Somatization, Factitious Illness, Movement Disorders, and Migraine Syndromes. Each chapter provides discourse on the general principles of underlying pathophysiologic mechanisms and current knowledge about the chapter topic under discussion. Specific clinical entities encompassed within the general topic are then discussed individually with particular attention to their clinical descriptions and presentations, natural history, particular pathophysiology, genetics, pertinent laboratory, and treatments. The text is amplified by pertinent tables highlighting diagnostic criteria where this applies and reference information where needed and is generously referenced to encompass the most relevant information available.

I hope that this text will assist in discerning the many identifiable nonepileptic paroxysmal behaviors encountered in children as well as serve to better categorize them. Clinicians are encouraged to continue to further identify and understand additional entities within this field of study. In order to understand we must first ask, in order to ask we must first observe. There is much we need to observe, ask and, understand.

Contents

Non-Epileptic Childhood Paroxysmal Disorders

1

General Principles and Epidemiology

INTRODUCTION

The non-epileptic paroxysmal childhood disorders are a group of disorders, syndromes, and phenomena that often mimic true epileptic seizures.[1-5] Many of these recognized entities are not pathologic at all but rather variations in normal childhood behavior or physiological functions. These are typically brought to medical attention by parents and caregivers who are surprised to witness a generally recurring, observable, discrete behavior not in context of that usually displayed by the child. When this is associated with an alteration in consciousness or level of alertness, or interferes with a normal sleep pattern, a more prompt and expeditious evaluation may be precipitated. Alternatively, a more insidious repetition of behaviors can develop often without recognition until a more intermittently available observer notes the behavior. These are more often not associated with alterations in consciousness or sleep and therefore tend not to intrude into the activities of the child or alter functions. Clearly, there are a number of phenomena in each of these categories that do interfere or are more dramatic in presentation and therefore difficult to overlook. Clinical experience and a clear description of the event in question will usually lead to a correct categorization. These encompass all ages, from neonate through young adulthood and older.[6] The individual clinical entities are apt to be among the most common diagnostic challenges clinicians regularly encounter in practice. The keys to diagnosis are a detailed history, careful observation, and judicious laboratory testing. No detail is unimportant! In fact, the more precise the details surrounding the event, the more precise the diagnosis will be (Table 1-1).[1]

Despite the large number of discrete entities enumerated herein, there are certain essential principles in a clinical approach, which can elucidate a diagnosis. Each specific entity can pose a significant clinical challenge in identification, etiologic pathophysiology, applicable genetic inheritance, and management. A number of classification schemas may be employed to aid organization and approach.[1-6] A simple division is offered here separating those episodes that are associated with a predominant alteration in mental status or occur during sleep and those that at initiation begin without a predominant alteration in mental status or occur while wakeful (Table 1-2).[1] There are some entities that straddle this arbitrary line of divide; however, each clinician may adapt this schema depending upon his or her own experience.

3

Table 1-1 Fundamental Queries for Patient History

- Age at onset?
- Is there more than one type of event?
- What is happening just prior to the event?
- Does the child seem to have a warning or recognizable behavioral prodrome?
- What is the exact sequence of events?
- Is the event stereotyped or does it vary?
- What are the child's posture, tone, respiratory pattern, color, and behavior before, during, and after the event?
- What is the relationship of the event to activity, attention, play, limit setting, temperament, sleep, and diet?
- What seems to ameliorate the phenomenon?
- What seems to precipitate the phenomenon?
- Are the events suppressible by the child?
- Can the child be distracted during the event?
- Are there any concurrent symptoms, clinical signs, or autonomic changes?
- What does the child do immediately afterward?
- How aware is the child of the preceding event?
- Can the observer estimate the duration of the event, the frequency of the events, and the periodicity of the events?
- Are there any family members with similar or related phenomena?
- Can the observer mimic the event or video record it?

Table 1-2 Classification Schema of Paroxysmal Non-epileptic Disorders

Paroxysmal Disorders Occurring with Alterations in Consciousness or Sleep

Syncopes
Severe breath-holding spells
Hyperventilation syndrome
Sleep-related phenomena
Apnea
Somatoform disorder
Munchausen syndrome
Others

Paroxysmal Disorders Occurring without Alterations in Consciousness or Sleep

Simple breath-holding spells
Movement disorders
Hyperekplexia
Stereotypies and self-stimulatory behaviors
Headache syndromes
Gastroesophageal reflux
Nasopharyngeal reflux
Severe Paroxysmal Pain Disorder (Familial Rectal Pain Syndrome)

Episodic behavioral syndromes
Paroxysmal extraocular gaze deviations
Somatoform disorder
Munchausen syndrome
Others

Elements that impact upon specific diagnostic considerations include age, specific provocative events, associated clinical findings, and familial and genetic influences. There is no substitute for observing the event first hand. In the absence of direct observation, parental video recordings can be immensely helpful. Occasionally, movement or only a partial recording captured or any number of other amateur mistakes made may obscure these. However, despite their shortcomings it is a glimpse at the event of interest. Although the parental home recordings do not incorporate simultaneous EEGs, they are recordings, nonetheless, of the actual events for which the evaluation is sought in 100%. Numerous reported series of pediatric video EEG telemetry recordings from epilepsy centers worldwide report some finite number of days dedicated to recording and capturing the events in question. Clearly, the duration of time spent recording increases the "diagnostic yield" of the test. Nonetheless, upwards of 17%–32% of the patients who undergo prolonged recording do so without capturing even a single event for which the referral was made.[4,7]

THE CLINICAL PROBLEM AND EPIDEMIOLOGY

The non-epileptic paroxysmal childhood disorders have by definition episodic periodicities, variable durations, and generally stereotyped characters. These qualities also describe true epileptic events. One may not be able to differentiate between epileptic phenomenon and non-epileptic phenomenon at first assessment. It is also possible that individual children will have more than a single phenomenon. There is considerable literature dedicated to the role for video EEG telemetry assessment and characterization of non-epileptic seizures (pseudoseizures, psychogenic seizures) from true epileptic seizures. This emphasis in differentiation stems from the fact that the predominant source of reported data is from surgical epilepsy centers, where correct diagnosis and seizure characterization is vital. These sources of data incur an inherent bias in the epidemiology of non-epileptic paroxysmal childhood disorders. In these settings, the identification of non-epileptic paroxysmal childhood disorders has ranged from 15% to 90% depending on the age range studied and the nature of the series and reason for referral, for example, sleep phenomenon, staring spells, infantile spasms, neonatal movements, compiled statistics, etc.[4,6–12] The attribute of the non-epileptic events can be further classified into nonorganic/nonphysiologic events from those that are organic/physiologic and epileptic seizures. Nonorganic/nonphysiologic events tend to be found most often both in the adolescent ages (12–18 years) and, to a greater degree, in older childhood (5–12 years) when compared with young children. Confirmed psychiatric diagnoses in these ages include Munchausen syndrome, intermittent explosive disorder, panic attacks, conversion disorders, and psychogenic events.[4,6,7,13–17]

Paroxysmal disorders of sleep have been best characterized through specific assessment with polysomnography. Paroxysmal motor behaviors and other phenomena in sleep have been carefully differentiated from nocturnal seizures by this means. This organized approach to study and definition has led to an international consensus defined in the International Classification of Sleep Disorders.[18] The major categories of importance are divided into parasomnias (disorders of arousal), sleep-related movements, and other sleep-related events.[18–20] The utility of polysomnography in this instance is to better qualify the exact sleep stage in which the behavior occurs. The clinician must bear in mind that especially during sleep the coexistence of true epileptic events can mimic otherwise identified non-epileptic behaviors.[21,22] Supplementary motor seizures and other epileptic frontal lobe ictal phenomena can, for example, give the appearance of psychogenic seizures.[21]

The vast majority of remaining entities are recognized clinically as physical movements and postures, brief alterations in consciousness, aberrations of patient perceptions, and periodic behavioral syndromes.[1–5] The tried and true classical approach to diagnosis with careful history and examination will arrive at an accurate identification of the problem in most instances. The perspective of time and periodic observation will allow the clinician sufficient opportunity to amass ample clinical data on the entity at hand. It must be remembered that as clinicians we work with children. By virtue of their various ages and maturity levels or additional underlying neurological impairments that exist, there will often be a lack of additional insight or descriptive embellishment. In some respects this allows for a more pure observation of the event at hand. However, in these circumstances so much of what we seek to answer from patient interview and individual portrayal of symptoms may go unanswered or misinterpreted. The acknowledgment of misdiagnosis, particularly of epilepsy, in these populations (infants, young children, and neurologically impaired children) may be substantial.[22–29] An even more important concept is that there may be ambiguity and clinical uncertainty for any specific diagnosis, epileptic or non-epileptic.[30] The occurrence of a misdiagnosis of epilepsy is recognized worldwide and may be more problematic when made by nonspecialists. The ratio of misdiagnosis to correct diagnosis has been found to be as high as 3:1 in some population studies.[28] Overall, epilepsy misdiagnoses in children range from 4.6% to 39% when definitive diagnoses (epileptic and non-epileptic) are ultimately arrived at.[7,24–29] Even when affirmed by specialists and epilepsy centers alike, the rates arrived at for uncertain or ambiguous diagnosis may be underestimated. The "uncertain" diagnostic category has been reported to be between 0% and 24%.[26,30] In a summary tabulation of a published series of diagnoses made from EEG telemetry studies in specialty centers, an overall rate of 15.6% of some 4237 subjects were identified as uncertain (Table 1-3). There may be several factors contributing to this likely underestimate, chief among them may be our own reluctance as clinicians to recognize and acknowledge diagnostic uncertainty. This is amplified when diagnostic interrater agreement studies for diagnosis and classification of first seizures are performed, where agreement may be only moderate at best.[31] The identification of "unclassified paroxysmal events" aids the patient in several ways: (1) It avoids unnecessary and potentially incorrect treatment, (2) reduces the inevitable stigma and negative impact upon the daily life activity of the patient, (3) encourages the family to continue to monitor for new and important signs and symptoms, and (4) may lead to the recognition of another important and clinically distinct diagnosis. This is not, however, to advocate for more intense or rigorous testing in order to "rule out" or "exclude" otherwise unlikely diagnoses but rather to be more observant and critical about the relevant details of the events at hand. Additional important aspects of diagnostic accuracy incorporate longitudinal observation and reassessment. There have been at least seven large studies, which have expressed these issues.[7,26–30] The initial diagnosis of epilepsy was felt to be "in doubt" upon referral in 16%–33% of the subjects studied, and it subsequently changed to specific non-epileptic paroxysmal disorders in up to a third of the subjects upon longitudinal review.[7,26–30] There was a variety of diagnostic entities ultimately arrived at, with staring behavior and reflex anoxic seizures most commonly reassigned.

A few population studies have added insight into the rates of misdiagnosis of epilepsy and prevalence data on non-epileptic paroxysmal events.[28,32–34] In these retrospective analyses, the terms are defined more precisely, diagnostic criteria applied equally, and the passage of time and observation act in favor of greater precision in diagnosis. In 1991, Somoza et al. ascertained the true prevalence of epilepsy in primary school children of Buenos Aires, Argentina, by carrying out a randomized, systematic cross-sectional survey of 10% of the entire (302,032 students estimated) primary school population ages 6–16 years. Data were collected on 26,270 students who responded (83.1% of the selected school population) out of 2,965,403 city district inhabitants.[28] The responders comprised those children attending both public (57.8%) and private (42.2%) schools. The first phase of the study was an analysis of a previously validated standardized epilepsy questionnaire given to the children at selected school sites. Those with positive responses to predetermined epilepsy criteria were further interviewed in person by a neurologist. The second phase of the study consisted of a concurring panel of three neurologists agreeing on the probable positive ($n = 1792$) and negative ($n = 24,478$) epilepsy diagnoses with predetermined criteria according to the International League against Epilepsy.[32] There were 1461 probable positive and 982 probable negative cases randomly chosen for subsequent interview. The resulting analysis after the interviews determined that there

Table 1-3 Summary of EEG Telemetry Series with Non-Epileptic Paroxysmal Events Identified*

EEG Telemetry Recorded Events	Kotagal[4] N=883	Bye[7] N=666	Gibbs[23] N=900	Stroink[26] N=881	Uldall[29] N=223	Beach[30] N=684	Totals N=4237[†]
Single Seizure	0	0	0	80	1	32	113 (2.6%)
Febrile/Acute Symptomatic Seizure	0	1	10	2	6	220	239 (5.6%)
Epilepsy	59 (18%)	269 (40%)	819 (91%)	494 (56%)	130 (58%)	131 (19.1%)	1902 (44.9%)
Non-Epileptic Paroxysmal Events	199 (22.5%)	397 (59.6%)	81 (9%)	175 (19.8%)	87 (39%)	272 (39.4%)	1211 (28.6%)[‡]
(EEG Recorded)	134	285	81	54	87	243	884 (20.8%)
(No EEG Recording)	65	112	0	121	0	29	327 (7.7%)
Syncope	1	3	11	14	4	60	93 (7.6%)
Severe Breath-Holding Spells	3	2	20	6	2	56	86 (7.1%)
Hyperventilation Syndrome	1				3		4 (0.3%)
Sleep-Related Phenomena*:	24	88	8	1	5	13	139 (11.4%)
(Neonatal Sleep Myoclonus)	3					5	8 (0.7%)
(Hypnic Jerks)	11	43	3				57 (4.7%)
(Disorders of Arousal)	10	36			4	1	51 (4.2%)

							Total
(Night Terrors)		9	1	4		6	20 (1.6%)
(Narcolepsy)			1	1		1	3 (0.2%)
Apnea	2	4	1			31	38 (3.1%)
Munchausen Syndrome	1	1				2	4 (0.3%)
Movement Disorders*:	18	77		8	6	20	129 (10.6%)
(Tics/Tourette's Syndrome)		32	1	6		18	57 (1.5%)
(Tremor)		3	1				4 (0.3%)
(Shuddering)	1	21					22 (1.8%)
(Myoclonus)		7					7 (0.6%)
(Dystonia/Posturing)		10		4			14 (1.2%)
(Paroxysmal Dyskinesias)		1		2			3 (0.2%)
(Stereotypies/Habit and Self-Stimulatory Behaviors)	12					2	14 (1.2%)
(Paroxysmal Torticollis)		1					1 (0.1%)
(Paroxysmal Tonic Upgaze)		2					2 (0.2%)
Migraine/Migraine Variants*:	1	14	2	11	3	7	38 (3.1%)
(Paroxysmal Vertigo)		4		3			7 (0.6%)
(Hemiplegic Migraine)		3					3 (0.2%)

continued

Table 1-3 continued

EEG Telemetry Recorded Events	Kotagal[4] N=883	Bye[7] N=666	Gibbs[23] N=900	Stroink[26] N=881	Uldall[29] N=223	Beach[30] N=684	Totals N=4237[†]
(Ophthalmoplegic Migraine)			2				2 (0.2%)
(Alice in Wonderland)							0 (0%)
Alternating Hemiplegia	1			1			2 (0.2%)
Gastroesophageal Reflux	4	9					13 (1.1%)
Episodic Behavioral Syndromes*:	81	116	7	28	55	57	345 (28.4%)
(Staring/Inattention)	14	98	4	6	46	20	188 (15.5%)
(Somatoform/Conversion Disorder)	61	12	3	15	9		100 (8.2%)
(Rage Attack)	4					12	16 (1.3%)
(Panic Attacks)	2			1		2	5 (0.4%)
(Gratification Disorder)		6					6 (0.5%)
Brainstem Release Phenomenon		4					4 (0.3%)
Normal Reflex Behavior		15					
Cardiac			1	1			2 (0.2%)
"Miscellaneous"		28					28 (2.3%)
Unknown/Uncertain	0	1	10	130	6	42	189 (15.6%)
Unaccounted For or Not Reported	684/883 (77%)						

* Subcategory of paroxysmal event not always specified. The final diagnosis is listed.
† Concurrent epilepsy and non-epileptic paroxysmal events noted.
‡ Some subjects had more than one type of non-epileptic paroxysmal event.

were 1380 false positive and only 3 false negative cases. Most striking was the fact that there was a 3.7:1 misdiagnosis of epilepsy. It underscores the importance of careful history taking, carefully applied diagnostic categorization, and less reliance on simplified questionnaires. These other non-epileptic diagnoses included episodic behavioral syndromes, "dizziness," and migraine that often resulted in inappropriate treatment and poorer school performance.[28]

In a prospective study of 5803 consecutive newborn infants from Australia, the etiology of "convulsions" in infants under 3 years of age is described.[33] There were 535 children lost to study, leaving 5268 (90%) of whom 325 had at least one convulsive episode during the first 3 years of life. They determined that 8.1 per 1000 experienced convulsions following breath-holding attacks and an additional 4 per 1000 had simple breath-holding attacks associated with transient loss of consciousness, but no convulsions.[33] Data such as this suggest that the incidence of epilepsy in childhood may be lower than thought, because of confounding and inappropriate identification of cases. The use of ambiguous terminology undoubtedly contributes to these misperceptions and diagnostic misinterpretations. Epilepsy is the tendency to have recurrent, unprovoked seizures caused by abnormal brain electrical activity is produced by diverse brain pathologies.[32] The epileptic seizure is thus a symptom (or clinical sign) of the underlying disorder. The qualification of "epileptic" implies a more specific mechanism of the seizure per se. Therefore, clarity of terms is important, and a few commonly used terms and definitions are presented in the adjoining tables (Tables 1-4 and 1-5).

Table 1-4 Terminology and Definitions

Term	Definition	Synonym
Epilepsy	The tendency to have recurrent, unprovoked seizures caused by physiologically abnormal brain electrical activity produced by idiopathic or diverse brain pathologies	Fits
Seizure	A sudden alteration in behavior, awareness, motor movement, body posture, autonomic function, and/or sensory or psychic perceptions from both physiological (epileptic, hypnic, chemical, anoxic, etc.) and nonphysiological (psychological) causes, which may be paroxysmal and stereotyped	Fits Convulsion Spell Drop attacks Funny turn
Convulsion	A sudden rhythmical motor behavior, body posture, or alteration in body tone from diverse physiological (epileptic, hypnic, chemical, anoxic, etc.) and nonphysiological (psychological) causes, which may be paroxysmal and stereotyped	Motor seizures Fits Attacks Drop attacks

continued

Table 1-4 continued

Term	Definition	Synonym
Syncope	A sudden physiological transient loss of consciousness due to acute cerebral hypoxia of short duration (sufficient duration may evolve into convulsive syncope or an anoxic epileptic seizure)	Faint Cyanotic breath-holding spell Falling out Blackout
Convulsive Syncope	A sudden physiological transient loss of consciousness due to acute cerebral hypoxia of sufficient duration to result in transient non-epileptic motor behavior characterized by brainstem release phenomenon of tonic extensor posturing, spasms, and/or irregular myoclonus	Syncopal convulsion Syncopal seizure Anoxic convulsion Anoxic seizure
Reflex Anoxic Seizure	A sudden physiological transient loss of consciousness due to acute cerebral hypoxia from brief reflex cardiac asystole causing a decrease in cerebral perfusion of sufficient duration to result in transient non-epileptic motor behavior characterized by brainstem release phenomenon of tonic extensor posturing, spasms, and or irregular myoclonus	Pallid breath-holding spell, Pallid infantile syncope, White breath-holding, Non-epileptic vagal attack, Neurally mediated syncope, Vasovagal syncope, Vagocardiac syncope, Neurocardiogenic syncope, Venipuncture fits, Reflex faint, Reflex fit
Anoxic Epileptic Seizure	An epileptic seizure produced by and following a profound syncopal event characterized by clonic motor activity	Anoxic seizure Anoxic convulsion
Dizzy	A premonitory sense of lightheadedness prior to syncope, or a sense of movement of oneself or the surroundings as in vertigo (these must be clarified by the subject)	Faint feeling Spins
Swoon	An apparent, sudden, nonphysiological transient loss of consciousness	Pseudosyncope, Psychogenic syncope, Psychogenic faint

In a recent epidemiological review, Cowan documents the real decline in the annual incidence of epilepsies in children across several different populations measured at different times.[34] A compilation of studies demonstrates an average annual incidence rate of 50–72 per 100,000 when epilepsy is defined as recurrent, unprovoked seizures.[34] There have been studies that demonstrated declining epilepsy rates in children from birth to age 14 years in Rochester,

Table 1-5 Examples of Common Lay Terms and Inferred Medical Meanings

Medical Inference*	Lay Terms Describing the Child's Appearance or Behavior
Epileptic Absence or Complex Partial Seizure, Narcoleptic Micro Sleep	*stare, blank-out, dazed, zone-out, looks through you, not there, out of it, oblivious*
Epileptic Atonic Seizure, Syncope, Cataplectic Attack	*faint, drop, fall out, crash, tripped over, hit the deck, smashed him/herself, swoon, blackout*
Epileptic Myoclonic Seizure/Spasm, Non-epileptic Myoclonus, Tic, Hypnic Jerk, Ballismus/Chorea	*jolt, jerk, jump, flail, slump, pitch forward, threw their head back, twitch, start*
Syncope, Presyncope, Vertigo, Opsoclonus, Ataxia	*dizzy, spins, lightheaded, head rush, unsteady, jiggles, buzzy, fuzzy*
Epileptic Tonic-Clonic Convulsion, Tremor, Stereotypy, Chorea/Ballismus	*shakes, unsteady hands, trembling, shivers, trembling*
Epileptic Tonic Seizure, Dystonia, Dyskinesia, Athetosis	*stiffening, twisting, arching, contorting*

* Medical inference is not always correct and needs to be further clarified or specified and defined.

MN, during 1935–1984 by 26%, and in England from 1974 to 1993 by 30% and from 1975 to 1985 by 60%.[35–37] A multitude of possible explanations may account for the results presented by these data, not least of all are a real decline, better early treatment after a first seizure, and better definition of epilepsy by means of technology and specialist interpretation. However, as it pertains to this discussion, possibilities also include a more clear recognition of "epilepsy-like" events or "epilepsy imitators." These non-epileptic paroxysmal events make a significant proportion of falsely identified subjects as epileptics. Their extraction from the epidemiological roles certainly accounts for a significant impact on the declining epilepsy rates. In a retrospective analysis of 324 adult case records referred to a single consultant within a regional epilepsy clinic and general neurology clinic in the United Kingdom, 184 subjects who were exposed to antiepileptic drugs—of whom 92 were refractory to treatment—were reevaluated and reclassified.[38] After reevaluation by means of careful history, examination, and observation of attacks, an overall misdiagnosis rate of 26.1% (46/184) was identified. Misdiagnoses were made by primary care physicians and referring specialists alike. Non-epileptic paroxysmal disorders identified included syncope, psychogenic events, migraine, paroxysmal positional vertigo, and hypnic jerks.[38] The authors concluded after analysis of the presenting clinical data that the chief reason for misdiagnosis was incomplete history taking, followed by misinterpretation of EEG findings.

There were significant consequences for the subjects due to incorrect diagnoses and unnecessary treatment, including driving restrictions, drug side effects, employment difficulties, and both socioeconomic and psychological impact.[38]

There exists few data examining the recognition of non-epileptic paroxysmal disorders presented by some children in settings where the initial emphasis is on the evaluation of children with apparently non-epileptic events at the outset. The report by Hindley et al. offers an opportunity to gain this insight.[39] They presented their findings of a prospective study, which summarized the diagnoses made in a secondary care referral clinic in the United Kingdom for children with paroxysmal disorders. They evaluated each of 380 consecutive children over an 8-year interval who presented with a first time event or for further classification and management of epilepsy. Diagnoses were made primarily on clinical information augmented by home video recording, and EEG and additional specialist opinion where needed. An important element of their history obtaining technique was the insistence of having at least one eyewitness to the event in question present at the evaluation. Epilepsy was diagnosed in only 89 (23%) of the cohort of 380 children. Syncope and reflex anoxic seizures were most common among the non-epileptic events in 100 children (42%) of the group, and in an additional 53 (14%) the events were unclassified. The specific entities are listed in Table 1-6 side by side with the totals column of Table 1-3 for easy comparison. These frequencies are in sharp distinction to those reported from EEG telemetry-based data. By nature of the referral base, the frequency of non-epileptic paroxysmal events was significantly greater than that of epilepsy (63% vs. 28.6%). Within the identified paroxysmal entities,

Table 1-6 Comparison of Specialty Clinic for Childhood Paroxysmal Events to EEG-Based Data

Clinical Evaluation Final Diagnoses	Hindley[39] N = 380	Table 1-3 Totals N = 4237
Single Seizure	0	113 (2.6%)
Febrile/Acute Symptomatic Seizure	0	239 (5.6%)
Epilepsy	89 (23%)	1902 (44.9%)
Non-Epileptic Paroxysmal Events	238 (63%)	1211 (28.6%)
(EEG Recorded)	23*	884 (20.8%)
(No EEG Recording)	215*	327 (7.7%)
Syncope	100 (42%)	93 (7.6%)
(Severe Breath-Holding Spells)	8 (2.1%)	86 (7.1 %)
Hyperventilation Syndrome	3 (0.8%)	4 (0.3%)
Sleep-Related Phenomena:	20 (8.4%)	139 (11.4%)
(Neonatal Sleep Myoclonus)	3 (0.8%)	8 (0.7%)
(Hypnic Jerks)		57 (4.7%)

(Disorders of Arousal)		51 (4.2%)
(Night Terrors)	17 (4.5%)	20 (1.6%)
(Narcolepsy)		3 (0.2%)
Apnea		38 (3.1%)
Munchausen Syndrome	6 (1.6%)	4 (0.3%)
Movement Disorders:	17 (4.5%)	129 (10.6%)
(Tics/Tourette's Syndrome)		57 (1.5%)
(Tremor)		4 (0.3%)
(Shuddering)	3 (0.8%)	22 (1.8%)
(Myoclonus)		7 (0.6%)
(Dystonia/Posturing)		14 (1.2%)
(Paroxysmal Dyskinesias)	2 (0.5%)	3 (0.2%)
(Stereotypies/Habit and Self-Stimulatory Behaviors)	8 (2.1%)	14 (1.2%)
(Paroxysmal Torticollis)		1 (0.1%)
(Paroxysmal Tonic Upgaze)	4 (1.0%)	2 (0.2%)
Migraine/Migraine Variants:	25 (10.5%)	38 (3.1%)
(Paroxysmal Vertigo)	9 (2.4%)	7 (0.6%)
(Hemiplegic Migraine)		3 (0.2%)
(Alice in Wonderland)	16 (4.2%)	
(Ophthalmoplegic Migraine)	2 (0.2%)	
Alternating Hemiplegia		2 (0.2%)
Gastroesophageal Reflux	2 (0.5%)	13 (1.1%)
Episodic Behavioral Syndromes:	51 (13.4%)	345 (28.4%)
(Staring/Inattention)	20 (8.4%)	188 (15.5%)
(Somatoform/Conversion Disorder)	31 (8.1%)	100 (8.2%)
(Rage Attack)		16 (1.3%)
(Panic Attacks)		5 (0.4%)
(Gratification Disorder)		6 (0.5%)
Brainstem Release Phenomenon		4 (0.3%)
Normal Reflex Behavior		0 (0%)
Cardiac	1 (0.3%)	2 (0.2%)
"Miscellaneous"	13 (3.4%)	28 (2.3%)
Unknown/Uncertain	53 (13.9%)	189 (15.6%)

* If not specifically enumerated, no EEG was assumed.

there was a nearly sixfold increase in syncope and anoxic syncopal convulsions identified and a threefold increase in migraine variants observed. Importantly, there were approximately one-half as many behavioral syndromes and movement disorders identified with nearly equal frequencies of sleep-related phenomena evaluated. It is rather striking as well that there were few movement disorders appreciated, especially tics/Tourette syndrome. This may again underscore the nature of the referral base rather than prevalence of specific disorders. Tics themselves may be fairly easily distinguished from epileptic events and recognized swiftly. The "uncertain" diagnosis group was similar in each referral population studied, which suggests that even with a specific focused expertise and referral bias, there are those children whose paroxysmal disorder requires longitudinal assessment. These same children with "uncertain" diagnoses can be managed expectantly provided a complete evaluation is made available and until the likely benign nature of the events becomes apparent. It has been suggested that misdiagnosis of epilepsy has been inadvertently aided by "overinterpretation" of EEG findings.[40] Useful features to distinguish these non-epileptic events from epileptic ones were the following: (1) common association to specific situations, (2) the events could often be interrupted, (3) repeated EEGs were normal, (4) there appeared to be a parental insistence of epilepsy, and (5) there remained continued clinical suspicion for a benign entity.[39] Taken in context, the data presented in Tables 1-3 and 1-6 are essential in that they emphasize that in children who present with paroxysmal disorders a majority do not have epilepsy, and that an important minority fraction of those previously diagnosed with epilepsy do not have it, whether studied in the United Kingdom or elsewhere.[41] This is especially true of epilepsy and of other non-epileptic paroxysmal disorders where a definitive test per se is not available and the diagnosis rests primarily upon symptom recognition and correct classification. The utility of ictal EEG recording (ambulatory EEG, EEG telemetry) and video recording have become crucial in many circumstances and certainly helpful in all.

The evaluation of children with concurrent cognitive and neurological impairments compounds the diagnostic clinical problem. There seems to exist the same spectrum of non-epileptic paroxysmal behaviors as seen in nonimpaired children who also not infrequently have coexistent epilepsy 39%–76%.[6,7,22,42,43] Despite this frequency, the behaviors that prompted EEG referral are epileptic in only 16%–40%.[6,7,22,42,43] However, an even higher prevalence of these non-epileptic paroxysmal disorders are found in this population of children compared to nonimpaired children, with frequencies ranging from 20% to greater than 60% having demonstrable non-epileptic events. In one series, 77% of subjects who had EEG-recorded events were identified as having more than one type.[22] Although the actual recorded events bare similarity to those identified in nonimpaired children, the percentage of specific types are skewed toward a greater proportion with abnormal movements of the head, neck, mouth, and eyes; behavioral staring; and various body posturing (see Table 1-7).[6,7,22,42,43] Tremulous behavior is fairly frequently encountered and can be distinguished from clonus and epileptic clonic activity clinically. One notable exception to the similar spectrum of non-epileptic paroxysmal behavior is the paucity of migraine phenomena identified. This is likely explained by the absence of a reliable history of associated headache, which is generally not clearly expressed in the more profoundly impaired individual and only inferred by parental suggestion at best.

Table 1-7 EEG-Based Paroxysmal Events in Neurological and Cognitively Impaired Children*

Clinical Evaluation Final Diagnoses	Desai[42] N=19	Donat[22] N=31†	Holmes[43] N=38	Neill[44] N=124	Bye[7] N=194	Hindley[39] N=380	Totals N=786
Epilepsy	0	12 (39%)	15 (38%)	20 (16.1%)	77 (40%)	89 (23%)	203 (25.8%)
Non-Epileptic Paroxysmal Events	19 (100%)	31 (100%)	24 (64%)	104 (83.9%)	116 (59.6%)	238 (63%)	532 (67.7%)
(EEG-Recorded Epileptic and Non-Epileptic Events)	19 (100%)	31 (100%)	38 (100%)	124 (100%)	194 (100%)	327 (86%)	733 (93%)
Syncope					2 (1%)	100 (42%)	102 (19.1%)
(Severe Breath-Holding Spells)					2 (1%)	8 (2.1%)	10 (1.9 %)
Hyperventilation Syndrome	1 (5%)	1 (%)				3 (0.8%)	5 (0.8%)
Sleep-Related Phenomena: (Neonatal Sleep Myoclonus)	2 (10%)	2 (6.5%)			46 (23.7%)	20 (8.4%)	70 (13.1%)
(Hypnic Jerks)		2 (6.5%)			21 (11%)	3 (0.8%)	26 (4.9%)
(Disorders of Arousal)							0 (0%)
(Night Terrors)					23 (12%)		23 (4.3%)
(Narcolepsy)					2 (1%)	17 (4.5%)	19 (3.6%)
Apnea		1 (%)		3 (2.8%)			0 (0%)
Munchausen Syndrome					3 (1.5%)	6 (1.6%)	7 (1.3%)
							6 (1.1%)

continued

Table 1-7 continued

Clinical Evaluation Final Diagnoses	Desai[42] N=19	Donat[22] N=31†	Holmes[43] N=38	Neill[44] N=124	Bye[7] N=194	Hindley[39] N=380	Totals N=786
Abnormal Movements:	11 (58%)		12 (32%)		64 (51.6%)	17 (4.5%)	104 (19.5%)
(Tics/Blink-Grimace-Vocalize)			1 (2.6%)	25 (24%)	16 (8.2%)		42 (7.9%)
(Head and Mouth Movements)		10 (32%)		22 (21.1%)			32 (6.0%)
(Tremor/Shuddering)		6 (20%)			16 (8.2%)	3 (0.8%)	25 (4.7%)
(Myoclonus)				12 (11.5%)	7 (3.6%)		19 (3.6%)
(Dystonia/Posturing/ Drops-Slumps)		13 (42%)		4 (3.8%)	19 (9.8%)		36 (6.7%)
(Paroxysmal Dyskinesias)					1 (0.5%)	2 (0.5%)	3 (0.6%)
(Stereotypies/Habit and Self-Stimulatory Behaviors)				8 (7.7%)		8 (2.1%)	16 (3.0%)
(Paroxysmal Torticollis)							0 (0%)
(Paroxysmal Nystagmus)		12 (40%)	3 (7.9%)	2 (1.9%)	2 (1%)	4 (1.0%)	23 (4.3%)
(Eye Deviations/Closure)				3 (2.9%)	3 (1.5%)		6 (1.2%)
Migraine/Migraine Variants:						25 (10.5%)	25 (4.7%)
(Paroxysmal Vertigo)						9 (2.4%)	9 (1.7%)
(Hemiplegic Migraine)							0 (0%)
(Alice in Wonderland)						16 (4.2%)	16 (2.0%)
(Ophthalmoplegic Migraine)							0 (0%)

Alternating Hemiplegia						0 (0%)
Gastroesophageal Reflux	1 (5%)				10 (5.1%)	2 (0.5%)	13 (2.4%)
Episodic Behavioral Syndromes:	6 (37%)	7 (22.5%)	8 (28.9%)	22 (17.7%)	91 (46.9%)	51 (13.4%)	185 (34.8%)
(Staring/Inattention)	5 (26%)	7 (23%)	3 (7.9%)	21 (20.2%)	84 (43%)	20 (8.4%)	140 (26.3%)
(Somatoform/Conversion Disorder)	1 (5%)				5 (2.5%)	31 (8.1%)	37 (6.9%)
(Rage Attack)			5 (13.1%)				5 (0.8%)
(Panic Attacks)							
(Gratification Disorder)					2 (1%)		2 (0.4%)
(Stutter)				1 (0.9%)			1 (0.2%)
Brainstem Release Phenomenon					8 (4.1%)		8 (1.4%)
Normal Reflex Behavior			1 (2.6%)		3 (1.5%)		4 (0.7%)
Cardiac						1 (0.3%)	1 (0.2%)
"Miscellaneous"	7 (23%)				26 (13.4%)	13 (3.4%)	46 (8.6%)
Unknown/Uncertain						52 (13.1%)	52 (9.8%)

* Multiple types of events may have occurred in a single child.
† Seventy-seven percent of the children had multiple types of recorded events.

REFERENCES

1. DiMario FJ. Paroxysmal non-epileptic events of childhood. Semin Pediatr Neurol 2006; 13; 208–221.
2. Fenichel GM. Paroxysmal disorders, In *Clinical Pediatric Neurology, A Signs and Symptoms Approach*, 5th edition. W.B. Saunders Co., Philadelphia, PA, 2005; 1–45.
3. DiMario FJ. The nervous system. In Rudolph's *Fundamentals of Pediatrics*. Eds: AM Rudolph, RK Kamei, KJ Overby. 3rd edition. Mcgraw Hill, New York, 2002; 796–846.
4. Kotagal P, Costa M, Wyllie E, et al. Paroxysmal nonepileptic events in children and adolescents. Pediatrics 2002, 110(4); e46–e51. http://www.pediatrics.org/cgi/content/full/110/4/e46.
5. Chaves-Carballo E. Syncope and paroxysmal disorders other than epilepsy. In *Pediatric Neurology: Principles & Practice*. Eds: Swaiman KF, Ashwal S, Ferriero DM. 4th edition. Mosby-Elsevier, Philadelphia PA, 2006; 1209–1223.
6. Paolicchi JM. The spectrum of non-epileptic events in children. Epilepsia 2002; 43(Suppl 3); 60–64.
7. Bye AM, Kok DJ, Ferenschild FT, et al. Paroxysmal non-epileptic events in children: a retrospective study over a period of 10 years. J Paediatr Child Health 2000; 36(3); 244–248.
8. Donat JF, Wright FS. Clinical imitators of infantile spasms. J Child Neurol 1992; 7(4); 395–399.
9. Nagarajan L, Bye AM. Staring episodes in children analyzed by telemetry. J Child Neurol 1992; 7(1); 39–43.
10. Carmant L, Kramer U, Holmes G, et al. Differential diagnosis of staring spells in children: a video-EEG study. Pediatr Neurol 1996; 14(3); 199–202.
11. Bye AM, Nunan J. Video EEG analysis of non-ictal events in children. Clinical and Experim Neurol 1992; 29; 92–98.
12. Scher M, Painter J. Controversies concerning neonatal seizures. Pediatr Clin North Am 1989: 36; 281–310.
13. Holmes G, Sckellares JC, McKiernan J, et al. Evaluation of childhood pseudoseizures using EEG telemetry and videotape monitoring. J Pediatr 1980; 97; 554–558.
14. Wyllie E, Friedman D, Rothner D, et al. Psychogenic seizures in children and adolescents: outcome after diagnosis by ictal video and electroencephalographic recording. Pediatrics 1990; 85; 480–484.
15. Wyllie E, Glazer JP, Benbadis S, et al. Psychiatric features of children and adolescents with pseudoseizures. Arch Pediatr Adolesc Med 1999; 153; 244–248.
16. Pakalnis A, Paolicchi J. Psychogenic seizures after head injury in children. J Child Neurol 2000; 15; 78–80.
17. Pakalnis A, Paolicchi J. Gilles E. Psychogenic status epilepticus in children: psychiatric and other risk factors. Neurology 2000; 54; 969–970.
18. ASDA (2005) *The International Classification of Sleep Disorders: Diagnostic and Coding Manual*, 2nd edition. American Academy of Sleep Medicine, Westchester, Il.
19. Derry CP, Duncan JS, Berkovic SF. Paroxysmal motor disorders of sleep: the clinical spectrum and differentiation from epilepsy. Epilepsia 2006; 47(11); 1775–1791.
20. Anders TF, Eiben LA. Pediatric sleep disorders: a review of the past 10 years. J Am Acad Child Adol Psychiatr 1997; 36(1); 9–20.

21. Kanner AM, Morris HH, Luders H, et al. Supplementary motor seizures mimicking pseudoseizures: some clinical differences. Neurology 1990; 40(9); 1404–1407.

22. Donat JF, Wright FS. Episodic symptoms mistaken for seizures in the neurologically impaired child. Neurology 1990; 40(1); 156–157.

23. Gibbs J, Appleton RE. False diagnosis of epilepsy in children. Seizure 1992; 1; 15–18.

24. Scheepers B, Clough P, Pickles C. The misdiagnosis of epilepsy: findings of a population study. Seizure 1998; 7; 403–406.

25. Shuper A, Mimouni M. Problems of differentiation between epilepsy and non–epileptic paroxysmal events in the first year of life. Arch Dis Child 1995; 73(4); 342–344.

26. Stroink H, van Donselaar CA, Geerts AT, et al. The accuracy of the diagnosis of paroxysmal events in children. Neurology 2003; 60; 979–982.

27. Leach JP, Lauder R, Nicolson A, et al. Epilepsy in the UK: misdiagnosis, mistreatment, and undertreatment? The Wrexham area epilepsy project. Seizure 2005; 14; 514–520.

28. Somoza MJ, Forienza RH, Brussino M, et al. Epidemiological survey of epilepsy in the primary school population in Buenos Aires. Neuroepidemiology 2005; 25; 62–68.

29. Uldall P, Alving J, Hansen LK, et al. The misdiagnosis of epilepsy in children admitted to a tertiary epilepsy centre with paroxysmal events. Arch Dis Child 2006; 91; 219–221.

30. Beach R, Reading R. The importance of acknowledging clinical uncertainty in the diagnosis of epilepsy and non-epileptic events. Arch Dis Child 2005; 90; 1219–1222.

31. Stroink H, van Donselaar CA, Geerts AT, et al. Interrater agreement of the diagnosis and classification of a first seizure in childhood. The Dutch Study of Epilepsy in Childhood. J Neurol Neurosurg Psychiatry 2004; 75; 241–245.

32. Commission on Classification and Terminology of the International League Against Epilepsy. Proposal for Revised Classification of the Epilepsies and Epileptic Syndromes. Epilepsia 1989; 30; 389–399.

33. Rossiter, EJ, Luckin J, Vile A, et al. Convulsions in the first year of life. Med J Aust 1977; 2(22); 735–740.

34. Cowan LD. The epidemiology of the epilepsies in children. Ment Retard Dev Disabil Res Rev 2002; 8; 171–181.

35. Hauser WA, Annegers JF, Kurland LT. Incidence of epilepsy and unprovoked seizures in Rochester, Minnesota: 1935–1984. Epilepsia 1993; 34; 453–468.

36. Cockerell OC, Eckle I, Goodridge DM, et al. Epilepsy in a population of 6,000 reexamined: secular trends in first attendance rates, prevalence, and prognosis. J Neurol Neurosurg Psychiatry 1995; 58; 570–576.

37. Sidenvall R, Forsgren L, Blomquist HK, et al. A community–based prospective incidence study of epileptic seizures in children. Acta Paediatr 1993; 82; 60–65.

38. Smith D, Defalla BA, Chadwick DW. The misdiagnosis of epilepsy and the management of refractory epilepsy in a specialist clinic. Q J Med 1999; 92(1); 15–23.

39. Hindley D, Ali A, Robson C. Diagnoses made in a secondary care "fits, faints, funny turns" clinic. Arch Dis Child 2006; 91; 214–218.

40. Benbadis SR, Tatum WO. Overinterpretation of EEGs and misdiagnosis of epilepsy. J Clin Neurophysiol 2003; 20(1); 42–44.

41. Ferrie CD. Preventing misdiagnosis of epilepsy. Arch Dis Child 2006; 91; 206–209.
42. Desai P, Talwar D. Nonepileptic events in normal and neurologically handicapped children: a video-EEG study. Pediatr Neurol 1992; 8; 127–129.
43. Holmes G, McKeever M, Russman B. Abnormal behavior or epilepsy? Use of long-term EEG and video monitoring with severely to profoundly mentally retarded patients with seizures. Am J Ment Ret 1983; 87(4); 456–458.
44. Neill JC, Alvarez N. Differential diagnosis of epileptic versus pseudoepileptic seizures in developmentally disabled persons. Appl Res Ment Ret 1986; 7(3); 285–298.

2

Differentiating the Diagnostic Considerations

INTRODUCTION TO THE DEDUCTIVE APPROACH

The approach to establishing a correct diagnosis when confronted with a child who appears to be experiencing events that could be epileptic in nature but are indeed non-epileptic is challenging. The appropriate identification will depend upon a careful extraction of the clinical history, confirmation of a supportive examination, observation of the critical events, and generally less reliance upon laboratory testing. These non-epileptic events by definition conform to a paroxysmal or intermittent character and are defined by key characteristics that allow identification. Unfortunately, not all entities are sufficiently well characterized at the outset to be confidently recognized. Repeated observations and precise descriptions accrued over time may be needed for clarification. Laboratory testing and EEG telemetry recording may be needed to exclude certain considerations and, a lesser likelihood, to identify a specific condition.

Certain clinical methods of diagnostic reasoning are worth reviewing. The deductive approach is the art of diagnosis in medicine and one that has a rich history.[1,2] The appropriate analysis of complex or particularly rare problems requires the cognitive formulation of a "road map" (Table 2-1). An application of the deductive approach can be gleaned from an analysis of the reasoning strategies behind arriving at a solution to the clinicopathological case presentation.[1,2] Critical to the process is an accurate statement of the problem. This is a succinct but fully complete description, which encompasses the entire scope of the chief complaint and an organized history of the present illness. The clinician must factor in the probabilities of certain diagnostic considerations as the history unfolds in order to elicit appropriate pertinent negative and positive elements of additional symptoms and signs. With these added elements, a mental exercise of comparisons and considerations will direct the clinician to a refined cluster of pertinent information and descriptions. This final compilation of facts serves as an aggregation of elementary features, which must be closely linked or embedded into a recognizable pattern. It is from this aggregation of elements identified as a cluster of related facts that the identification of a nodal point or points, those that are unique and distinctive, can be extracted.

Table 2-1 Road Map for the Deductive Approach

Elements of Deductive Reasoning:
- Accurate statement of the problem
- Aggregation of the facts
- Identification of the nodal point(s)
- Generate a list of possible causes
- Trim the list of possible to probable causes
- Identify the most probable cause
- Validate the identified probable cause

Source: Modified from References.[1,2]

Only exceptionally will more than one nodal point be identifiable. This point or points, however, will serve to drive the deductive reasoning process forward. As it relates to non-epileptic events of childhood, a pathognomonic description (e.g., a positive nose tap sign inducing hyperekplexic attacks) may be ascertained. Absent this, a consideration of causes to explain the nodal point(s) will serve to focus the diagnostic considerations. This can be further amplified by considering the examples of causes of intermittent hemiplegia. This could represent a hemiplegic migraine syndrome, alternating hemiplegia of childhood or, in the appropriate context, a paroxysmal dyskinesia or SMART syndrome (strokelike migraine syndrome after radiation therapy). Once a list of potential causes is developed, then a comparison of probabilities can be accomplished by assessing the likelihood of encountering the presented symptoms and signs from among the diagnostic considerations and specific features found upon additional systems review. This comparative exercise allows for trimming the list of causes into those that best characterize the clinical presentation. Those causes under final consideration (differential diagnoses) must not only embody the presence of critical elements of the clinical event under evaluation but also not miss any of the critical components that are included. The deductive exercise continues such that those considerations that reach some ethereal threshold set at by the clinician are retained and those that do not are, at least temporarily, excluded. In the final steps, a selection of favored causes then can be contrasted with each other such that the one that most closely matches those of the event under consideration is mentally highlighted. This diagnostic choice must withstand validation. If possible an objective measure or laboratory test may be applied in order to secure the diagnosis. Many times, however, this choice is at best a clinical judgment, which must ultimately endure the test of time.

Although the deductive approach may serve the clinician well in terms of differentiating the diagnostic possibilities, others have highlighted its limitations as a teaching method.[3] Nonetheless this road map can both identify and eliminate categories of diagnostic considerations. Other approaches often enlisted by clinicians and used in medical problem solving include four basic approaches: (1) pattern recognition, (2) the process of "ruling everything out," (3) use of algorithms, and (4) hypothesis generation and testing.

Pattern Recognition

Pattern recognition requires that clinicians have sufficient familiarity with many diseases or, as it pertains to non-epileptic events, many presentations of these events in order to cluster features into recognizable groups for identification. This approach requires experience and astute observation skills. As a result, it is an acquired skill set and strategy more usually relied upon by the seasoned clinician.

Ruling Everything Out

The process of ruling everything out is fraught with peril and waste. This approach assumes that there is test for each entity under diagnostic consideration that is both specific and sensitive. There is a further implicit assumption that one can simply test enough to exclude all incorrect possibilities and ultimately arrive at the correct diagnosis. In reality, this is a faulty premise. Not only is it a costly and time-consuming strategy, but it also demands that the child endure an increasingly greater number of unnecessary discomforts with even lesser likelihood of benefit as the endless possibilities are (never really) ruled out. Testing can be best utilized when directed toward validating the deduced cause rather than eliminating everything else.

Algorithmic Approach

Algorithms have some intrinsic value when one considers that these are in large part, a forced logical analysis. These often require a binary approach (yes or no) in order to flow from one decision section to the next. Their directedness and stepwise progression help organize data and compel implicit reasoning at each junction. However, the lack of nuance and inability to accept ambiguity into the schemas sometimes limits usefulness. Similarly, not all considerations can be easily and discretely incorporated into the decision process. One must always rely upon clinical judgment and reasoning to adapt the algorithm appropriately. In some respects the process of hypothesis generation and testing incorporates elements of each of the prior mentioned approaches. The use of the deductive reasoning approach described above allows for the generation of hypotheses and mental hypothesis testing. These are generated based on a critical appraisal of the elements from history and physical examination with an important interpretive step. Some basic principles, including the following, help to guide the utility of this reasoning strategy: (1) Common things are common, (2) one cause to explain most findings is advocated (parsimony), (3) generated hypotheses should be based upon probability, and (4) all hypotheses can be modified or rejected over time.

Hypothesis Generation

In studies comparing individuals with different levels of clinical experience (third and fourth year medical students to clinical faculty) and their clinical reasoning skills using standardized clinical vignettes, hypothesis generation errors decrease as clinical expertise increases but identification of important data and interpretation errors increase.[4] This may be due in part to an inappropriate use of, or too heavy a reliance upon, pattern recognition as a strategy or to a limitation in the knowledge base of the most experienced clinicians. Of greater interest is the fact that, although hypothesis generation errors increased in proportion to increases in problem difficulty, the identification and interpretation of data errors decreased.[4] This has been explained by the fact that as problem difficulty increases, clinicians at all levels of expertise are less able to differentiate between relevant and irrelevant clinical data and thus give equal consideration to all information contained within a case history. It has been suggested that the development of clinical reasoning during preclinical and clinical medical education may be enhanced by both an analysis of the clinical reasoning process and a specific focus on each of the stages at which errors commonly occur.[4] An important direct corollary of this is the imperative to value lifelong learning as an important means to improve clinical reasoning skills in concert with the acquisition of clinical experience.

As was stated at the outset of this chapter, an accurate statement of the problem is a necessary first step in deciphering the events at hand. The quality of the information obtained during the interview will clearly depend upon the quality of the observations and the observer's descriptions. These in turn rely upon the frequency of the observations, the totality of the observed event, and the state of the observer to notice and recall detail. Often the fabric of the history is disjointed and in need of repair. Important is the fact that certain non-epileptic events are characterized by multiple hallmark symptoms any of which may present at different ages. This is particularly true of migraines and psychosomatic illness where migraineurs have an average of three or more symptoms and children with psychosomatic illness complain of two or more, when compared to healthy controls (one complaint) or those children with chronic medical conditions (one or two complaints).[5] The effect of age upon the symptom presentation cannot be overstated. A single pathogenesis may express itself variably at different ages. Migraine, again, is expressed in a succession of symptoms and periodic syndromes evident only in young children (car sickness, cyclic vomiting, paroxysmal vertigo, paroxysmal torticollis, and perceptual distortions of Alice in Wonderland phenomenon), which eventually evolve into more typical migraine symptoms (visual scotoma, nausea, and throbbing unilateral headache) at later ages.[5] Thus, the impact of age at presentation, underlying pathophysiology, and quality of the observations and comprehensiveness of the details will all be elements that the clinician needs to consider and contend with when developing the diagnostic hypotheses for validation.

THE CLINICAL PRESENTATIONS

The primary considerations in obtaining a correct identification of the non-epileptic paroxysmal disorders of childhood are to apply the strategies discussed in the forgoing sections and assess their likelihoods. This approach can be applied to the recognized possible diagnostic entities that occur with some reasonable frequency within the specific age range of the subject under evaluation.[6,7] In the succeeding chapters, details concerning specific diagnostic entities within more broad categories can be found. Although somewhat arbitrary, it may be useful to initiate consideration of the entities best characterized as those with alterations of consciousness or occurring in sleep versus those that do not (Table 2-2). It should be recognized, however, that overlap between these two groups exists; nonetheless this division does allow a useful paradigm with which to begin. Discrete entities may have dominant and unique clinical characteristics ("nodal points") that allow it to be recognized as distinct, whereas other entities have specific and necessary combinations of clinical features that allow characterization.[8,9] As a general approach, nodal points may be the most useful clinical keys to focus upon (Table 2-3). Familiarity with them

Table 2-2 Initial Diagnostic Paradigm for Non-Epileptic Disorders of Childhood

Alteration of Consciousness or Occurrence in Sleep?	
Yes	No
Syncopes	Movements disorders
Rage and panic attacks	Migraines
Sleep disorders	Paraneoplastic
Toxic/metabolic/medical disorders	Toxic/metabolic/medical disorders
Somatoform disorders	Somatoform disorders
Factitious disorders	Factitious disorders
Factitious disorders by proxy	Factitious disorders by proxy

Source: Modified from References.[6,7]

Table 2-3 Hallmark Clinical Characters Differentiating Non-Epileptic Paroxysmal Events in Childhood

What Is the Dominant Clinical Characteristic Observed?

- Paralysis
- Collapse or drop attacks
- Generalized posturing, jerking, or twitching
- Focal or segmental posturing, jerking, or twitching
- Ocular movements or deviations
- Autonomic phenomenon (diaphoresis, color changes, altered respiration)
- Sensory phenomena (paresthesias, pain, vertigo, visual and auditory obscurations/distortions)

Source: Modified from References.[6,7]

will be gained only after considerable clinical experience and an augmented fund of knowledge. It should also be stated that many medical diseases, toxic ingestions/injections/inhalations, and medical and metabolic disorders can produce paroxysmal phenomenon—hypoglycemia, pheochromocytoma, and hyperthyroidism, for example. These as well as true epileptic seizures are considerations that must always be kept in mind especially when there appears to be no clear explanation for the protracted duration of an unde-fined symptom complex. More importantly, however, somatoform disorders and factitious illness (by proxy) need to be considered early and promptly con-cluded when diagnostic criteria are satisfied and/or specific evidence becomes clear.[10,11] By its very nature, the latter disorder, factitious illness (by proxy), can be life threatening and clearly criminal, fostering a certain urgency and need for expedient identification when suspected.[11] By the same token, reconsideration of a diagnosis previously made should be undertaken when there is an evolu-tion in symptoms or an unexpected alteration in its natural history. Lastly, one must be mindful that subjects with epilepsy may additionally and concurrently suffer from non-epileptic events and visa versa. A few relevant points will be highlighted in the sections that follow.

PAROXYSMAL PARALYSIS OR COLLAPSE

Paroxysmal paralysis or collapse may be the most dramatic presentation of the paroxysmal non-epileptic events seen in childhood (Table 2-4). These presenta-tions can occur in any age group and may or may not be associated with altered consciousness or sleep. Clearly, syncope and the progression from syncope to

Table 2-4 Paroxysmal Paralysis or Collapse as a Hallmark Presenting Feature

Age Range	With AC or Sleep	Without AC or Sleep
Neonatal	Apnea	Myasthenia syndromes
	GE reflux	Factitious disorder by proxy
	Reflex anoxic syncope	
	Cyanotic breath holding	
	Pallid breath holding	
	Factitious disorder by proxy	
	Suffocation	
Infants (<2 years)	Apnea	Hemiplegic migraine
	Central hypoventilation syndrome	Alternating hemiplegia of childhood
	GE reflux	Factitious disorder by proxy
	Reflex anoxic syncope	
	Cyanotic breath holding	
	Pallid breath holding	
	Benign familial alternating hemiplegia of childhood	
	Factitious disorder by proxy	
	Suffocation	

Children	Syncopes	Hemiplegic migraine
	Reflex anoxic syncope	Alternating hemiplegia of childhood
	Cyanotic breath holding	Hyperekplexia
	Pallid breath holding	Coffin-Lowry syndrome drops
	Benign familial alternating	SMART syndrome
	hemiplegia of childhood	Periodic paralyses
	Forced valsalva	Somatoform disorder
	Somatoform disorder	Factitious disorder (by proxy)
	Factitious disorder (by proxy)	
Adolescents	Syncopes	Hemiplegic migraine
	Reflex anoxic syncope	Alternating hemiplegia of childhood
	Sleep paralysis	Hyperekplexia
	Benign familial alternating	Coffin-Lowry syndrome drops
	hemiplegia of childhood	SMART syndrome
	Forced valsalva	Periodic paralyses
	Hyperventilation syndrome	Somatoform disorder
	Somatoform disorder	Factitious disorder (by proxy)
	Factitious disorder (by proxy)	

Notes: AC = altered consciousness, GE = gastroesophageal, SMART = strokelike migraine after radiation therapy.

anoxic syncope with convulsive activity occur with such frequent regularity that the clinician evaluating a child who presents with "seizures" must always seriously consider this an alternative explanation.[12, 13] It is particularly important to extract a clear history of triggers, premonitory symptoms, auras, and a gradual collapse into loss of consciousness. When this sequence is identified, further investigation will only be needed when ominous (cardiogenic) or unclear etiologies are considered.

Hemiplegic migraine and alternating hemiplegia of childhood are quite striking clinical entities that are often arrived at after the exclusion of other causes, although in retrospect each has clear and characteristic descriptive symptoms and signs.[14] The diagnosis of hemiplegic migraine is made easier when there is the existence of a firm family history of the same. Nuances may be easily overlooked especially if in younger children periodic syndromes are not well appreciated as precursors and if there are infrequent recurrences. A similar but less common and even more clinically devastating syndrome begins in children under 18 months of age, alternating hemiplegia of childhood.[15] This has all of the hallmarks that characterize non-epileptic disorders of childhood, each manifesting at various time points throughout childhood. The disorder combines a progressive character that impairs cognition, language, voluntary coordination, and motor skills. Paroxysmal complex nystagmus, autonomic phenomenon, tonic/dystonic posturing, bouts of alternating hemiplegia, and concurrent epilepsy generally develop over time.[15] Thus, it is the evolution and combination of features that allows identification. The proper diagnosis of a non-epileptic disorder may also depend upon a proper context. The SMART syndrome is a paroxysmal alternating hemiplegia syndrome identified only in subjects who had received prior cranial irradiation as a prerequisite.[16] Although the hemiplegic events are readily identifiable, the underlying etiology may not be as readily ascertained. A typical investigative approach to rule out other known causes of hemiplegia in subjects who had been previously treated for central nervous system tumors (vascular stroke, tumor recurrence, epileptic seizure) may be necessary before settling upon this etiology. Diagnosis is important not only for prognosis but also for instituting appropriate treatment. Unfortunately, many entities herein described have few treatments with proven efficacy. This will undoubtedly change as we not only clinically better characterize subjects but also pathogenetically better understand their disorder mechanisms.

PAROXYSMAL POSTURING, SHAKING, JERKING, TWITCHING, AND BEHAVIORAL SYNDROMES

Paroxysmal generalized or focal posturing, shaking, jerking, or twitching and behavioral syndromes are the most commonly presenting non-epileptic disorders of childhood (Table 2-5). These encompass a vast array of involuntary movement disorders. Many of these are benign and self-limited; however primary progressive and secondary causes may also exist. Several also share qualities noted with epileptic seizures, those being rhythmic, stereotyped, and unpredictable. There are various entities that are unique to childhood and have no counterpart in adults, such as bobble-head doll syndrome and transient paroxysmal dystonia of infancy.[17, 18] Conversely, there are numerous others that have an adult equivalent in terms of physiologic mechanism and character,

Table 2-5 Paroxysmal Generalized or Focal Posturing, Shaking, Jerking, or Twitching as a Hallmark Presenting Feature

Age Range	With AC or Sleep	Without AC or Sleep
Neonatal	Reflex anoxic syncope	Neonatal jitteriness
	Benign neonatal sleep myoclonus	Hyperekplexia
	Hypnic jerks	Paroxysmal dyskinesias
	Binkie flutter	Chorea associated with BPD
	Factitious disorder by proxy	Cardiac surgery-associated choreoathetosis
		Factitious disorder by proxy
Infants (<2 years)	Reflex anoxic syncope	Hyperekplexia
	Benign infantile sleep myoclonus	Paroxysmal dyskinesias
	Hypnic jerks	Sandifer's syndrome
	Benign familial alternating hemiplegia of childhood	Shuddering spells
		Benign myoclonus of infancy
	Binkie flutter	Transient paroxysmal dystonia of infancy
	Hereditary chin trembling	Gratification disorder

| | | Hypnogogic paroxysmal dystonia
Factitious disorder by proxy | Chorea associated with BPD
Cardiac surgery-associated
   choreo athetosis
Tonic reflex seizures of infancy
Stool holding syndrome
Paroxysmal torticollis
Stereotypies
Bobble-head doll syndrome
Opsoclonus-myoclonus-ataxia
   syndrome
Other movement disorders
Factitious disorder by proxy |
| Children/
   Adolescents | | Reflex anoxic syncope
Benign sleep myoclonus
Hypnic jerks
Benign familial alternating
   hemiplegia of childhood
Excessive fragmentary sleep
   myoclonus
Restless leg syndrome
Rhythmic movement disorder of
   sleep
Non-REM and REM-associated
   parasomnias
Hypnogogic paroxysmal dystonia
Rage attacks/panic attacks
Somatoform disorder
Factitious disorder (by proxy) | Alternating hemiplegia of
   childhood
Hyperekplexia
Paroxysmal dyskinesias
Tics/Tourette's syndrome
Sandifer's syndrome
Gratification disorder
Stool holding syndrome
Paroxysmal torticollis
Non-epileptic head nods
Myoclonus-dystonia syndrome
Stereotypies
Fever-precipitated movement
   disorder
Diaphragmatic flutter
Palatal tremor
Head tremor
Opsoclonus-
   myoclonus-ataxia
   syndrome
Other movement disorders
Panic attacks
Somatoform disorder
Factitious disorder (by proxy) |

Notes: AC = altered consciousness, BPD = broncho-pulmonary dysplasia, REM = rapid eye movement.

such as non-REM parasomnias, REM-associated sleep behavior, and Tourette's syndrome.[19,20] Although specific disorders such as the paroxysmal dyskinesias are genetic in origin and persist throughout life once manifest, there are others that are sporadic, transient, and seen only in children (e.g.) gratification disorder.[21,22] Occasionally the presentation of one movement could be misinterpreted by the observer and lead to an incorrect assessment of the underlying problem. Head shaking, for example, may be an intrinsic head movement such as tremor or bobbing or alternatively could be a secondary and compensatory movement for underlying nystagmus.[23] Careful longitudinal evaluation of the subject should help elucidate these points especially if the observed behavior is paroxysmal in nature. The essential elements of the phenomenon may not be immediately apparent and only after serial observations will clarification be made. Certain of these disorders incorrectly suggest one etiologic mechanism, whereas the actual underlying cause is not intuitive. This is the case with paroxysmal torticollis.[24] The child will assume a torticollis posture suggesting a type of paroxysmal dystonia when in actuality it is a precursor to migraine. Thus, the clinician must be mindful of prior events as part of the history of present illness and integrate them into the current context. Similarly, events occurring in the present may be harbingers of the future and allow anticipation of the development of new symptoms in time.

OCULAR MOVEMENTS AND DEVIATIONS

Ocular movements or deviations and autonomic and sensory phenomenon all have particular importance in non-epileptic event identification (Tables 2-6 and 2-7). These specific symptoms and signs should prompt recognition of particular entities because they are fairly unique and uncommon presentations of neurological disorders. Fortunately, many of the disorders identified in neonates and young children are benign; however, several can also be associated with significant underlying pathology. Sunsetting sign, for example, may be associated with an increased intracranial pressure and downward compression of the midbrain by hydrocephalus or mass.[25] Exclusion of these possibilities allows the acceptance of the benign explanation pertaining to immature

Table 2-6 Ocular Movements or Deviations as a Hallmark Presenting Feature

Age Range	With AC or Sleep	Without AC or Sleep
Neonatal	Reflex anoxic syncope REM sleep Factitious disorder by proxy	Ocular motor gaze phenomenon Tonic upgaze Tonic downgaze (sunsetting sign) Ocular nystagmus associated with alternating hemiplegia of childhood
Infants (<2 years)	Reflex anoxic syncope REM sleep Factitious disorder by proxy	Ocular motor gaze phenomenon Tonic upgaze Tonic downgaze (sunsetting sign) Ocular nystagmus associated with alternating hemiplegia of childhood Otitis media spells Spasmus nutans Benign paroxysmal vertigo Opsoclonus-myoclonus-ataxia syndrome Other movement disorders Factitious disorder by proxy

Children/ Adolescents	Reflex anoxic syncope REM sleep	Ocular nystagmus associated with alternating hemiplegia of childhood
	Somatoform disorder	Functional habit
	Factitious disorder (by proxy)	Otitis media spells
		Tics/Tourette's syndrome
		Opsoclonus-myoclonus-ataxia syndrome
		Other movement disorders
		Somatoform disorder
		Factitious disorder (by proxy)

Notes: AC = altered consciousness, BPD = broncho-pulmonary dysplasia.

Table 2-7 Autonomic and Sensory Phenomenon as Hallmark Presenting Features

Age Range	With AC or Sleep	Without AC or Sleep
Neonatal	Severe paroxysmal pain disorder Reflex anoxic syncope Cyanotic breath-holding spells Pallid breath-holding spells Dysautonomia Factitious disorder by proxy	Severe paroxysmal pain disorder Simple cyanotic breath-holding spells Simple pallid breath-holding spells Alternating hemiplegia of childhood Dysautonomia Hypoglycemia Factitious disorder by proxy
Infants (<2 years)	Severe paroxysmal pain disorder Reflex anoxic syncope Cyanotic breath-holding spells Pallid breath-holding spells Dysautonomia Factitious disorder by proxy	Severe paroxysmal pain disorder Simple cyanotic breath-holding spells Simple pallid breath-holding spells Episodic spontaneous recurrent hypothermia Alternating hemiplegia of childhood Dysautonomia Hypoglycemia Benign paroxysmal vertigo Factitious disorder by proxy
Children	Reflex anoxic syncope Non-REM parasomnias Night terrors Confusional arousals Panic attacks/rage attacks Somatoform disorder Factitious disorder (by proxy)	Severe paroxysmal pain disorder Episodic spontaneous recurrent hypothermia Dysautonomia Migraine Sensory tics/Tourette's syndrome Mastocytosis Rett's syndrome

continued

Table 2-7 continued

Age Range	With AC or Sleep	Without AC or Sleep
		Benign paroxysmal vertigo
		Abdominal migraine
		Cyclic vomiting
		Factitious disorder (by proxy)
Adolescents	Reflex anoxic syncope	Severe paroxysmal pain disorder
	Non-REM parasomnias	Dysautonomia
	Night terrors	Sensory tics/Tourette's syndrome
	Confusional arousals	Abdominal migraine
	REM parasomnias	Cyclic vomiting
	Panic attacks/rage attacks	Basilar artery migraine
	Somatoform disorder	Factitious disorder (by proxy)
	Factitious disorder (by proxy)	

Notes: AC = altered consciousness, BPD = broncho-pulmonary dysplasia, REM = rapid eye movement.

visual pathway development. Nystagmus of all forms typically signifies important disturbances potentially within the visual pathways, cerebrum, and/or brainstem-cerebellum circuitry. The specific quality of the movement has specific relevance with regard to diagnosis and possible etiology. Opsoclonus in particular may be subtle at onset but may be associated with underlying occult neuroblastoma.[26] When coupled with the gradual and progressive development of myoclonus and ataxia, the syndrome, opsoclonus-myoclonus-ataxia syndrome, can be easily recognized.[26] Therefore, in the absence of immediate recognition of the eye movements, an appreciation of the accumulation of symptoms over time is an absolute requirement of the clinician. Alternatively, a less easily characterized and sometimes confusing form of "complex nystagmus" may be identified paroxysmally. Parental reports of intermittent unilateral eye movement should prompt consideration of at least two specific syndromes in childhood, spasmus nutans and alternating hemiplegia of childhood.[15,27] In the former (spasmus nutans), unilateral horizontal movements of fine quality, best described as evanescent shimmering, may be noticed. This unilaterality may eventually give rise to bilateral nystagmus or alternatively a complete remission. Although in many children (29%) this may be a benign condition, that is, true spasmus nutans, when neuroimaging and visual assessment are normal (with qualifications), there is also an even higher frequency of retinal, visual pathway, and other CNS abnormalities appreciated.[27] Correspondingly, unilateral nystagmus may take on variable qualities such as rotatory, fine, and coarse horizontal jerking and alternating types within the same eye or between eyes. This history of rather bizarre, confusing, and seemingly improbable forms of nystagmus in a single child should signal the likely diagnosis of alternating hemiplegia of childhood as an explanation.[15]

AUTONOMIC AND SENSORY PHENOMENON

Autonomic and sensory disturbances can be recognized as part of several periodic syndromes and as an accompaniment to a number of other important non-epileptic phenomena (Table 2-7). Pallor and flushing are the commonest presentations of vasomotor instability appreciated among the disorders. These changes are but one characteristic of an activated or disrupted functioning autonomic nervous system. Vasomotor changes may be noted as a terminal component of a sequence of clinically appreciated steps that allow for a diagnosis of pallid breath holding (pallid infantile syncope) or can be appreciated as the initial attribute in the sequence identifying the extreme paroxysmal pain disorder.[28,29] In extreme paroxysmal pain disorder, the extreme pain attacks are precipitated by innocuous mechanical triggers to individualized sensitive body zones.[29] Infants may display harlequin vasomotor changes in response to specific stimuli at the initiation of a sequence leading to tonic arching posture with resultant apnea, bradycardia, and loss of consciousness (syncope) without crying.[29] Of interest is that water immersion for bathing may be a particularly potent trigger of these attacks. A similar triggering from bathwater has been identified in children aged 2–15 months who suffer from aquagenic urticaria.[30] In this disorder, bathwater immersion precipitates the sudden onset of pallor, hypotonia, and unresponsiveness, which may further proceed to syncope.[30] Therefore even the circumstance and specificity of the triggers may hold particular relevance in diagnosis of these particular syndromes.

Episodic spontaneous recurrent hypothermia with inappropriately activated diaphoresis is but one other periodic syndrome encountered in both children and adults recognized under the eponym Shapiro's syndrome when associated with agenesis of the corpus callosum.[31] The hypothermia must be measured at or below 34°C–35°C to qualify. Periodic bouts (two to four per year) of hypothermia are less consistently accompanied by bradycardia, pallor, hypertension, somnolence, abdominal pain, and headache.[31] Children as young as 2 months old may present with this unusual clinical combination, but the more typical ages are 2–5 years old.[31]

As a final comment, it is incumbent upon the clinician to not only diagnose the problems presented by the patient but also to follow up and assure its veracity. It is not infrequent that an underlying medical problem is the etiology for the non-epileptic disorder encountered. In this circumstance, treatment of the underlying problem should help ameliorate the presenting neurological disorder. This is certainly true for a medical problem such as gastroesophageal reflux when associated with the presentation of Sandifer's syndrome.[32] This too can be a case when otitis media is ultimately identified as the underlying cause of spells resembling absence and complex partial seizure episodes.[33] Adequate treatment of this medical problem resolves the behavioral events prompting neurological evaluation. But more to the point, further evaluation and unnecessary treatment are averted when a correct identification is secured. Occasionally the correct diagnosis even leads to an unexpected identification of a previously unmasked and unidentified non-epileptic disorder. This has been true in rare instances when absence epilepsy has been appropriately identified and treated with valproate, only to unmask a paroxysmal tonic upgaze disorder when seizures were abated.[34]

REFERENCES

1. Eddy DM, Clanton CH. Solving the clinicopathological exercise. N Engl J Med 1982; 306; 1263–1268.
2. Elstein AS, Schulman LS, Sprafka SA. *Medical Problem Solving: An Analysis of Clinical Reasoning.* Cambridge MA: Harvard University Press, 1978.
3. Engel GL. The deficiencies of the case presentation as a method of clinical teaching. N Engl J Med 1971; 284; 20–24.
4. Groves M, O'Rourke P, Alexander H. Clinical reasoning: the relative contribution of identification, interpretation, and hypothesis errors to misdiagnosis. Med Teach 2003; 25(6); 621–625.
5. Lanzi G, Zambrino CA, Balottin U, et al. Periodic syndrome and migraine in children and adolescents. Ital J Neurol Sci 1997; 18; 283–288.
6. Andermann F. Neurologic aspects of non-epileptic seizures. In *Non-Epileptic Seizures*, Eds: JR Gates, AJ Rowan, Boston MA, Butterworth-Heinemann, 2000; 51–69.
7. DiMario FJ. The nervous system. In Rudolph's *Fundamentals of Pediatrics.* Eds: AM Rudolph, RK Kamei, KJ Overby. 3rd edition. Mcgraw Hill, New York, 2002; 796–846.
8. Paolicchi JM. The spectrum of non-epileptic events in children. Epilepsia 2002; 43(Suppl 3); 60–64.
9. Obeid M, Mikati MA. Expanding spectrum of paroxysmal events in children: potential mickers of epilepsy. Pediatr Neurol 2007; 37; 309–316.
10. Eminson DM. Somatising in children and adolescents. 1. Clinical presentations and aetiological factors. Adv Psychiatr Treat 2001; 7; 266–274.
11. Galvin HK, Newton AW, Vandeven AM. Update on Munchausen syndrome by proxy. Curr Opin Pediatr 2005; 17(2); 252–257.
12. McLeod KA. Syncope in childhood. Arch Dis Child 2003; 88; 350–353.
13. Stephenson JBP. Anoxic seizures: self-terminating syncopes. Epilep Dis 2003; 3; 3–6.
14. Thomsen LL. Familial hemiplegic migraine: update. Cephalalgia 2008; 28; 415–470.
15. Mikati M, Kramer U, Zupanc ML, et al. Alternating hemiplegia of childhood: clinical manifestations and long-term outcome. Pediatr Neurol 2000; 23(1); 134–141.
16. Shuper A, Packer RJ, Vezina LG, et al. "Complicated migraine-like episodes" in children following cranial irradiation and chemotherapy. Neurol 1995; 45; 1837–1840.
17. Wiese JA, Gentry LR, Menezes AH. Bobble-head doll syndrome. Review of the pathophysiology and CSF dynamics. Pediatr Neurol 1985; 1; 361–366.
18. Deonna T, Ziegler AL, Nielson J. Transient idiopathic dystonia in infancy. Neuropediatrics 1991; 22; 220–224.
19. Malow BA. Paroxysmal events in sleep. J Clin Neurophysiol 2002; 19(6); 522–534.
20. Tourette's Syndrome Classification Group. Definitions and classification of tic disorders. Arch Neurol 1993; 50; 1013–1016.

21. Nechay A, Ross LM, Stephenson JBP, O'Regan M. Gratification disorder ("infantile masturbation"): a review. Arch Dis Child 2004; 89: 225–226.
22. Demkirkiran M, Jankovic J. Paroxysmal dyskinesias: clinical features and classification. Ann Neurol 1995; 38; 571–579.
23. Gottlob I, Zubkov AA, Wizov SS, et al. Head nodding is compensatory in spasmus nutans. Ophthalmol 1992; 99(7); 1024–1031.
24. Giffin NJ, Benton S, Goadsby PJ. Benign paroxysmal torticollis of infancy: four new cases and linkage to CACN1A mutation. Dev Med Child Neurol 2002; 44; 490–493.
25. Yoshikawa HB. Benign "setting sun" phenomenon in full-term infants. J Child Neurol 2003; 18(6); 424–425.
26. Pranzatelli MR. The neurobiology of the Opsoclonus-myoclonus syndrome. Clin Neuropharm 1992; 15(3); 186–228.
27. Gottlob I, Zubkov AA, Catalano RA, et al. Signs distinguishing spasmus nutans (with and without central nervous system lesions) from infantile nystagmus. Ophthalmology 1990; 97(9); 1166–1175.
28. DiMario FJ. Breath-holding spells in childhood. Am J Dis Child 1992; 146; 125–131.
29. Fertleman CR, Ferrie CD, Aicardi J, et al. Paroxysmal extreme pain disorder (previously familial rectal pain syndrome). Neurology 2007; 69; 586–595.
30. Mouterde O, Mallet E, Spriet J. Syncope during bathing in infants, a pediatric form of water-induced urticaria? Arch de Pediatrie 1997; 4(11); 1111–1115.
31. Ruiz C, Gener B, Garaizar C, et al. Episodic spontaneous hypothermia: a periodic childhood syndrome. Pediatr Neurol 2003; 28; 304–306.
32. Sutclife J. Torsion spasm and abnormal postures in children with hiatus hernia Sandifer's syndrome. Prog Pediatr Radiol 1969; 2; 190–197.
33. Soman TB, Krishnamoorthy KS. Paroxysmal non-epileptic events resembling seizures in children with otitis media. Clin Pediatr (Phila) 2005; 44; 437–441.
34. Luat AF, Asano E, Chugani HT. Paroxysmal tonic upgaze of childhood with co-existent absence epilepsy. Epilep Dis 2007; 9(3); 332–336.

3

Syncope

INTRODUCTION TO SYNCOPE

Generalized convulsions are recognizable by a sudden loss of consciousness, collapse, rhythmic motor behaviors, and gradual recovery. This sequence of clinical events may be mistakenly concluded if the additional precise details of the initiating triggers, prodromal symptoms, more gradual development of lost consciousness, and prompt recovery are not specifically sought after in order to identify syncope. The ease at which these distinct clinical entities, syncope, and epileptic seizure are inadvertently confused can be easily understood but with careful attention to the clinical history may as easily be distinguished. The nuances in the clinical expression of syncope can deepen the potential confusion with epileptic seizures. Those nuances being the fact that both convulsive syncope and syncope with resultant epileptic convulsions can each be evident as a terminal event of a syncopal episode. These and many other facets of syncope are discussed below.

THE CLINICAL PROBLEM AND EPIDEMIOLOGY

Syncope is a symptom defined as a sudden, transient, self-limited loss of consciousness that leads to an alteration of postural tone. It is produced by the interplay of several physiologic mechanisms, which culminate in cerebral hypoperfusion/hypoxia.[1,2] There is usually a prompt, spontaneous, and complete recovery. The word *syncope* is derived from the Greek verb "koptein," to cut or disrupt, which in this circumstance implies cerebral perfusion.[2] As with all clinical encounters, the precision of clinical detail and description begets the accuracy of ultimate diagnosis.[1] This is particularly true of syncope especially when there is a convulsive component, where, in the heat of the moment, even observers to the event may block out memory for these details until the astute clinician jogs them lose and identifies their importance. In this instance, certain figures of speech, vernacular and colloquial language with their specific connotations, need clarification (see Tables 1-4 and 1-5). When the subject or observers simply describe collapsing or falling, it is important to establish whether or not there was a clear and concurrent loss of consciousness. Without this specific feature there is no syncope.

Most forms of syncope have an identifiable provocation and warning or aura that accompany the early phase prior to the loss of consciousness.[1] Should the event terminate prior to the loss of consciousness, identifying "pre-syncope" symptoms offers a suggestive understanding but not a definitive one. Subjects undergoing other phenomena (e.g., psychogenic syncope or partial seizures) may experience the same or similar symptoms. Similarly, "collapsing" without loss of consciousness implies a different etiology, such as possible cataplexy, atonic/myoclonic epileptic seizures, non-epileptic myoclonus, tics, or psychogenic events, etc. The "diagnosis" of pre-syncope is therefore fraught with peril such that repetition of events and clarification over time may be needed for assuredness. The patient with clear syncope may experience a sudden "graying out" of vision described as a gradual constriction of their visual fields, a fading out of sounds, echoing or tinnitus, and/or some vague abdominal upset, followed by an impending sense of collapse and loss of consciousness. Observers may identify certain pallor to the subject's color and associated diaphoresis. These are typical premonitory symptoms (subjective feelings) and signs (observed phenomenon) particularly in reflex syncope (Table 3-1). The subject may attempt to protect himself or herself while falling limply to the ground, but sudden stiffening and "collapse to the floor like a board" may also transpire. The observation of sudden tonic extensor posture while standing may have the more specific implication of a brainstem release posture associated with anoxic syncope rather than an epileptic tonic convulsion, which most often occur in sleep and in cognitively impaired children with Lennox-Gastaut syndrome.[1–6] Eye rolling, urinary incontinence, and vocalizations are each possible during the syncopal event and thus do not imply epilepsy. Prompt resolution (<30 seconds) with return of consciousness upon recumbency is usual, but a short lingering sense of confusion, fatigue, and dysarthria upon speaking may be appreciated. There are many elements of syncope that share commonality with epileptic seizures; however, certain precipitating factors,

Table 3-1 Premonitory Symptoms Prior to Syncope

Subjective

- Lightheadedness, dizziness
- Generalized wave of heat or cold sensation
- Visual field constriction
- Auditory reverberations, tinnitus
- Gustatory bitterness, nausea, gastric discomfort
- Knee buckling, weakness

Objective

- Facial pallor
- Sweaty and clammy damp skin
- Pupillary dilatation
- Hypophonic speech
- Frail effort to protect oneself or prompt collapse

Table 3-2 Shared and Discriminating Features of Epileptic-Generalized Convulsions and Syncope

Shared Features	Discriminating Features of Syncope
• Aura	• Specific provocative factors and specific trigger mechanisms
• Loss of consciousness	
• Tonic postures	• Convergence of premonitory symptoms
• Myoclonic movements (proximal & distal)	• Unforced brief tonic head & trunk extension (opisthotonus with breath-holding spells)
• Eye deviations	
• Automatisms	
• Vocalizations	• Early downbeat nystagmus or upgaze
• Hallucinations	• Rare, short, solitary automatisms
• Tongue bites	• Rare tongue biting
• Incontinence	• Prompt postictal mental clarity
• Traumatic injury	
• Postictal confusion & fatigue	

Source: Modified from References.[5, 66]

premonitory symptoms, and postictal features will help to clinically discriminate between the two (Table 3-2). It is of interest to note that when the videotaped eye movements in a volunteer cohort of 14 healthy young adults who induced self-syncopes upon tilt testing were systematically studied, 6/14 demonstrated downbeat nystagmus, which evolved into upgaze deviation, 7/14 showed tonic upgaze gaze deviation from the start, and 1/14 remained in the primary position.[7] These eye movement behaviors have been commented upon in recorded childhood syncopes as well. Many focal onset epileptic seizures are accompanied by eye deviations laterally; however, sustained gaze in primary position or brief upgaze deviation at onset is not uncommon in generalized seizures at onset. The observation of downbeat nystagmus or tonic upgaze may have some distinguishing value between syncope and epilepsy. The utility of identifying tongue biting has also been prospectively and retrospectively studied and reported from an adult EEG monitoring unit.[8] Of 108 events recorded (34 epileptic seizures, 29 non-epileptic seizures, 45 syncopes), only epileptic (8) events and syncope (1) had tongue lacerations noted. These were only on the lateral surfaces in epileptic events (8), and in the single syncope subject who had a tongue laceration it was found on the tip.[8] Therefore, tongue biting per se is much more suggestive of epileptic events and when identified on the lateral margins of the tongue appear to be more specific.

Concurrent EEG recording has defined the actual electrographic correlate of this phenomenon. Clearly, there are many patients who additionally manifest an anoxic convulsion (convulsive syncope). Clinically these are generally composed of an extensor posturing of the head and trunk, with arms held either slightly flexed or extended for a short burst of activity (<15–30 seconds), often (90%) with arrhythmic multifocal myoclonic jerks that can be focal (16%) or generalized (1%).[1,3] This clinical evolution is characterized by an

EEG, showing 1–3 Hz slow wave patterns evolving to extreme attenuation, or flat and then a gradual rebound in the terminal phase of the syncope.[1,9–13] Several authors have thoroughly reviewed the data concerning the EEG pattern correlates of syncope by all such triggers and ages.[1,9,13] Sudden, complete interruption of cerebral oxygenation leads to what are referred to as classical EEG changes of a slow-flat-slow pattern. There exists a point, an individual's anoxic threshold, which, if crossed, produces the anoxic convulsion. This threshold will be crossed earlier in a child and progressively later at older ages.[1] There is by direct extension and direct clinical observation a linear relationship between the durations of anoxia (asystole) and the EEG signal flattening.[1] The anoxic convulsion has been cited to occur as frequently as 70%–90%.[1,4,5,9–11] By definition and EEG evaluation, these are non-epileptic and are thought to represent brainstem release phenomena. In addition, there are rare reported instances in which an anoxic epileptic convulsion (EEG with concurrent spike-wave discharges) evolves at the terminal phase of the syncope, altering the classic slow-flat-slow EEG pattern to become slow-flat-spike EEG pattern.[1,12,14–16] Prior early descriptions and more recent video recordings demonstrate a variety of clinical seizure expressions, in part dependent upon the concurrent EEG discharge, and include absence, rhythmic clonic activity with or without irregular myoclonus and vocalizations, and vibratory tonic posturing behaviors.[1,14–18] The type of motor behavior observed may differentiate the more common anoxic (non-epileptic) seizure from the less frequently observed anoxic epileptic seizure type. The development of rhythmic clonic convulsive activity of varying durations is most distinctive for anoxic epileptic seizures, which can continue for many minutes. A brief (<30 seconds) combination of extensor posturing with arrhythmic myoclonus is most commonly exhibited with anoxic seizures. The so-called reflex anoxic seizure (with or without evolution into an anoxic epileptic seizure) is characterized by an associated and causative "reflex" or neurally mediated cardiac inhibition that results in profound bradycardia or brief periods of asystole (6 seconds).[1,19] Other common synonyms include pallid breath holding, pallid infantile syncope, vagocardiogenic attacks, etc. (see Table 1-4). Unique among the reflex mechanisms are childhood cyanotic breath-holding spells, in that these are mediated by a primary "reflex" respiratory inhibition without concurrent bradycardia.[19]

Syncope in children is common. Epidemiological studies identify population frequencies ranging from 0.3%–15% of children before 18 years of age.[2,20] Surveys of specific young age groups such as military recruits, and college and medical students report frequencies of 20%–25%, with up to 50% reporting having experienced a single episode.[21,22] Syncope results in about 3% of emergency room visits annually and up to 6% of hospitalizations in the adolescent age group.[23,24] These figures should, but generally do not, include breath holding as one of the specific syncopes of childhood, and thus the actual prevalence would additionally increase. A population-based study in Geelong, Australia (The Geelong Study), reported by Rossiter, determined the population incidence of breath holding in a sample of 4988 children born from April 1970 to April 1972 and followed from birth through age 11 years to be 14.6 per 1000 live births.[25] Other well-child clinic and practice-based prevalence figures of children with severe breath-holding spells (i.e., those children who lose consciousness) suggest a range of 0.1%–4.6%.[19]

The long-term outcomes for subgroups of subjects with syncope can be stratified. Young healthy individuals with no heart disease and normal EKG—many of whom have neurally mediated syncope syndromes—show no evidence of increased mortality. (see below).[2] There may be added morbidity, however, with lacerations, bruises, and fractures reported in up to 12%–29% of adult cohorts.[2,26] This may be significantly lower in younger populations, which include preschool and school-aged children. The number of unintentional syncope-related injuries after immunization reported to the FDA for the years 1990–2004 was 3168, with 35% among children aged 10–18 years.[27] For the most recent period, 2000–2005, the number of reported injuries was 107, with one additional fatal report.[28,29] The fatality was in a 15-year-old boy who died from consequent cardiac arrhythmia after sustaining an initial head injury from falling.[28,29] The most severe injuries of those reported were from cases of head trauma suffered after falling or from a delayed onset of symptoms that caused motor vehicle accidents. The majority (89%) of syncopes reported occurred within 15 minutes after immunization.[27] These and other reports prompted formal recommendations for a 15-minute observation period after immunization administration.[27]

OVERVIEW: PATHOPHYSIOLOGY AND MECHANISMS

What is it that produces the syncopal event? In order to understand this we must first review the factors required to maintain normal consciousness. This requires both intact and functioning brain, cardiovascular, and autonomic nervous systems. The normal cerebral blood flow of 45 mL/100 g tissue/minute is seen in healthy term newborns, which increases to 105 mL/100 g tissue/minute in children, and then reduces to 50–60 mL/100 g tissue/minute in adolescents and young adult subjects.[2,30,31] In order to sustain this flow, about 10%–15% of resting cardiac output is required. From this a minimum of 3–3.5 mL O_2/100 g tissue/minute is required to sustain consciousness.[2,31] Cerebral perfusion is dependent upon systemic blood pressure, which is responsive to physiological alterations in vascular resistance and heart rate, which are in turn effected by blood volume, oxygenation, forces of gravity and posture, emotional state, and ambient temperature among others. These alterations in systemic blood pressure are mediated through circulating humoral factors and autonomic nervous system reflex activity affecting neurocardiovascular homeostasis. The brainstem, in particular, integrates afferent inputs from the cerebral cortex and hypothalamus, peripheral cardiovascular baroreceptors and oxygen chemoreceptors (aortic and carotid bodies), fourth ventricular carbon dioxide chemoreceptor cells, integument and mucosal pain and temperature receptors, respiratory tract, mechano-/irritant-/j- and stretch-receptors, as well as inputs from internal viscera (bladder, intestines, etc.).[19] In turn, there is an intricate network of efferents, which mediate both instantaneous and gradual net surges of sympathetic or parasympathetic outflow to the heart and vascular beds, diaphragm and respiratory tree, and intestinal and genitourinary tracts. This is coupled with a commensurate release and metabolism of neuroactive and vasoactive compounds. Syncope will be induced when the final common effect is a critical reduction cerebral perfusion through an excessive or inadvertent but appropriate reflex activation, or via an inappropriate or inadequate response to a presented stimulation.

The major mechanistic categories of syncope are listed in Table 3-3. Within each category are listed subheadings of possible trigger mechanisms (neurocardiogenic) or specific presumptive etiologic causes. Neurally mediated or neurocardiogenic syncope is a heterogeneous group, which have a dominant primary nervous system induced mechanism resulting in reduced cerebral perfusion.[32,33] This mechanism may be initiated by a number of primary

Table 3-3 Mechanisms of Syncope

(i) Primary neurally-mediated reflex syncope/neurocardiogenic syncope
  A. Reflex "situational"/"vasovagal" types
    1. Cyanotic breath holding
    2. Swallow
    3. Tussive
    4. Hair grooming
    5. Stretch
    6. Postexertional
    7. Micturiction/defecation
    8. Pallid breath holding
    9. Emotion (fear/pain evoked)
    10. Venipuncture/acupuncture
    11. Photic induced
    12. Laughter induced.
  B. Carotid massage/carotid sinus syndrome
  C. Neuralgia (trigeminal/glossopharyngeal)
  D. Cerebral cortex-induced arrhythmia
  E. Reflex "postural" type
    1. Prolonged standing/orthostasis
  F. Paroxysmal extreme pain disorder
(ii) Orthostatic
  A. Forced valsalva/hyperventilation ("fainting larks")
  B. Postural orthostatic tachycardia syndrome
  C. Hypovolemia/anemia
  D. Vasodilatation
  E. Venous insufficiency
  F. Dysautonomia (primary, secondary)

  (iii) Primary cardiogenic
      A. Structural cardiac lesions with decreased cardiac outflow
      B. Valvular disease
      C. Cardiac arrhythmia (intrinsic, drug induced, pacemaker failure, etc.)
      D. Cardiomyopathy
      E. Cardiac tumors
      F. Exertional

  (iv) Secondary cardiogenic
      A. Aortic dissection
      B. Pericardial disease/tamponade
      C. Pulmonary hypertension/embolus

  (v) Cerebrovascular insufficiency
      A. Vasculopathy (dissection, atheroma, shunts, dysplasias, etc.)
      B. Vascular steal

  (vi) CNS malformations
      A. Chiari malformation
      B. Syringobulbia

  (vii) Suffocation

  (viii) Unknown/medical causes

---

events or "situations" that result in an inadvertent, inappropriate, or excessive activation of normal reflex pathways (central and peripheral) to produce bradycardia (absolute or relative) and/or vasodilation that summate to a reduction in systemic blood pressure and, ultimately, cerebral perfusion. The typical "situational" reflex triggers appear to overactivate reflex afferent feedback loops from the periphery: irritant, stretch, baroreceptors, and mechanoreceptors within the aortic arch and carotid bodies; the respiratory/gastrointestinal/genitourinary tracts or muscle stretch receptors within the cervical neck and shoulder girdle.[32–35] When activated, these excessive but appropriate afferent volleys result in sustained autonomic efferent outputs, which primarily affect a rapidly responsive vagally mediated bradycardia and an accompanying slowly activated decreased sympathetic vasoconstrictor effect. The vagally mediated reflex component exerts a dominant influence in the absence of an adequate sympathetic response; a reduction in systemic blood pressure and ultimately cerebral hypoperfusion results.[32–35] When evaluating the situational reflex triggers, the syncope occurs during or immediately after the trigger is activated. The underlying pathophysiology in other forms of reflex syncope, on the other hand, is incompletely understood and controversial in some instances.[32] In the case of prolonged standing and orthostasis, there is postulated to be an individual predisposition allowing excessive venous pooling and reduction in venous return to the heart.[32–34] This state allows for inadvertent upregulated afferent signals to the CNS from peripheral vascular mechanoreceptors mimicking the feedback provided under the situation of hypertension. This "dysfunctional" feedback results in an efferent volley back to the peripheral vascular beds producing a "paradoxical," (under this circumstance) vasodilation via a reduction in sympathetic outflow and systemic blood pressure. This aberrant mechanoreceptor response is augmented by the necessary and inappropriate redistribution of blood volume. These situations will be clinically experienced and described by the patient with the accompanying subjective premonitory symptoms enumerated in Table 3-1. Vasovagal reflex-mediated syncope refers to those triggers, which directly produce a vagally mediated bradycardia, or asystole.[1,35] These are most often emotionally induced—for example, with the experience of sudden fear, pain, or surprise, as with immunization. An important pediatric entity precipitated by this mechanism is pallid breath holding (reflex anoxic syncope) (see below). The cyanotic breath-holding spells (cyanotic infantile syncope, prolonged expiratory apnea) are similarly autonomic reflex mediated, but rather than a predominant centrally mediated vagal cardioinhibition, there is a centrally mediated respiratory inhibition with attendant hypertension and absence of glottic closure (i.e., no valsalva).[1,19] Each type is associated with more subtle underlying autonomic dysregulation, which appears to be modified with maturation and age. Carotid massage induces an appropriate baroreceptor-mediated reflex bradycardia and resultant hypotension. In older individuals, there may be an inappropriate hypersensitivity to carotid stimulation, which produces profound hypotension and orthostatic intolerance.

Orthostatic mechanisms refer to those factors that fail to enact peripheral vasomotor constriction in order to maintain and adjust systemic blood pressure enough to sustain upright posture. As with the reflex autonomic response to prolonged standing, arising from recumbency initiates all the afferent feedback mechanisms described above. However, when there is a critical reduction in venous return to the heart from faulty autonomic regulation of circulatory responses secondary to vascular or neuropathic causes or an inadequate volume of normally oxygenated blood within the circulation for whatever reason, the inadequacy of these responses will result in a critical decrease in cerebral perfusion and oxygenation resulting in syncope upon postural change. Forced valsalva (true breath holding) or inspiratory apnea (apneusis) may precipitate syncope especially if combined with ocular compression, carotid massage, or occlusion, which will induce added bradycardia.[1,13,36] In this instance, forced expiration against a closed glottis results principally in a reduction of venous return and diminished cardiac output. Another important but less well defined entity in children, postural orthostatic tachycardia syndrome (POTS), produces chronic orthostatic intolerance characterized by tachycardia with decreased cerebral blood flow upon upright posture. This can result in a severe disabling sense of lightheadedness and syncope despite an appropriate increase in cardiac rate.[37–39] There is an accompanying inadequate vasomotor response with signs of increased peripheral sympathetic nervous system outflow, particularly in supine posture, coupled with catecholamine excess from surges of adrenomedullary hormones when studied in adult subjects.[38–40]

Primary cardiac causes include rhythm disturbances and structural heart diseases that impair cardiac output.[2,3,41,42] Arrhythmias result in diminished cardiac output regardless of whether there is a physical or physiologic demand placed on pumping function. Structural heart disease on the other hand results in syncope when the demand on the heart is surpassed by its ability to keep pace with it. The secondary cardiac causes each result in a net decrease in blood volume delivery to the target tissues and brain in particular. This blood flow impairment will again reduce cerebral perfusion and result in a syncopal propensity. The specific pathologies may in turn produce consequent heart pumping failure over time.

Acquired cerebrovascular diseases, vascular dysplasias, dissections, fistulas, and steals, all potentially impair blood delivery to the brain depending upon their location within the vascular tree and physiological effect. Although these vascular disorders are more frequently identified in the adult population, certain vulnerable childhood populations exist as well. Sickle cell disease may be accompanied by atheroma and aneurysmal formation within the cerebral arteries. These vascular abnormalities coupled with intermittent sickling may impede regional and global cerebral blood flow to produce transient ischemia, recognized clinically as a transient ischemic attack.[43,44] Seizures may ultimately herald the impending cerebral infarction. This may be provoked in susceptible vascular territories by provocation with hyperventilation. Syncope theoretically may result, should multiple vessels be affected, impacting bilateral cerebral circulation, or major flow to the brainstem is curtailed. Similar susceptibility may be seen in children who have been exposed to ionizing radiation to the brain and cerebral circulation as a treatment for certain cancers.[45]

As should be clear from the foregoing discussions on mechanisms of syncope, the brainstem serves a critical role in the reception, referral, and relay of afferent and efferent-autonomic responses. These functions are critical and continual throughout the individual's life. Structural disease of the brainstem, developmental or acquired, particularly in the ponto-medullary region, will affect the integrity of this integrating function. The effects upon the brainstem's intrinsic pacemaker properties, which emanate from the respiratory and cardiovascular drive centers, and potential interference with the accurate interpretation and response from the chemoreceptor region, may be devastating.

TESTING

The evaluation of syncope in pediatric patients should be aided by our collective experiences. In a prospective evaluation of 58 consecutive pediatric subjects aged 6 months to 15 years (mean age 8.2 years, 1.9 years for breath holders) presenting to an emergency room, 43% presented after a single event, and 57% after multiple.[46] The vast majority had neurally mediated syncope (91%), with reflex vasovagal as a primary mechanism.[46] Diagnosis was established in 45/58 by history alone and in 15 others, aided with additional testing

(11 ocular compression, 4 head-up tilt test). Among the group, 10 children had a history of breath holding, and 19 had a positive family history of syncope. In a more recent study of 226 consecutive pediatric subjects presenting to the emergency room with syncope (0.41%) out of 60,754 patient visits, 80% had a diagnosis of neurally mediated syncope (mean age 11 years), and 9% other neurological diagnoses (18 epileptic seizure, 1 meningitis, 1 stroke, 1 narcolepsy).[47] Girls were significantly overrepresented (111:70) among those with neurally mediated syncope. The children with neurally mediated syncope underwent a total of 425 tests, with only 24 (5%) identifying diagnostically significant findings. Once again history, particularly the identification of specific triggers, and a normal examination were 98% predictive of correct diagnosis with this etiology.[47] Those with cardiac disease (5/226, i.e., 2%) were most often identified when there was an abnormal cardiac auscultation, exercise-induced events, lack of prolonged upright posture, or variable position at time of syncope.

Steinberg and Knilans performed a cost analysis of diagnostic testing yields in a retrospective cohort of 169 pediatric patients presenting for outpatient evaluation of syncope.[48] A total of 663 tests were performed at a cost of $180,128.00, with only 26 tests (3.9%) proven to be of diagnostic value in 24 patients (14.2%). The average cost was $1055.00 per patient and $6928.00 per diagnostic result in 1999 dollars.[48] Loop memory cardiac event recording was the most cost-effective test in their study amounting to 1 diagnostic yield in 13. This yield was a normal sinus rhythm during syncope excluding arrhythmia as a cause. In fact, no arrhythmias were identified. Electrocardiograms were most frequently ordered (221/663), with only one diagnostic result.[48] In another study determining the diagnostic yield of screening echocardiography in a cohort of 480 pediatric patients, 458 had noncardiac causes.[49] There were only 20 (4.1%) with an arrhythmia or long QT syndrome of the 449/480 (94%) who underwent EKG.[49] Echocardiograms were performed in 322/480 (67%) cases and were abnormal in 12%. When the authors considered the sensitivity/specificity of a screening protocol consisting of a history of exercise-induced events, family history positive for cardiomyopathy, syncope, long QT, or sudden death, and an abnormal examination or abnormal EKG, a positive screen was 96% sensitive and 36% specific, with a positive predictive value of only 7% but a negative predictive value of 99%.[49]

The use of Holter monitoring in pediatric patients has been further studied in a group of 1500 children undergoing 2017 Holter records.[50] In the infant to 24-year age range, 67% underwent screening evaluation for symptoms of palpitations, chest pains, or syncope.[50] There were patients with known cardiac disease who were investigated for effects of antiarrhythmic therapy in 17%, postoperative findings in 5%, and pacemaker control in 4%. Overall, only 5.3% of all patients studied had an identified symptomatic arrhythmia during monitoring, and asymptomatic arrhythmia was more common. Palpitation was the most frequently associated symptom with arrhythmia, not syncope. Arrhythmias were highest among patients who had undergone cardiac repair exhibiting supraventricular extrasystole, supraventricular tachycardia, and complete heart block.[50] The authors concluded this was a low-yield diagnostic tool especially in patients without palpitation or prior cardiac repair.[50]

The utility of head-up tilt (HUT) testing in the evaluation of pediatric syncope has been debated.[2,3] Positive test results imply that there was an induction of syncope during the test, although some laboratories define the development of near-syncope as a positive test.[51] In an adult series of 694 patients, 8% had neurological events observed, which included anoxic convulsions, tonic posturing, focal seizures, aphasia, dysesthesia, and syncope.[52] The test has been helpful to distinguish epileptic seizures from syncope and anoxic convulsions in children.[53] There has been a small series of pediatric patients with positive tests who have undergone repeat testing within the same day.[54] Fifteen of seventeen patients with a positive initial test had a positive test upon repetition (88%), inferring a positive probability of 70% at a confidence interval of 95%.[54] Overall, these "positive" results has been appreciated in up to 40%–70% of tested children with neurally mediated syncope.[51,53–56] Remarkably, it has been noted that just placement of an intravenous line prior to the procedure has resulted in syncope/near-syncope in up to 40% of these otherwise healthy children and teenagers.[51] Importantly, most series previously identified a significant false positive and false negative rate, reducing diagnostic specificity associated with HUT. Shorter tilt duration has been suggested as an adaptive strategy with improved specificity >85%.[57] The general protocol and responses are listed in Table 3-4.[2,3] These are adapted from adult procedures and may

Table 3-4 Head-Up Tilt Table Protocol Outline[3]

- Supine pre-tilt phase: 5 minutes (20 minutes after IV insertion)
- Tilt phase: angle 60°–70° upright
- Passive phase: 10 minutes tilted (20–45 minutes adults)
- Drug challenge phase:15–20 minutes with isoproterenol IV or sublingual nitroglycerin if passive phase is negative
- The end point is defined as the induction of syncope or completion of the planned duration of tilt

Positive if syncope occurs or

- I-Mixed type: Heart rate falls but >40 bpm or <40 bpm for less than 10 seconds with or without asystole <3 seconds, or BP falls before HR
- II-A Cardioinhibition without asystole: Heart rate falls <40 bpm for more than 10 seconds with asystole <3 seconds, or BP falls before HR
- II-B Cardioinhibition with asystole: Asystole >3 seconds. BP falls with or before HR fall
- III Vasodepressor: Heart rate does not fall more than10% from its peak at time of syncope

Exceptions: No HR raise during tilt, excessive HR rise at onset upright and throughout duration before syncope.

Notes: bpm = beats per minute, HR = heart rate, BP = blood pressure.

not be as specific for pediatrics. Another suggested approach to studying syncope in pediatric patients has been to use an active standing test (AST) instead of HUT in the investigation of children with orthostatic syncope.[58] The AST simply entails noninvasive physiologic measuring modes of the subject during and after each maneuver, the person arising to a standing posture after lying supine over standard durations of time. In a comparative study of the two techniques and a review of the literature, Matsushima et al. found similar positive test rates (AST 43%, HUT 47%) and similar, although low, syncope induction rates (AST 27%, HUT 18%).[58] Curiously, in a questionnaire study of the daytime distribution of syncopal episodes in a cohort of children (mean age 13.7 years; 19 boys, 30 girls) who underwent HUT, the authors found a significant ($p < 0.001$) positive correlation between time of syncope and result of tilt testing.[59] The children with positive tests (28/49) had syncopal episodes clustered in the mornings (10 AM–12 PM), whereas the children with negative tests (21/49) had syncopal episodes more typically in the afternoons (2 PM–6 PM).[59] The findings suggest an inherent circadian rhythm in the functioning of the autonomic nervous system, which favors higher sympathetic function earlier in the day, and hence positive HUT testing in those subjects with a sympathetically mediated syncope more likely in the morning. This has been shown to be true for plasma noradrenaline levels and sympathetic effects on QTc dispersion.[60–62]

Tilt testing may have its greatest utility, however, in the patient with an "unknown etiology" to the syncope. In a recent adult series of 640 consecutive patients aged 8–85 years (mean age 45 years) with unexplained syncope/pre-syncope despite careful history and examination, who underwent HUT testing, 54% (344/640) had positive tests.[63] There was an age-related gradient in hemodynamic responses, such that older patients had vasodepressor (type 3) and late responses, whereas younger patients more commonly experienced cardioinhibitory or mixed responses (types 1 or 2).[63] This is in contrast to a recent pediatric series where 155/208 (74.5%) of children aged 3–19 years (mean age 11 years) with unexplained syncope undergoing HUT testing had a positive test.[64] However, the hemodynamic pattern was predominantly vasodepressor (type 3) in 34.6%, postural orthostatic tachycardia syndrome in 28.8%, cardioinhibitory or mixed (types 1 or 2) in 2.4% and 8.7%, respectively, and normal in 25%.[64] There are clearly difficulties with extrapolating data from adult series to the pediatric age range. Beyond age, the incidence of significant heart disease in the adult series makes the populations fundamentally incomparable with a bias toward orthostatic mechanisms. A more fundamental mechanism of syncope may be induced from brain perfusion studies using 99mTc-ECD SPECT in pediatric patients with neurally mediated syncope.[65] Ilgin and colleagues performed SPECT scans with injections done during HUT testing in order to determine hemodynamic responses and correlates to regional brain perfusion in twenty subjects.[65] Pooled data analysis showed decreases in perfusion were more widespread regionally in the left hemisphere (left anterior fronto-parietal > prefrontal posterior > other regions) than concomitant decreases in the right hemisphere.[65] However, they also found that when tilt-positive subjects (10/20) were compared to tilt-negative subjects, brain perfusion was significantly lower in the right periinsular posterior parietal and temporal regions ($p < 0.05$) in the tilt-positive subjects than in any other region.[65] This area of the brain, the periinsular cortex, has been shown to be important as a lateralized cerebral region of cardiac autonomic control. The right periinsular cortex has been suggested to produce sympathetically mediated tachycardia, an increased diastolic pressure, whereas the left periinsular cortex has been implicated in parasympathetically mediated bradycardia and vasodepressor effects.[66–68] The decrease in regional brain perfusion of these areas allows for the imbalance of centrally mediated autonomic reflex cardiovascular functions.[66–68] The right insular control of sympathetically mediated function appears to have been transiently affected in these tilt-positive subjects.[65] The use of near-infrared spectroscopy (NIRS) during HUT-induced vasovagal reflex syncope has demonstrated changes in cerebral oxygenation prior to the syncope. In a study of sixty-nine adult subjects, forty-two had syncope induced during the tilt procedure.[69] Changes in oxyhemoglobin concentration as measured by NIRS were noted >3 minutes before the syncope. These reductions in oxyhemoglobin concentration were visible about 1.3 minutes before pre-syncope symptoms, 2.2 minutes before a drop in heart rate and blood pressure, and 2.6 minutes before a drop in arterial blood oxygen saturation.[69] These changes suggest that the reflex mechanisms responsible for syncope are actuated and begin to affect regional blood flow prior to symptoms developing. This has implication in that the first recognition of syncope may well be within a critical time period for the responder or the subjects themselves to alter the initiated sequence.

In summary, many tests of cardiovascular function may be employed in the evaluation of patients who present with syncope. The most important evaluative procedures remain the carefully extracted history and physical examination with orthostatic blood pressure/pulse measurements. In cases where syncope occurs during exercise, the subject has a sensation of cardiac palpitations, abnormal examination findings exist (hearing loss, neck-cranial bruits, steal phenomenon, etc.), or there is a family history of sudden cardiac death/arrhythmia, then the use of paraclinical testing such as EKG may not only aid in diagnosis but will be necessary. The use of HUT testing, Holter recording, and other laboratory measures should be reserved for individual cases where etiology or mechanism is unclear. These evaluations have particular importance where the risk for significant injury exists with or without heart disease and where specific identification of mechanism would alter treatment. Head-up tilt table testing may have utility in differentiation of epilepsy from convulsive syncope, dysautonomic syndromes, and in patients without heart disease in whom postexercise syncope cannot be reproduced with exercise stress testing.[2, 3]

Specific syndromes and etiologies of syncope are discussed below.

PRIMARY NEURALLY MEDIATED REFLEX SYNCOPES: THE CLINICAL CONDITIONS AND TREATMENTS

Cyanotic and Pallid Breath-Holding Spells

Breath-holding spells (BHS) in childhood are, not as the name implies, a prolonged expiratory apnea.[19,70,71] The diagnosis relies primarily upon the distinctive history of an initial provocation that produces an emotional upset or crying by the child, soon followed by a noiseless pause, mouth open, and a change in color (pale or cyanotic).[19,70,71] Simple BHS will terminate here, after the change in color and gasp of breath. The severe spells evolve to a state in which there is a progressive loss of consciousness and postural tone. The child will often assume an initial opisthotonus posture (body arched and resting on head and heels), with brief myoclonic jerks and a dazed trancelike appearance on the face. When the spell terminates, there is a period of relief and sighing, with a general sense of reconnoitering before registering their whereabouts and activity. These observations are identical to those noted during prolonged syncope from other provocations with incurred brainstem release phenomenon of reflex anoxic seizures and are accompanied by the EEG pattern of "slow-flat-slow." As other reflex syncopes, provocation to induce the spells is usual. The commonest inducers are minor traumas such as falls and bumps to the head. However, these spells can also be induced by simple frustration, anger, fear, and, perhaps more potent, the sudden sense of surprise that can occur with any of these other provocatives. Up to 15% of children with severe BHS experience a generalized anoxic epileptic seizure at the terminal phases of the spell, characterized by more prolonged clonic jerking and an EEG pattern of "slow-flat-spike."[1,17-19,72-77] The spell terminates with a sudden gasp and prompt return to consciousness if not prolonged by an anoxic epileptic seizure. Pallid BHS (PBHS) are much more rapid in their symptom development. Usually, a few whimpers will trigger sudden pallor or gray color, followed promptly by noiselessness and loss of consciousness. There may be a hint of facial flushing as the child recovers. Cyanotic BHS (CBHS) usually have a protracted period of crying accompanied by evolving cyanosis before loss of consciousness occurs. BHS may have been identified as early as day one of life but usually develop between ages 6–12 months and gradually escalate in frequency over the second year of life.[19,70,71] The prevalence of CBHS, PBHS, and mixed types has been fairly consistent over time and is approximately 5:3:2 (50%–60%, 20%–30%, 10%–20% ranges), as identified by recent authors.[1,19,71,73] The average frequency of spells is one or more per week by 18 months to 2 years of age, with a declining frequency thereafter.[19,70,71] About half of the children have the spells terminate by 36–42 months of age, with the remainder resolving by 7–8 years of age.[71,78] A strong family history is obtained in as many as 34%, with an autosomal dominant inheritance with reduced penetrance.[79] The presence of a maternal family predominance suggests the possible additional role of genomic imprinting. The reported prevalence of severe BHS is 0.1%–4.6%.[19,26]

Fortunately, serious sequelae from BHS have not been routinely observed. Nonetheless, a few fatalities in the midst of a severe BHS have been reported.[19,70,80–82] Each of two deaths was compounded by airway obstruction from food in the mouth during CPR administration, coexistent respiratory tract anomalies, and a cardiac arrest in a single child.[80–82] There have been no clearly demonstrated adverse neurodevelopmental outcomes attributed to BHS as a causative factor.[25,71,73,83–85] The association has been noted but not shown to be a result of the spells. The ultimate development of epilepsy has been variously reported to occur in 0.5%–11% of breath holders.[71,73,84–87] In the population-based study in Geelong, Australia (The Geelong Study), from the population sample of 4988 children born in the early 1970s and followed from birth through age 11 years, 73 developed severe BHS.[25] From this subset of children (51/73 had complete follow-up), there was a higher incidence of febrile convulsions noted (9.6%) compared to non-BHS children (5.2%) as also a higher incidence of non-febrile epileptic convulsions (11% compared to 3.2%).[25] Other abnormal outcomes specific to this group were not noted.[25] Syncope, particularly in children with pallid spells, may later develop in 17% of adolescents.[71,73]

The underlying pathophysiology of BHS involves interplay among CNS maturity, breathing control mechanisms, cardio-pulmonary mechanics, blood oxygen carrying capacity, and the autonomic nervous system. Autonomic dysregulation is the common underlying physiologic mechanism causing BHS. This appears to be maturationally dependent, with a gradual resolution of this dysregulation propensity over time. Reflex sympathetic overactivity is associated with cyanotic spells, and reflex parasympathetic overactivity is associated with pallid spells.[19] A number of additional physiologic factors also may impact upon the expression of these spells in the child predisposed to have them (see Table 3-5). Early investigations of autonomic responses were prompted by the observations of a parent who noted a slowed heart rate in her infant during a pallid spell, "vagotonia."[83] The oculocardiac reflex has been studied through means of ocular compression by many investigators. Application of pressure to both closed eyeballs simultaneously over 10 seconds triggers afferent signals via the ophthalmic branch of the trigeminal nerve back to the brainstem cardioinhibitory vagal nerve cell bodies within the nucleus ambiguous. This in turn results in a prompt efferent signal via the vagus nerve to the sinoatrial node of the heart, which results in cardiac slowing or transient asystole as measured by the progressive lengthening of the R-R interval. The intention would be to induce a syncope or anoxic seizure for diagnostic purposes; however, an asystole of >2 seconds has often been used as a positive test. Stephenson has amply reviewed the normative data and responses observed.[1] A period of >6 seconds of asystole is required to achieve specificity and sensitivity >98%. It can be questioned whether or not there exists any clinical utility at this time to merely induce some period of asystole (<6 seconds) during EEG recording.[1] Unless the procedure induces an anoxic seizure that is recognized as the exact type of event the parents have been viewing, the procedure becomes

Table 3-5 Pathophysiologic Mechanisms Leading to Severe Breath-Holding Spells

Autonomic Dysregulation

- Inappropriate pulmonary vascular bed shunting (CBHS)
- Inappropriate orthostatic vasomotor responses (CBHS)
- Excessive centrally mediated sympathetic responses (CBHS)
- Excessive centrally mediated parasympathetic responses (PBHS)
- Brief airway obstruction with increased sweating during sleep and wakefulness
- Transiently diminished ventilatory chemosensitivity
- Altered RSA tracings (PBHS)

Iron Deficiency

- Augments CNS serotonin due to decreased aldehyde oxidase activity
- Augments CNS norepinepherine due to decreased monamine oxidase activity
- May induce behavioral irritability
- Decreased blood oxygen-carrying capacity, with significant anemia

Respiratory Mechanics

- Overly compliant rib cage in neonates/infants
- Inappropriate overstimulation of normal respiratory reflexes

Alveolar Collapse

- Decreased surfactant quantity
- Decreased surfactant surface tension properties.

Source: Modified from Reference.[20]

largely an academic exercise. If the result of the maneuver is a confirmed event, then the diagnostic certainty of syncope can be assured. This centrally mediated parasympathetic stimulus is more readily elicited in children who have vagally mediated BHS (i.e., pallid breath holding) but can be induced from both CBHS subjects and nonselected controls in decreasing frequency rates: PBHS 61%–78%, CBHS 25%–36%, syncope subjects without BHS 26%–46%, and nonselected consecutive EEG subjects 13.5%–24%.[1,73,88–92] More recent examination of the maneuver in 116 patients with syncope or breath holding compared to 46 with epileptic seizures were retrospectively reviewed.[92] The authors used a duration of 2 seconds asystole as a positive response and found that there was only a 26% sensitivity yet 100% specificity in identifying syncopal/breath holder from epileptic patients.[92] Of course both epilepsy and syncope may occur concurrently in the same child. Similar too is that there are many children who display mixed patterns of breath holding, that is to say, a predominant of either cyanotic or pallid type but expressing both types at different times or some indeterminate mixture of the two at once. The prevalence of CBHS, PBHS, and mixed types has been fairly consistent over time and is approximately 5:3:2 (50%–60%, 20%–30%, 10%–20% ranges), as identified by several authors.[1,19,71,73,85,93] Maulsby and Kellaway recognized that the effect of ocular compression was to induce the now familiar sequence of prominent forced expiration and accompanying bradycardia or asystole during concurrent EEG changes of slow to flat.[93] They referred to CBHS as a type 1 hypoxic crisis and PBHS as a type 2 hypoxic crisis and posited that each type could occur in the same individual child.[93] Demonstration of this would occur such that if a stimulus such as ocular compression was maintained during the period of bradycardia to asystole, then forced expiration would be reflexively continued despite flattening of the EEG and loss of consciousness.[93] The major points to be taken from these investigations is that there is the strong propensity to experience reflex asystole via a vagally mediated mechanism in breath holding and other forms of neurally mediated syncope in addition to forced expiration and a lesser degree of inappropriate reflex vasodilation.

In the classic work done by Gastaut and Gastaut, physiological monitoring with an accompanying EEG was done during ocular compression precipitated severe breath holding spells in 24 subjects.[94] Groups were divided into those children exhibiting intense cardiac inhibition (asystole) with little respiratory effect (the pallid group), intense respiratory inhibition and little cardiac effect (the cyanotic group), and a third group displaying both cardiorespiratory inhibition (the mixed group). In each group, at the onset of color change and bradycardia and/or bradypnea, the EEG demonstrated a burst of slow waves, followed by deepening color changes, and loss of consciousness and postural tone, lastly followed by EEG flattening, and concurrent opisthotonus and myoclonic jerks.[94] Similar findings have subsequently been demonstrated by a number of investigators.[73, 88, 91, 94–96] This sequence was expanded upon by Gauk et al., who recorded events in twenty children to last up to 40 seconds, with clinical evolution occurring in full respiratory expiration.[96] They determined that cyanotic spells developed over a series of four distinct phases: provocation, expiratory apnea, rigidity, and stupor.[96] The final result was from a fall in oxygen saturation from 98% to a nadir of 40%, which was postulated to be from rapid oxygen utilization but later shown to be from intrapulmonary shunting of deoxygenated blood, causing cyanosis and ultimate cerebral hypoxia.[96, 97] Cyanotic breath holders demonstrated concurrent hypertension without a change in pulse rate in the absence of glottic closure (no valsalva), thereby negating diminished venous return as a prominent pathophysiologic factor.[97, 98] The observation of opisthotonus followed by an inspiratory gasp signaled the termination of the cyanotic spell. This contrasts to children with pallid spells, which evolve symptoms principally from reflex asystole, resulting in prompt cerebral hypoperfusion/hypoxia.[1, 96] The confirmation of "prolonged expiratory apnea" with hypertension without glottic closure as the underlying respiratory sequence was initially provided by Southall et al. in a physiological monitoring study of 8 subjects and later expanded upon to include 28/51 subjects.[97, 99] The forced expiration resulted in low lung volume and lung collapse compounded by overly compliant rib cages not remedied by tracheostomy.[97] Low phosphatidylcholine (surfactant) measures prompted the use of continuous positive airway pressure (CPAP).[97]

They were able to extinguish cyanotic spells with the use of CPAP in two subjects who underwent tracheostomies.[97] Ventilation scans during recorded cyanotic breath-holding spells in seven subjects led to the conclusion that intrapulmonary shunting produced the rapid deoxygenation observed in these children.[99] Other investigators have also found abnormalities in the surface tension properties of surfactants in children with CBHS.[100] Although the authors postulated a possible mechanism for neurodevopmental sequelae, this was disputed and ultimately not borne out in longitudinal studies.[25, 71, 73, 83, 85, 100] An important aspect deserving emphasis with respect to the underlying physiology of BHS is the profound, persistent, and involuntary brainstem-mediated bradycardia-asystole and/or forced expiration observed in these children. The sum total of all peripheral receptor stimulation results in this pronounced autonomic reflex syncope.[19] Triggered upper respiratory tract mechanoreceptors serve to mediate elevations in blood pressure, whereas lower respiratory tract stretch receptors and j-receptors serve to stimulate reflex-forced exhalation with simultaneous inhibition of active inspiration.[19] The cardiac inhibition results from excess and persistent parasympathetic vagal efferent outflow, whereas the effects of excess sympathetic efferent output mediate hypertension.[19] Even in CBHS there may be a brief (<6 seconds) asystole prior to the more pronounced expiratory apneic phase of respiratory inhibition and concurrent EEG flattening.[83, 93]

Given the foregoing discussions as regards the evidence that a centrally mediated autonomic reflex mechanism produces as well as prolongs BHS (both cyanotic and pallid), investigations concerning the state of autonomic functioning at times other than during a spell have been fruitful. Central and peripheral autonomic responses to orthostatic maneuvers (arising to stand from supine rest) have demonstrated distinctions between pallid and cyanotic breath holders among measures of vasomotor and orthostatic responses.[101, 102] Children with pallid spells show a marked drop in mean arterial pressure and an unsustained increase in pulse rate, whereas children with cyanotic spells, in contrast, demonstrate elevated and maintained mean arterial pressures with an initial excess increase in pulse rate when compared to age- and gender-matched controls. The results of EKG analyses and measured ratios, of 30 : 15, have also shown statistically significant differences between breath holders and controls.[101, 102] This measure is a numeric value, which represents the degree of normally provoked relative bradycardia after standing (30th RR interval) and the immediate tachycardia upon arising to stand (15th RR interval). Ratios of <1.03 are representative of the absence or blunting of the expected vagally mediated decrease in heart rate upon standing. This measure was found to be abnormal in cyanotic breath holders but not in pallid when compared to each other and matched controls.[101, 102] These data emphasize the centrally mediated excess sympathetic response and delayed parasympathetic response in the cyanotic group in contrast to the excess parasympathetic response in the pallid group. There have been no measurable differences in the expiratory : inspiratory (E:I) ratio, plasma norepinepherine levels, cutaneous vasodilator responses to applied cutaneous heat, or pupillary responses to the instillation of dilute pilocarpine as measures of peripheral autonomic disturbances.[101, 102] Several investigations have measured respiratory sinus arrhythmia (RSA) in breath holders. RSA is a measure of centrally modulated vagal (parasympathetic) tone, which was defined as the variability in time over a frequency range corresponding to respiratory rates 6–30 breaths per minute. Because a normal resting heart rate is dependent upon the individual's intrinsic cardiac rate and the net effect of cardioexcitatory (sympathetic) and cardioinhibitory (parasympathetic) neural influences, alterations in heart rate (sinus rhythm) reflect a change in their net balance or modulation. The major contributor to the oscillation in resting heart rate at rest is respiration. Exhalation is associated with a slight decrease in heart rate as parasympathetic influence increases. Conversely, heart rate increases during inhalation as parasympathetic influence decreases. This modulation is mediated principally through cardioinhibitory vagal efferents such that the greater and more tonic the cardioinhibitory influence, the less variability in RSA is observed. This parasympathetic modulation is reflected in the high frequency ranges in particular, whereas multiple inputs in addition to sympathetic influences are reflected in low frequency domains.[103, 104] There were no differences in cyanotic breath holders when compared to age- and gender-matched controls, whereas pallid breath holders had a significant difference in RSA, confirming centrally mediated parasympathetic reflex excess in the face of an elevated tonic sympathetic effect.[105, 106] This tonic cardioinhibitory effect is somewhat enhanced in breath holders with concomitant anemia, thereby reducing RSA.[107] The net effect of correcting underlying anemia in breath holders has been to normalize the RSA.[107, 108]

Accompanying anemia can exacerbate BHS. This was first proposed by Holowach and Thurston, when 23.5% of 102 breath holders were found to have mean hemoglobin concentrations less than 8 g/100 mL compared to 6.9% of 572 hospitalized children and only 2.6% of 192 epileptic children examined.[109] These findings could not initially be replicated.[85, 93] Recently, however, Bhatia et. al. found the mean hemoglobin concentration of 50 children with breath holding to be 8.12 g/dL compared to 9.92% g/dL in a randomly selected control group ($p < 0.01$).[110] All children (96% CBHS, 4% PBHS) were given iron supplementation (5–6 mg/kg/d elemental iron) until they had achieved a hemoglobin of >11 g/dL. All children were reported to have experienced a reduction in their BHS frequency, although the precise quantification was not elaborated on.[110] More recently Daoud et al. completed a randomized placebo-controlled trial of iron therapy (5 mg/kg/d) for 16 weeks in 67 breath holders.[111] The results disclosed complete or partial response (>50% reduction in frequency) in 29/33 assigned to therapy.[111] Those with favorable responses had significantly lower mean hemoglobin concentrations compared to nonresponders (8.6 g/L vs. 10.6 g/L).[111] Mocan and colleagues treated 63 of 91 breath holders aged 6–40 months (60 cyanotic, 31 pallid) who had iron deficiency anemia (hemoglobin <105 g/L, MCV < 75 fl) with elemental iron (6 mg/kg/d) for 3 months.[112] There was a significant reduction in spells for children treated with iron compared to those who were not. The reduction in breath-holding spells was by 84% in the treated group compared to 21% of those untreated ($p < 0.02$).[112] Clearly, iron deficiency has an additional impact on the frequency of BHS exhibited in these children. BHS will be ameliorated in those children with anemia and possibly improved in those without anemia. There are both children with anemia who do not respond to iron supplementation and those without anemia who do. Iron supplementation appears most helpful for the iron deficient anemic child. This becomes most evident in children who suffer from transient erythroblastopenia of childhood, where supplementation with iron and/or correction of the anemia by transfusion has resulted in resolution of both concurrent anemia and BHS.[70, 113, 114] It has been speculated that the iron deficient state may impart higher CNS levels of serotonin because of a relative deficiency or reduced activity of its iron-dependent degrading enzyme, aldehyde oxidase.[115] A similar increased availability of additional sympathetomimetic neurotransmitters due to a reduction of their degrading enzyme, monoamine oxidase, also reduced in iron deficiency states, potentially exacerbates centrally mediated sympathetic outflow excess.[116] A final important corollary to iron deficiency in children is the added degree of greater accompanying behavioral irritability.[117] This by itself may enhance a greater likelihood of spells if the propensity to become frustrated, emotional, or to cry is also heightened.

Further investigations into the central autonomic function of breath holders during sleep have identified limited and subtle findings. An initial study of 21 breath holders comparing 9-hour sleep recordings to controls found no abnormalities.[118] The authors found that the mean number of sleep apneas was actually lower than that of the control group. A subsequent study of sleep in 71 infants (34 simple spells, 37 severe spells), with a mean age 14 weeks, when compared to controls found more frequent sweating with a significantly elevated evaporation rate of $20.5 \, g/L/m^2/h$ versus $1.6 \, g/L/m^2/h$ ($p < 0.001$).[119] The investigators also identified more frequent airway obstructions, more frequent arousals, more sleep-stage changes, increased slow-wave stage III sleep, and increased fragmentation of sleep compared to controls.[119] There were no differences in central apnea frequencies between groups. However, although the overall differences measured between breath holders and controls were not physiologically compromising, these did suggest a subtle immaturity and dysregulation of central respiratory control.[120] These control mechanisms were further investigated by assessing the ventilatory chemoreceptor responsiveness to progressive hypoxia and hypercarbia in former breath holders compared to controls by Anas et al.[121, 122] Their overall responses were within normative ranges; however, the breath holders had greater variances of responses and, as a group, had significantly less response to hypercapnia ($p < 0.05$), with a similar trend but not statistically significant to hypoxia.[121, 122] It was postulated that earlier in life these responses may be more significantly disturbed, and undergoes maturation and normalization with age.[121, 122] Of interest are the findings of Cintra et al. who studied heart rate variability (both sympathetic and parasympathetic effects) during sleep in adolescent and adult patients with vasovagal syncope compared to controls with and without positive head-upright tilt tests.[123] They found similar outcomes in those subjects with syncope as in breath holders in that all sleep parameters were normal, except an increase in slow-wave sleep. They also found no differences in a 24-hour time domain heart rate variability analysis; however, there was a decrease in the low frequency range of heart rate variability during rapid eye movement sleep compared to controls ($p < 0.03$), which suggests an alteration in sympathetic activation.[123]

Treatment of BHS incorporates parental education about the underlying physiology and expected natural course in addition to several therapeutic options (see Table 3-6).[19,71,124] Most interventions have been borne from anecdotal reports of response with the exception of iron treatment. An often-overlooked source of hidden morbidity is parental stress, particularly in mothers of breath holders. The parental stress level in mothers of children with breath holding is significant and requires specific intervention. When the Parenting Stress Index with questions regarding how mothers coped with their

Table 3-6 Treatment Approaches for Severe Breath-Holding Spells

Demonstrated Benefit

- Parental education regarding underlying pathophysiology and natural course
- Parental support for their care-providing capability
- Iron therapy (5–6 mg/kg/dose elemental iron), especially if concurrent iron deficiency anemia

Pallid Type

- Anticholinergic therapy (atropine sulfate 0.01 mg/dose BID or TID; scopolamine transdermal patch 0.25–0.5 mg/72 hour)
- Theophylline
- Cardiac pacemaker insertion

Cyanotic Type

- Central α-adrenergic agonists (clonidine 0.01 mg/d divided BID or TID)
- Central α-adrenergic antagonists (tetrabenazine 1 mg/d divided TID or QID)
- Continuous positive airway pressure (neonate infant)

Suggested or Speculative Benefit

- Piracetam (20 mg/kg/dose BID)
- Levetiracetam
- Selective serotonin reuptake inhibitors
- Acetazolamide
- Naltrexone
- Medroxyprogesterone

breath-holding children was administered to 34 mothers of individual children with BHS, 16 different mothers of children with epilepsy and 16 mothers of children with no medical conditions (controls), the results showed significant disruptions in breath-holder mothers' sense of competence as a parent, ability to maintain self-identity, and a lack of positive reinforcement from their child.[124] Mothers of the BHS group alone had these responses, which were not related to maternal health or feelings of depression/isolation, insufficient spousal support, child's mood, or other life stresses.[123] These findings were emphasized in a recent Turkish cohort of 30 mothers of breath holders who were compared to a group of mothers of healthy control children, which investigated maternal stress factors, sociodemographic characteristics, and iron deficiency on the development of BHS.[125] The investigators found that iron deficiency rather than any behavioral or psychosocial problems of mothers played a role the development of BHS in these children.[125] As an intervention strategy, a succinct description of the underlying physiology of this type of reflex syncope is what parents will need to understand. An emphasis on the nonvolitional nature of the spells, the emotional trigger which sets in motion the cascade of autonomic effects that result in syncope are the important concepts to convey.

Therapy for pallid breath holders would be aimed at reducing the anticipated reflex bradycardia/asystole or augmenting resting cardiac rate. Commonly prescribed anticholinergic drugs have been used with some benefit as has theophylline.[19,73,93,95,126–129] Select patients with pallid BHS may require cardiac pacemakers in order to prevent prolonged asystole and reflex anoxic seizures.[130–135] Children who have prolonged bradycardia or asystole associated with extended convulsions, a need for resuscitation, or prolonged apnea may be considered for pacemaker implantation. These qualifications would typically apply to a limited population.[134,136] There has been a few series of patients treated successfully in this manner with varied devices and limited adverse effects.[130–134]

Cyanotic breath holders have had some limited benefit from interventions aimed at reducing reflex central sympathetic activity with central α-adrenergic agonists (clonidine) and antagonists (tetrabenazine), or similar cogners (e.g., levetiracetam).[99] In addition, piracetam, a compound similar to γ-aminobutyric acid, has been used in a small placebo-controlled trial with some stated benefit but with poorly quantified outcomes.[136] CPAP had been used in two young infants (<7 weeks old) with success, but the use of a tracheotomy has not been typically helpful.[97]

Given the potential interactions of iron deficiency on neurotransmitter concentrations, speculative consideration to selective serotonin reuptake inhibitors and opiod antagonists may hold promise.[19] Similarly, the enhancement of respiratory drive via augmentation of the chemosensitive reflex reactivity to CSF pH and CO_2 concentrations with carbonic anhydrase inhibitors (acetazolamide, topiramate) or medroxyprogesterone may also be worthy of trial.[19]

Swallow Syncope

This form of reflex syncope, also known as deglutition syncope, has been rarely recognized and reported in children. Woody et al. reported a child 4 years of age who had a total of 345 episodes observed and recorded by her parents.[137] They reported these syncopes to occur with increasing frequency associated with swallowing, eating, or the thought of food. Only after EEG monitoring captured an event during the syncopal provoking activity of eating, with brady-cardia to forty beats per minute associated with loss of consciousness, was the diagnosis made. Subsequent Holter monitoring disclosed second-degree atrioventricular (AV) heart block precipitated by swallowing. Treatment with a permanent cardiac pacemaker placement eliminated the events. Prior reports of swallow syncope in children have also been in 4–5 year olds.[138–140] One child with infrequent events, also associated with AV block precipitated by swallowing, received conservative treatment with parental explanation and reassurance. A second child was observed to experience significant reflex bradycardia and syncope after esophageal fistula repair in association with swallowing. This child underwent ablation of vagal fibers to the sinus node, which cured the reflex events.

The syncopal event itself is precipitated by an increase in afferent inputs to brainstem cardiorespiratory centers via the glossopharyngeal nerve during esophageal stimulation (similar mechanism in glossopharyngeal neuralgia). This in turn produces an increase in vagal efferent effects upon cardiac rate and rhythm. There is a sudden drop in heart rate, precipitating AV block and peripheral vasodilatation. This culminates with a drop in cerebral perfusion and syncope. This reflex mechanism may be similarly precipitated by abnormal esophageal peristalsis.[141] The production of cardiac arrhythmias has been observed with swallow syncope in adults and has been attributed to carcinomatous meningitis infiltrating the glossopharyngeal nerve, with demyelination of the vagus nerve in one autopsied case.[142] Stimulation of the posterior pharyngeal wall by hot liquids has also been documented in adult patients.[143] One adult subject experienced swallow syncope for over 13 years before diagnosis.[144]

Tussive Syncope

Tussive or cough syncope is a form of reflex syncope most often identified in adult subjects with coexistent pulmonary and cardiovascular disease. In childhood, this is rarely encountered but is recognized in the context of coughing paroxysms associated with cystic fibrosis, asthma, and pertusis infection.[145, 146] Its original description is credited to Charcot in a report dating 1876.[147] In a unique survey of all pediatric patients aged 10 years or older seen at a single cystic fibrosis center, each was screened for the past experience of a predefined "coughing paroxysm."[145] A paroxysm was defined as at least two series of repetitive coughs with only one intervening breath, progressing to near total expiration and a subjective sense of breathlessness. Of 273 eligible subjects,

68%, or 186 subjects, had experienced these. Details about specific accompanying symptoms were elicited, which included alterations in consciousness, headache, visual disturbances, sensory changes, and involuntary movements. Syncope occurred in only three subjects, none younger than 24 years. However, lightheadedness (near-syncope) and confusion occurred in 36/186 (19%).[145] The frequency of associated neurological disturbances with coughing bouts is equal between genders in children, both in the asthmatic and cystic fibrosis populations.[145, 146]

The mechanism of syncope during cough has been infrequently and incompletely evaluated in a few adult studies, with several underlying pathophysiologies postulated. Those forwarded include impairment of venous return and decreased cardiac output, activation of a hypersensitive carotid sinus, increased intracranial pressure with resultant cerebral ischemia, and reflex bradycardia and vasodilatation.[148–152] Although typically considered benign, death has been rarely reported as a consequence in adults.[148, 153] There are two distinct types of clinical scenarios noted. The first is a brief coughing series, with a syncopal event promptly initiated. This more rapid induction of syncope has been attributed to an abrupt and transient elevation of intra-arterial pressure, triggering arterial baroreceptor-mediated bradycardia and venous stretch receptor-mediated vasodilation, similar to other forms of neurally mediated reflex syncope.[149, 154] Other trigger sites may exist in the larynx and bronchopulmonary tree.[152, 155, 156] The second clinical scenario is a more prolonged paroxysm with the evolution of neurological premonitory symptoms and eventual syncope. This latter sequence has been recently examined in a group of nine subjects with cough syncope compared to thirty-one subjects, with and without positive HUT testing, without cough syncope by having subjects cough with continual EKG and cardiovascular monitoring.[154] The cough induced an abrupt rise and a subsequent statistically greater drop in systolic pressure, with prolonged duration of hypotension observed in the cough syncope group. This was accompanied by a statistically lower rise in heart rate change relative to blood pressure fall and slower blood pressure recovery.[154] These same subjects did not demonstrate more sensitivity to carotid massage than the non-cough syncope subjects, which suggests that in this group of subjects the reflex bradycardia was an accompanying mechanism. An additional study of eighteen cough syncope adult subjects was conducted by means of transcranial Doppler to monitor middle cerebral artery blood flow velocity in addition to concurrent EKG and cardiovascular measures during forced valsalva maneuver.[157] They found that two distinct subject groups emerged. Similar to that noted previously, 8/18 subjects (44%) had a prolonged drop in blood pressure with concurrent reduction in blood flow velocity over several phases of valsalva, whereas the remainder of subjects had an appropriate blood pressure overshoot response with preserved cerebral blood flow velocity.[157] The subjects were not distinguished clinically as having brief or prolonged coughing paroxysms, however. Similar severe reductions in cerebral blood flow velocity had been demonstrated during coughing, with recorded syncope within

10–18 seconds.[158] The results again suggest that there are at least two distinct mechanisms that can induce syncope during cough. Clinical observations of rhythmic limb movements and jerking have been appreciated during these syncopal events as with other forms of syncope.[159, 160] Concurrent EEG recording of diffuse slowing during the syncope mirrors that in other forms as well.[160] Gastroesophageal reflux-induced cough with resultant syncope has also been reported in an adult.[161] Symptoms were completely resolved after Nissen fundoplication.[161]

Hair-Grooming Syncope

Hair grooming is a relatively common trigger of syncope. There are, however, few descriptive series and no physiological studies invoking these trigger mechanisms. In one of the two most complete series published in children, fifteen subjects were identified over a 10-year span at a children's hospital neurology clinic.[162] There were fourteen girls and one boy, with ages ranging from 5 to 13 years (mean 11 years).[162] Each subject had experienced syncopal convulsions in temporal association with hair grooming. The actual activity was varied and consisted of hair brushing (40%), combing (26%), blow drying (20%), and braiding (13%). The hair-related activity occurred with the subject standing in the majority of instances (80%), seated in 13%, and kneeling in one case.[162] An important observation was that the posture of the head was in a neutral position in 12/15 (80%), extended in 2 (13%), and flexed in 1. Each child experienced some premonitory symptoms, with dimming of vision noted by all, lightheadedness in 12/15, diaphoresis in 8/15, and nausea in 3/15.[162] Syncopal convulsions consisted of tonic posturing, tonic-clonic or clonic jerking, and atonic posture lasting from 5 seconds to 3 minutes, with longer events witnessed by parents in those who were supported upright rather than placed supine.[162] Observations by Stephenson of six additional subjects are described similarly, with the additional observation of significant pallor in a few.[1] Many of the subjects prone to this form of reflex syncope have been identified as having other types of reflex precipitants and orthostatic syncope as well.[162, 163] In the series of twenty children reported by Igarashi et al., syncope was additionally precipitated by events other than hair grooming in more than half.[163] Typical precipitants included events that caused pain, such as minor lacerations, splinters, head bumping, and wiggling a loose tooth.[163] Vagally mediated bradycardia has been the accepted mechanism likely triggered by trigeminal sensory afferent stimulation (similar mechanism in trigeminal neuralgia). A concurrent valsalva maneuver could be additionally operative depending upon the state of the child.

Stretch Syncope

The trigger for stretch syncope was once thought to more prominently employ a strong valsalva maneuver.[1] This forced expiration against a closed glottis reduces cardiac venous return and cardiac output in the face of increased cerebral venous pressure. However, during a stretch, the neck is typically held in hyperextension, and previous cardiovascular responses in six stretch syncope subjects during stretch were no different from controls.[164] These results suggest an additional mechanism that has been postulated to be vertebral artery compression. More recent transcranial Doppler and four-vessel angiography in two additional subjects were performed during neck stretch maneuvers.[165] These identified reproducible and rapid reductions in cerebral blood flow velocities to an average of 28%–41% of baseline associated with the development of syncopal symptoms, demonstrating the importance of posterior circulation compromise during the act of stretching.[164] This propensity may be more likely to occur in teenage boys, especially in whom there is a familial tendency to faint.[163]

Postexertional Syncope

This is the recognition of a syncopal event immediately after exercise when the individual is at rest and recuperating.[2] This is a form of reflex syncope that has been identified in adults but has potential to be recognized in adolescents. It rarely may be associated with autonomic failure or, more commonly, with associated reflex bradycardia and accompanying hypotension that occurs in otherwise healthy individuals without heart disease as a result of a reduced sympathetically mediated vasomotor responsiveness.[166–168] This has been shown to be due to a failure of reflex vasoconstriction during exercise of the splanchnic capacitance vessels and forearm resistance vessels. The importance of identifying this likely etiology of syncope is to separate this from the more ominous forms of primary cardiac syncope, which occur during exercise or also immediately thereafter.[166–168] When the timing of the event is uncertain, then exercise testing may be needed.[2]

Micturition/Defecation Syncope

These are rarely recognized as reflex syncopes in children. Activation of autonomic responses required to empty the bladder or pass a bowel movement may inadvertently trigger reflex bradycardia, hypotension, and ultimate syncope.[169,170] Micturition syncope is most prominent in men approaching their sixth decade of life, initiated by standing while urinating. Defecation syncope can be experienced in the act of defecating, especially if there is the addition of valsalva effect with passage of hard stool. The autonomic coordination of sphincter and intestinal activation along with colonic peristalsis may activate additional hypotension-producing mechanisms upon arising from a seated position shortly after stool passage. Avoidance of the trigger is not feasible, and therefore minimizing the potential for syncope by sitting during micturition or arising more slowly after defecation may help lessen the likelihood of occurrence.[2] The use of stool softeners or avoidance of excessive fluids prior to sleep may accomplish the same end.

A rarely recognized entity, familial rectal pain syndrome, presents in the neonatal period with sudden paroxysmal attacks initiated by a startle, resulting in a terrified appearing infant inconsolably screaming and displaying a harlequin color.[171] A number of triggers, such as feeding, bathing, sneezing, loud noises, and defecation, may bring on the clinical sequence of (1) pain on defecation, (2) flushing over the buttocks/harlequin appearance, and (3) bradycardia.[171] The infants will arch into a tonic posture, with associated bronchospasm and sometimes syncope. This begins within the first 3–4 months of age.[171]

Venipuncture/Acupuncture Syncope

Syncope as a result of venipuncture, blood drawing, immunization, and needle sticks has been well recognized in all age groups.[1,27,28,51,172–174] These specific triggers induce a strong and prompt vagally mediated bradycardia/asystole within 6 seconds in some individuals.[1] Approximately 35% of all immunization-related syncopes reported to the CDC over the years 1990–2004 were in the age range 10–18 years (1109 children from among 3168 persons who were reported to have had a syncopal event).[27] Fourteen percent of all these syncopes resulted in hospitalization.[27] A recent fatality was reported in a 15-year-old boy who died after suffering a cardiac arrhythmia subsequent to sustaining an initial head injury from falling.[28,29] By comparison, in a prospective study of blood donors aged 18 years and older, the incidence of syncopal events was 0.3% (824/262,935 blood donations).[172] From among these adult blood donors with syncope, 0.03% experienced non-epileptic convulsive syncope, and its occurrence was twice as frequent in men than women.[172] Convulsive syncope has also been reported in a healthy 25 year old individual volunteer who underwent acupuncture in both legs below the tibial tuberosity after thermal sensory stimulation as part of a research trial.[175] The event occurred while seated and was accompanied by pallor, upward eye rolling, and tonic-clonic activity for 30–40 seconds.[175]

An interesting psychological construct in adult subjects finds that there are strong positive associations between blood-injection-injury fears and syncope.[176] These associations have been enumerated into three mutually exclusive categories: (1) "escape fainters," those who express fear prior to syncope, report constraints that make it impossible to escape, and experience syncope in the presence of the blood-injection-injury stimulus; (2) "relief fainters," those who report fear prior to syncope but do not experience syncope until after the threatening stimulus has passed; and (3) "essential fainters," those who report no fear or anxiety during the blood-injection-injury stimulus.[176] Anxiety itself did not add to the prediction of syncope associated with blood-injection-injury fears.[176] One can only imagine that there exists similar if not more potent emotional components in children.

Visually Induced Syncope/Laughter-Induced Syncope

A rarely reported and probably underappreciated trigger for reflex bradycardia-induced syncope is visual stimuli. There is general and immediate recognition for the induction of epileptic seizures with the application of various visual stimuli such as strobe-light flicker, video monitor screens, and certain static images in predisposed individuals. However, a few reports of children have now documented visually induced bradycardia with concomitant convulsive syncope.[177–179] Syncopal events such as these have been most often prompted by television viewing, but video game playing has also been recognized. These episodes of convulsive syncope can be repeatedly induced with the proper intermittent photic stimulation rate. They are accompanied by a progressive bradycardia/asystole associated with the typical tonic posture and eventual clonic seizure simultaneous with a slow-flat-slow EEG tracing and eventual recovery. It has been suggested to use polarizing lenses outdoors and in bright light, view television and video games on an LCD screen, and to avoid stroboscopic stimulation.[177]

Laughter as an inducer of syncope has now been recognized in four children with Angelman syndrome.[180–182] Simultaneous EKG recording has captured the progressive bradycardia/asystole up to 11 seconds induced by spontaneous laughter coinciding with the development of syncope. Attacks were abolished with the administration of atropine and diphemanil (anticholinergic agents) during subsequent bouts of laughter.[181,182] One child later died after a cardiorespiratory arrest during a "seizure" 2 months after discontinuing medication.[182]

CAROTID MASSAGE/CAROTID SINUS SYNDROME

In adult populations with atherosclerotic vascular disease within the carotid vessels, if manipulated properly, carotid sinus stimulation will produce reflex bradycardia of variable degree.[1,13] In the hypersensitive individual this stimulation may prompt syncope much like ocular compression can induce the equivalent result. This is typically not a concern in the pediatric population but could in theory result with volition, overly tightened neckwear, or tracheal collars as examples. Volitional carotid stimulation coupled with forced valsalva causing syncopal events has been reported in a child.[183]

CEREBRAL CORTEX-INDUCED ARRHYTHMIAS

The induction of arrhythmias from a cortically mediated brain region has been identified infrequently. These are more apt to occur during the course of an epileptic seizure when specific cortical regions are activated (i.e., temporal and frontal lobes).[184–186] Ischemia to regions surrounding the insular cortex bilaterally but most prominently on the left hemisphere has been clearly implicated as have the posterior temporal and parietal lobes, anterior cingulate cortex, and amygdala in producing autonomically mediated cardiac rate and rhythm changes.[66–68] Sympathetically mediated tachycardia, an increased diastolic pressure, has been the result of right periinsular cortex ischemia, whereas parasympathetically mediated bradycardia and vasodepressor effects have arisen from the left periinsular cortex albeit rarely.[66–68]

POSTURAL ORTHOSTASIS

Prolonged standing invokes a number of specific compensatory physiologic changes to adjust and maintain blood pressure. Upon standing, contractions of leg and abdominal muscles increase peripheral vascular resistance by the compression of capacitance and resistance vessels, and activation of sympathetic vascular tone, thereby shifting blood volume to the heart.[34, 35, 187] This increased venous return to the heart results in augmented cardiac output and later activation of baroreceptors within the heart. Their stimulation signals brainstem cardiovascular relays to reduce peripheral vascular resistance and ultimately drop systemic blood pressure. As an adjustment, there is an immediate increase in heart rate, which gradually declines with continued upright posture. These shifts in blood volume can amount to a 30% reduction in the thorax and an equal 30% increase in cardiac output.[34, 35, 37, 187] Neuro-hormonal changes are actuated upon continued upright posture to the degree that volume depletion exists. This includes activation of the renin-angiotensin, aldosterone, and vasopressin systems. Because blood volume is greatest within the venous system (60%), inability to activate these steps will result in decompensation, cerebral hypoperfusion, and syncope.[35, 187] Adolescents are particularly prone to perturbations in these reflex mechanisms and commonly experience the end result. This is particularly accentuated in the tall individual, especially with an asthenic body habitus or with lesser well-developed musculature.[35, 37, 188] Arising too fast can precipitate symptoms rather quickly if compensatory mechanisms are not entrained rapidly enough. Similarly, volume depletion will accentuate decompensation that will be enhanced by attendant overheating and emotionality, such as with fear or claustrophobia. The prior sections on reflex situational/reflex vasovagal forms of neurally mediated syncope were primarily induced by centrally mediated vagal bradycardia/asystole with noted exceptions. Postural orthostatic syncope involves a reflex vasodepressor effect by which there is venous pooling and resultant lack of cardiac output, although the exact mechanisms are yet to be definitively determined.[35, 187, 189]

A corollary to the foregoing discussion is the entity of instantaneous orthostatic hypotension in children. Stewart and colleagues found this in American children with symptoms described as chronic fatigue syndrome after earlier descriptions in Japanese children.[190] Children complained of recurrent dizziness, fatigue, headache, and syncope, among other symptoms, to the degree that impairment of life activities ensued. The symptoms seemed to closely parallel a drop in blood pressure upon arising to stand and appeared to be due to an impairment of sympathetic activation of resistance vessels. Tanaka and colleagues evaluated 228 consecutive children and adolescents with a diagnosis of suspected orthostatic intolerance with cardiovascular and autonomic monitoring during an orthostatic maneuver.[191] There were forty-four children (19%) who demonstrated abnormal orthostatic circulatory responses, defined as a marked instantaneous drop in blood pressure at the onset of standing with delayed recovery (mild form), and a prolonged reduction in blood pressure in the severe form.[191] The abnormal circulatory response cutoff was >25 seconds for recovery of a <60% decrease in MAP (mean arterial pressure), or a recovery time >20 seconds with a 60% or greater decrease in MAP from rest, which corresponds to a ≥ 45 mm Hg for mean blood pressure reduction.[191] Immediate heart rate elevations were 22–67 beats per minute, with the severe group remaining significantly higher at 1–3 minutes of standing.[191] The specificity of these criteria was 95.7% and conforms closely to criteria in adults.[187] The measured plasma catecholamine levels in supine and upon standing were normal.[191] It has been postulated that the underlying mechanism involves centrally mediated inhibition of sympathetic nervous system function.

Strategies for intervention of orthostatic syncope should include patient education regarding the typical posturally induced triggers. Avoidance of sudden head-upright changes in posture and prolonged standing are most important. Less well appreciated triggers that deserve attention for minimization include avoidance of prolonged recumbency during wakeful periods; straining during defecation and micturition; hyperventilation; high ambient temperatures, especially as with saunas, hot tubs, and showers; large meals; and drugs with potential vasodilator/depressor properties. Augmentation of vascular volume with increased fluid and salt intake, support stockings to reduce gravity-dependent venous pooling, and the use of physical countermaneuvers can be individually suggested (see below).

FORCED VALSALVA MANEUVER

As described in previous sections, forced expiration against a closed glottis results in (1) an immediate rise in intrathoracic pressure, (2) a reduction in cardiac output, producing a reflex acceleration in heart rate with an increase in cerebral venous pressure, and (3) an ultimate fall in systemic blood pressure. If the reduction in cardiac output continues over 10–20 seconds, cerebral hypoperfusion ensues, and the process is eventually accompanied by the gradual appearance of EEG slowing, pallid color, and loss of consciousness (syncope).[36, 192] This behavior has been identified in cognitively impaired and autistic children who have engaged in this compulsive activity.[36, 192, 193] The syncopes evolved into anoxic convulsions, anoxic epileptic convulsions, and anoxic absence epileptic seizures. The concomitant EEG patterns of slow-flat-slow, slow-flat-spike-wave, and slow-flat-3 cycle per second spike-wave were recorded.[192, 193] Treatment with fenfluramine alleviated the syncopes; however, separate concurrent epileptic seizures persisted in some.[192]

An unusual 12-year-old subject has been described who engaged in the perilous behavior of simultaneous hyperventilation and forced valsalva to induce syncopes for fun. The effect was heightened with a final trial on the playground incorporating hyperventilation, forced valsalva, carotid self-massage, and the reception of a bear hug to induce a bradycardia-induced syncope, from which he later died.[194] The combination of hyperventilation while squatting and suddenly arising to induce syncope has been described as a "mess trick," with the combination of hyperventilation and forced valsalva a "fainting lark."[195]

POSTURAL ORTHOSTATIC TACHYCARDIA SYNDROME (POTS)

This is a type of orthostatic intolerance whereby excessive tachycardia is accompanied by decreased cerebral perfusion upon assuming an upright posture.[38, 187, 189]

Disabling symptoms of lightheadedness, fatigue, palpitations, and syncope mainly affect women of childbearing age, but childhood affliction has been recognized. The diagnosis of POTS requires an orthostatic heart rate acceleration in excess of 120 beats per minute, or an absolute increase of ≥ 30 beats per minute in the absence of hypotension.[187, 196, 197] This appears to be a less severe form of autonomic failure where two mechanistic forms exist: (1) a peripheral failure to increase vascular resistance by the sympathetic vasomotor fibers resulting in excess venous pooling and reflex heart rate increase in the face of orthostasis, and (2) a central form where, after triggering, the baroreflex responds such that the initial appropriate increase in heart rate to upright posture is adequate, but there is a faulty feedback mechanism to halt the stimulus.[187, 196–200] In the latter form, there is additionally an orthostatic hypertension exhibited.[187, 196–200] Subjects with the central form will be plagued by hyperadrenergic symptoms of migraine headache, sweating, and tremor in addition to the symptoms common to both the peripheral and central forms: lightheadedness, fatigue, and syncope. At least one family has been identified with an inherited genetic defect in a protein responsible for the recycling of norepinepherine within the peripheral intrasynaptic clefts. This thus allows for an accumulation of excess plasma norepinepherine.[201] There is a gender bias of POTS occurring in a greater prevalence in females. This greater prevalence has been correlated to an intrinsic difference in muscle sympathetic nerve fiber burst frequency and amplitudes between males and females in response to orthostatic stimuli.[202] This fiber burst discrepancy would be exploited by the natural loss of sympathetic fibers over time and renders females more vulnerable to the development of POTS.[202]

Treatment for POTS has met with variable success, and results includes excess water loading, volume expansion with salt and fludrocortisones, and the only drug shown to be beneficial in placebo-controlled trials, midodrine, an α-adrenergic agonist.[187, 196–200, 203–206] The more recent use of acetylcholinesterase inhibition has been a major advance.[203–206] The rationale for its use stems from the fact that the baroreflex arc is composed of two neurons synapsing at the autonomic ganglion, where acetylcholine is the neurotransmitter between the first and second neuron. It is degraded by the enzyme acetylcholinesterase. Thus inhibiting the degrading enzyme will augment the availability of acetylcholine to trigger the respective second neuron (both sympathetic and parasympathetic) in the reflex arc at the site of the synapses. This in turn would increase the peripheral vasoconstrictor effects more completely and efficiently at the sympathetic nerve terminal endpoint, where norepinepherine is secreted, and inhibit heart rate via the augmented acetylcholine secretion at the paparasympathetic nerve terminal endpoint. It has recently been used in a 16-year-old adolescent girl with POTS, and in adults, with good efficacy and tolerance, supported by cardiovascular monitoring and physiologic tilt testing.[203–206] The report by Filler et al. provides pharmacokinetic data on pyridostigmine in the adolescent subject as well.[206] Given the drug's short half-life in adolescents (2.29 hours), a daily dose (90 mg) divided three times a day provided good effect similar to that used in subjects with myasthenia gravis.

Treatment considerations for neurocardiogenic syncope are directed to the specific triggers and their avoidance. When neurocardiogenic mechanisms incorporate both unavoidable specific triggers and orthostatic mechanisms, other treatment options merit consideration (Table 3-7). A number of options listed in Table 3-7 have been studied in controlled trials in adult subjects (marked with asterix). Most of the interventions have been utilized in the adolescent age group. The utility of tilt training programs has been studied in a nonrandomized controlled trial of forty-seven consecutive adolescents with recurrent syncope and refractoriness to—one to three medical therapies.[207] All

Table 3-7 Treatment Options for Orthostatic Intolerance

Intervention	Dose or Method	Potential Adverse Effects
Head-up tilt of bed	45° Head-up/with footboard	Sliding down
Head-up tilt training*	Hospital head-up tilt training 10–50 minutes/d, Home: 40 minute intervals against wall BID	Syncopal symptoms resume
Physical counterpressure maneuvers*	Leg-crossing with abdominal & buttock tensing, handgrip rubber ball, arm tensing with interlocking hands — abduct arms apart, squatting, crash position	Syncopal symptoms persist
Elastic support hosiery	Ankle pressure (30–40 mm Hg)	Uncomfortable
Fluid & salt intake*	2–2.5 Lt/d, Na+ 150–250 mEq/d	Peripheral edema, supine hypertension
Exercise	Mild aerobic	Too vigorous may lower BP
Fludrocortisone	0.1–0.2 mg/d titrate to 1.0 mg/d	Hypomagnesemia, weight gain, edema, hypokalemia

Methylphenidate	5–10 mg/dose TID	Agitation, tremor, anorexia, headache, tics, insomnia
Midodrine*	2.5–10 mg q 2–4 hours to 40 mg/d	Nausea, supine hypertension
Clonidine	0.1–0.3 mg/d/BID/TID	Dry mouth, bradycardia, hypotension, fatigue
Yohimbine	8 mg BID/TID	Diarrhea, anxiety, agitation
Ephedrine sulfate	12.5–25 mg/TID	Tachycardia, tremor, supine hypertension
Erythropoieten	8000 IU SC q wk	Injections, stokes/thromboses
Fluoxetine	10–20 mg/d	Nausea, anorexia, agitation
Paroxetine*	10 mg/d	Nausea, tremor, agitation
Propranolol	25–50 mg/BID/TID	Hypotension, fatigue, bradycardia, nightmares
Metoprolol	25–50 mg/BID/TID	Hypotension, fatigue, bradycardia
Pyridostigmine	10–30 mg/TID	Nausea, diarrhea, cramping

Source: Modified from Reference.[187]
Notes: Consult pharmacy for appropriate drug dosages; BID = twice a day, TID = three times a day, d = dose.
* Denotes controlled trial assessment.

had positive syncope with HUT testing and were divided into two groups self-selected to tilt training ($n = 24$) or no tilt training (control $n = 23$), where orthostatic training consisted of in-hospital tilt training on a tilt table for a 10–50-minute session per day for five sessions on serial days to the point of symptoms development. The subjects were discharged home and instructed to continue tilt training over the subsequent month, for up to 40 minutes twice a day by standing against a wall supervised by a family member.[207] No other instructed interventions were made. All subjects returned after 1 month for repeat tilt testing. There was only a single subject from the training group who experienced syncope (4.2%) compared to eighteen subjects in the control group (73.9%) ($p < 0.0001$). The subjects who underwent training and had long-term follow-up at 15 months revealed 56% (13/23) spontaneous recurrence compared to none of the training group ($p < 0.0001$). There was a considerable level of self-motivation in the tilt training group, however, and this does suggest that there is a degree of placebo effect contributing to positive outcomes.[207] In a subsequent study of counterpressure maneuvers (leg crossing, muscle tensing, squatting, and crash position) as interventions against vasovagal reactions, continuous cardiovascular monitoring during performance of these maneuvers was done in a series of 26 subjects (16–80 years old) who had positive syncope during HUT testing.[208] The subjects underwent training in performance of these maneuvers and applied them in a specific sequence for 40–60 seconds upon command during repeat tilt testing and on arising from recumbency at onset of symptoms. Results demonstrated that all maneuvers effectively caused an increase in systolic blood pressure, with onset of increase within 3 seconds.[208] All maneuvers increased cardiac output without a change in total vascular peripheral resistance. Furthermore, all maneuvers prevented impending syncope. Leg crossing or abdominal muscle tensing could be used as a first measure, followed by squatting, then the crash position, in sequence, for an impending syncope.[208] The authors further studied the effectiveness of these techniques in a prospective randomized clinical trial of 223 subjects (16–70 years old) with recurrent syncope.[209] Tilt testing confirmed syncope, and subjects were randomly assigned: $n = 117$ to counterpressure maneuvers plus conventional therapy, and $n = 106$ to conventional therapy alone.[209] Of the 208/223 remaining in study, there was a significant decrease in syncope recurrences, with 31.6% of those in the counterpressure maneuvers plus conventional therapy group versus 50.9% conventional therapy alone group ($p < 0.004$) experiencing recurrence over 14 months of follow-up.[209] These seem to be effective, low risk, and cost-effective measures to employ in patients with neurocardiogenic syncope who experience prodromal symptoms.

There exists real doubt as regards the efficacy of many of the pharmacological and nonpharmacological interventions available for the treatment of neurocardiogenic syncope. Randomized, double-blinded, placebo-controlled trials of fludrocortisone and salt versus placebo, atenolol versus placebo, fludrocortisone and atenolol versus placebo, active versus inactive pacemakers, counseling versus placebo counseling, metoprolol versus placebo, and sertraline versus placebo have shown no difference in efficacy in some pediatric and adult studies.[199,210–215] This increases the value of the placebo effect for the treatment of some young patients.[216] Interestingly, a capsule color other than white may be more effective than a traditional little white pill.[217] In children, the utility of midodrine, methylphenidate, and selective serotonin reuptake inhibitors have been shown to be helpful.[199,218,219]

DYSAUTONOMIA

The major causes of primary childhood dysautonomia are the hereditary autonomic sensory neuropathies (HSAN types I–IV), which are made up of several identified genetic syndromes.[220,221] Most are autosomal recessive disorders presenting in infancy, (HSAN types II–IV), whereas hereditary sensory radicular neuropathy (HSAN type I) is a dominant disorder that becomes symptomatic in early adulthood. Familial dysautonomia (Riley-Day syndrome, HSAN type III) and congenital insensitivity to pain and anhidrosis (HSAN type IV) are better characterized with specific genetic mutations identified.

All HSAN types have a characteristic failure of the axon-flare response to intradermal histamine injection.[221]

Familial dysautonomia is nearly exclusively found in families of Eastern European Jewish extraction and presents with neonatal hypotonia and feeding difficulties. It is caused by mutations in the gene is *IKBKAP* (I$\kappa\beta$ kinase–associated protein gene), which has been postulated to be important in neurotransmitter expression.[222] Evolution of symptoms into early childhood discloses more definitive reduction in pain and temperature sensitivity, particularly in the feet, with gradual loss of joint position and vibratory sensation in conjunction with arreflexia. These abnormalities are not as profound as the associated autonomic disturbances such as faulty blood pressure regulation producing alternating periods of postural hypotension and hypertension, syncope, gastroesophageal reflux with aspiration, breath-holding spells, increased sweating, and an absence of tears with emotional crying. These autonomic disturbances are a result of underdevelopment and loss of predominantly peripheral sympathetic neurons and fiber tracts. Examination of these children discloses an absence of the fungiform papillae of the tongue and diminished taste. These are medium-sized papillae found along the lateral edge of the tongue, whose absence is a hallmark of the condition. Other clinically identifiable signs of dysautonomia include corneal scars in the face of absent corneal reflexes, pedal edema, and trophic skin changes. Autonomic testing in addition to the absent histamine response often identifies abnormal sympathetic skin responses, HUT testing, pupil reactivity, and respiratory sinus arrhythmia.[220,221] These children experience periodic prolonged bouts of vomiting and autonomic crises manifesting tachycardia, blotching, hypertension, and agitation, with a high risk for aspiration.[220,221] Many episodes are triggered by physical or emotional stress. Patients have been found to exhibit a relative insensitivity to hypoxemia.[223] This failure to enact the appropriate autonomic responses to hypoxic conditions as found in pneumonia or at high altitude results in uncompensated bradycardia, hypotension, and syncope.[223]

Secondary dysautonomia is autonomic dysfunction acquired from a number of primary medical conditions (diabetes mellitus, kidney and liver failure, etc.), drugs (tricyclic antidepressants, phenothiazines, antihistamines, levodopa, MAO-inhibitors, etc.), toxins and heavy metals, or postinfectious acute demyelinating polyneuropathy (Guillain-Barre syndrome).

PRIMARY CARDIAC

The specific primary cardiac causes of syncope are potentially legion. Important discrete categories include structural cardiac lesions that impair cardiac outflow from the left ventricle. These lesions may be intrinsic complex cardiac malformations and septal defects, great vessel transpositions ("tet" spells), aortic valvular incompetence/stenosis, and others.[2,224,225] Left ventricular inflow obstruction can also but more rarely be a cause of syncope from mitral valve incompetence/stenosis, right ventricular outflow obstruction, and right-to-left intracardiac shunts due to pulmonary valve stenosis or pulmonary hypertension.[2,224,226] Atrial myxomas and rhabdomyomas of the ventricles or atria may similarly impair outflow from either atrial or ventricular chambers depending upon location and lesion size.[2,224] Hypertrophic cardiomyopathy and a number of the previously noted cardiac lesions are often additionally compounded by both concurrent arrhythmias and a propensity to induce neurally mediated syncopal events.[2,224]

Probably the most important indicators of a cardiac cause of syncope in a child is the induction of syncope during exertion (possibly, although much less commonly postexertional), the presence of palpitations during the event, prior cardiac disease, and family history of sudden cardiac death or arrhythmia.[2,4,49,50,224,227–229] In the absence of structural heart disease, the identification of an arrhythmia causing syncope is an important step in the evaluative process. Arrhythmias can be broadly sorted into bradyarrhythmias and tachyarrhythmias, where palpitations are more commonly associated with tachyarrhythmia. Bradyarrhythmic events are more sudden with onset of lightheadedness. An important pediatric entity predisposing to an arrhythmia producing syncope is the long QT syndrome (LQTS). This is a disorder of transmembrane ion channels affecting repolarization of the cardiac conducting system, which causes a prolongation of the cardiac action potential duration. This prolongation is manifest in the duration of the heart rate corrected QT (QTc) interval. This syndrome is clinically and genetically heterogeneous with both acquired and congenital genetic causes. There are several identified genetic mutations coding for potassium and sodium ion channels. Symptomatic individuals have been found to have QTc intervals of >470 ms (males) and >480 ms (females). Symptoms develop when the normal sinus rhythm converts into brief bursts of a ventricular tachyarrhythmia (torsades de pointes).[230] This can ultimately deteriorate further into ventricular fibrillation and sudden death.[230]

The predisposition to a long QT interval may be congenital or acquired. The acquired causes include the effects of various drugs (antiarrhythmics, antipsychotics, psychoactives, tricyclic antidepressants, antimicrobials, antihistamines, and others), electrolyte disturbances (e.g., hypokalemia), protein-sparing starvation, illicit drugs, HIV, hypovolemia, and bradycardia.[2,230,231] Congenital forms with a multitude of mutations have been linked to seven specific genes (LQT1-7).[232] There are congenital mutations causing two well-defined clinical syndromes: Romano-Ward syndrome (autosomal dominant) and Jervell and Lange-Nielsen syndrome (autosomal recessive with associated deafness).[232] Genetic testing has been positive in up to 64% of screened patients; however, three genetic mutations account for the vast majority (95%) of identified patients: LQT1, LQT2, and LQT3.[233,234] Identified triggers for significant arrhythmia production have been found to be distinctive between these genotypes, with exercise or stress a trigger commonly associated with LQT1. Loud noise and emotion are significant triggers in LQT2 patients, and LQT3 are at risk in sleep or rest.[232] These trigger distinctions suggested an inherent difference among genotypes (LQT1 and LQT2 from LQT3) in regard to catecholamine sensitivity and therefore sensitivity to treatment differences.[235] LQT1 and LQT2 (potassium ion channel) have been responsive to B-blockers, whereas the LQT3 genotype (sodium ion channel) has been treated with mexiletine or flecanide, sodium channel blockers, and/or pacemakers because of the higher incidence of events during sleep and a greater likelihood of dying from them.[230, 235, 236] Cardiac events have a high predisposition to occur during adolescence with each of these genotypes.[232, 235] Recent investigations have demonstrated that the maximum QTc duration measured at any time before age 10 years was the most powerful predictor of cardiac events during adolescence, regardless of any other measured QTc during any other age or time period.[237] Certain EKG characteristics may have additional prognostic value for poor outcome (recurrent cardiac events and sudden death) such as notched T-waves, T-wave alternans (alternating high and low amplitude T-wave forms), and markedly prolonged QT intervals (>500 ms), in addition to family history of sudden death.[235]

Other important arrhythmia producing syndromes with some propensity to syncope but a greater risk of sudden death, particularly in infancy, includes the short QT syndrome (SQTS) with QT <300 ms and the Brugada syndrome with >2 mm elevation of the ST segment in leads V_1–V_3. Genetic mutations in the potassium channel genes KCNH2, KCNQ1, and KCNJ2 have been identified in SQTS, although only in a small number of patients. The Brugada syndrome has been associated with the SCN5A sodium channel gene mutation.[238, 239]

CEREBROVASCULAR STEALS

These are anatomic obstructive abnormalities in specific arteries, in consequence of which there is a diversion of blood away from the cerebral circulation in order to supply the demands from an extracranial circulation. These are distinctly uncommon but have been recognized in children with particular underlying syndromes.[240] The typical vascular steal involves the obstruction of one of the subclavian arteries proximal to the takeoff of the vertebral artery and distal to the takeoff of the internal carotid. This then allows for the diversion ("stealing") of blood when the appropriate arm is exercised by reversing the direction of flow across the posterior circulation from the carotid-supplied anterior cerebral circulation and down the vertebral artery to the arm on the affected side. This in turn produces cerebral insufficiency and syncope. Theoretically, this proximal subclavian obstruction could occur after traumatic injuries to this region of the subclavian artery or with intrinsic vascular disease in the same location by atheroma, dysplasia, thrombus, or dissection.[240, 241]

Cervical aortic arch syndrome is a congenital vascular anomaly where the aortic arch is abnormally situated in a more cranial direction within the neck above the clavicle.[242–246] About 160 patients have been reported.[242] Additional abnormalities of the aorta coexist in these patients, such as coarctation, kinks, aortic wall necrosis, and aneurysms.[242–246] The syndrome may occur in isolation but can be accompanied by other ventricular outflow abnormalities such as tetralogy of Fallot, pulmonary atresia, and ventricular septal defects.[242, 247] The static clinical picture is a pulsatile neck mass with bruit, with or without symptoms of tracheal and esophageal compression.[248] Of course the patients can induce syncope if there is an adequate activation of the "steal." There has been an association with the deletion syndrome of chromosome 22q11 (DiGeorge syndrome).[242, 249] This is characterized by cardiac anomalies, facial dysmorphism, thymic and parathyroid hypoplasia/aplasia, renal and skeletal anomalies, and cognitive impairment. Spells associated with tetralogy of Fallot ("tet spells") may in part be attributed to cerebral ischemia when there is an accompanying cervical aortic arch. The spells, however, are generally ascribed to anoxia associated with the left-to-right shunting and inadequate systemic oxygen saturation. This phenomenon has been well documented with Doppler flow imaging of the hypoxic spell during anesthesia and surgery.[226]

Posterior circulation, vascular malformations, fistulas, and basilar artery aneurysms, each have the potential to produce syncope by virtue of brainstem ischemia as a tissue "steal" phenomenon. This has been reported in a 2-year-old girl who presented with congenital heart disease and cyanotic breath-holding spells but later succumbed to rupture of a distal basilar artery aneurysm.[250]

CNS MALFORMATIONS

The Arnold-Chiari malformations with and without myelomeningocele (types II and I, respectively) and hydrosyringomyelia have each been associated with obstructive apnea as a result of palatal and bilateral adductor cord palsy and or laryngomalacia. This form of apnea is amenable to intubation and tracheostomy. However, a centrally mediated prolonged expiratory apnea with cyanosis (PEAC) and repeated syncopes may instead dominate the clinical picture in Arnold-Chiari type II. These spells are similar in description to severe cyanotic breath-holding spells in otherwise normal children in that there is typically a trigger to commence crying followed by prompt evolution to cyanosis, loss of consciousness, tonic limb extension, clonic jerks, and opisthotonic posturing. In contrast to cyanotic breath-holding spells, concurrent bradycardia and asystole occurs with PEAC. In a series of 9 children with Arnold-Chiari type II malformations, 6/9 experienced the central form of PEAC, with the onset of apneic syncopes noted on the 1st day of life in 3/6 of the subjects, and on the 9th day, end of the 1st month, and at 6 years in the remaining 3 subjects.[251] Neither ventriculoperitoneal shunting nor posterior fossa decompression corrected the spells in these children. Tracheostomy did not ameliorate them, and unfortunately 5/6 subjects ultimately died during these spells.[251] There is a high likelihood that intrinsic brainstem cardiorespiratory control center dysgenesis and, therefore, dysregulation existed in these patients. Autopsy material in three cases disclosed no uniform abnormalities but unilateral absence of the olivary nucleus or neuronal loss within the olivary nucleus were found in two.[251] This was in addition to hydromyelia, neuronal loss within the nucleus ambiguus, and paramedian clefts within the floor of the fourth ventricle in one child.[251] Similar spells (PEAC) have been reported in a patient with a medullary tumor.[252]

In contrast to the cases described above, an older child age 10 years, who presented with recurrent syncope, Chiari I malformation, and hydrosyringomyelia had no identifiable etiologic association between syncopes and the malformations identified.[253] This was despite innumerable attempts to provoke syncope by means of valsalva, cough, and postural changes. There were no neurological abnormalities on examination to suggest either autonomic dysfunction or myelopathy.[253] An additional adult subject was reported with similar findings, and the author concurred that the associations were coincidental.[254] However, autonomic assessment in 9 subjects, ages 7–49 years old, with Arnold-Chiari malformations (7 subjects type I, 2 subjects type II) and in 5/6 subjects before and after posterior fossa decompression surgery demonstrated reversible changes in identified abnormal orthostatic heart rate and blood pressure responses as well as correction in abnormalities of heart rate variability and respiratory sinus arrhythmia power spectral analysis.[255] Most of these subjects experienced their syncope associated with cough (7/9), two others had associated vertigo or incontinence.[255] These findings suggest that transient medullary brainstem compression altered predominantly sympathetic cardiorespiratory reflex mechanisms producing syncope in these subjects. The presence of intrinsic brainstem dysgenesis seems unlikely in that these were reversible but cannot be entirely excluded. Support for this concept of progressive compression of the medullary region producing progressive alterations in autonomic reflex functioning is provided by the series of subjects studied by DiMario et al. Heart rate variability and respiratory sinus arrhythmia power spectral analysis in three subjects with radiologically more severe degrees of cervico-medullary brainstem compression disclosed progressively more abnormal power spectrum in frequency domain analyses.[256]

In related brainstem-mediated syncope, respiratory apneusis (marked prolongation of inspiration) has its genesis in pontine damage and dysfunction.[257] This has been rarely reported but has been encountered in a 2-year-old pediatric subject after partial surgical resection of a pontine glioma.[258] The apneustic episodes gradually increased in frequency and severity to the point of causing extreme bradycardia and hypoxemia. The authors of the report treated the child with buspirone ($5-HT_{1A}$-receptor agonist) to a maximum of 12 mg/day with resolution of the apneustic events.[258] Over a period of 12 weeks there was sustained remission, and the drug was withdrawn without recurrence.[258] This author has treated another infant (3 months old) with

Arnold-Chiari type II and PEAC with buspirone after posterior decompression and ventriculoperitoneal shunting were ineffective. There was sustained resolution of PEAC events over the subsequent 3 years while continuing on the medication.

SUFFOCATION

Published accounts of four cases of covert video surveillance has documented child abuse by mothers of children being evaluated for cyanotic apneic spells—the mothers smothered their children.[259, 260] The initiation of surveillance was prompted by police requests to substantiate or exclude suspicions of smothering by the mothers of two of these children.[259] While in the hospital, with the mother rooming in with her child in each case, concurrent EEG, oxygen saturation, arterial pulse recording, abdominal movement, and nasal airflow monitoring were recorded. A characteristic combination of recorded features were recognized: (1) the regular breathing pattern of sleep was abruptly interrupted by sudden large body movements, reflecting physical struggle; (2) about 1 minute after the start of the large body movements, a series of large, slow, and prolonged expiratory breaths developed, the "gasping" respirations in response to arterial hypoxemia; (3) the entire episode was accompanied by a severe degree of sinus tachycardia; and (4) 60–70 seconds after the initiation of the event, EEG slow waves evolved to an isoelectric tracing, indicative of cerebral hypoxemia.[259] The physiological correlates were videotaped for clear examination. Earlier methods without covert videotaping identified the same physiologic patterns of respiration, body movement, and EEG changes.[260] It is important to recognize the relatively slow development of the slow-flat-slow EEG pattern in this circumstance compared to the rapid (<30 seconds) evolution of this EEG pattern in typical cyanotic breath-holding spells. This pattern of child abuse is referred to as Munchausen syndrome by proxy.[259, 260] Self-asphyxiation is an even more rare cause of induced syncope and anoxic seizure.[183]

OTHER COMMENTS

Mastocytosis is a collection of disorders characterized by increased numbers of circulating mast cells, where the cutaneous form, urticaria pigmentosa, is the most prevalent type in pediatrics. The excess number of these cells allow for the availability of a large quantity of hisatamine to be spontaneously degranulated from these cells into the circulation. The sudden exposure of circulating histamine produces a number of systemic effects, with syncope prominent among them. Concurrent flushing, diaphoresis, diarrhea, cramping, vomiting, and anaphylaxis may be encountered. There are limited reports of this constellation of symptoms with recurrent syncope as a primary and presenting manifestation in children.[261]

Aquagenic urticaria is a rare and vaguely described entity where immersion of an infant into bathwater precipitates the sudden onset of pallor, hypotonia, and unresponsiveness.[262] If the infant is not removed from the water promptly, the sequence, once initiated, proceeds to syncope. This has been described in a series of eight infants aged 2–15 months at onset of symptoms.[262] Extended family members in each case as well as the infants themselves suffered from dermatographism and photosensitivity with skin eruptions upon exposure to specific thresholds of water temperature (hot) or bright sunlight. Two of the infants had elevated levels of serum histamine measured after bath immersion. Over a follow-up period of 2–7 years, four of the seven had attacks remit and the other three infants had attacks continue.[262] In what perhaps represents a similar phenomenon, but without supportive details (histamine levels), four other infants have been reported independently as a form of reflex epilepsy, and were further discussed by Stephenson.[1, 263–266] Each was an infant of 5–7 months of age who, upon immersion into hot water, experienced either sudden eye rolling, pallor, and limpness or stiffening associated with cyanosis and generalized convulsing. Concurrent EEG recording during a bath-induced attack in two infants recorded diffuse slowing consistent with cerebral hypoxia and no epileptiform activity. Interictal EEG recordings were normal, as were the ultimate developmental outcomes.[1, 263–266] These also appear to represent immersion-induced (reflex situational) syncope as opposed to reflex epilepsy.

Pseudosyncope (psychogenic syncope), much like psychogenic phenomena of all kinds, also occurs in the pediatric age group. In reality, these are events that express a reaction to chronic or acute stress, which exceeds the capacity of the individual to adapt to it.[267] Thus, this is not malingering. These stressors are often overlooked or denied by the patient and their family. The more common non-epileptic seizure behavior can coexist in this circumstance as well. There have been several reports of pediatric and young adult subjects experiencing syncopal events during HUT testing in the context of up to 8 years of recurrent psychogenic syncopal events.[268–272] These have also been recorded within families (sisters) and have been predominantly in females.[271] A report of a cluster of ten cases in a school setting (mass hysteria) has also been evaluated.[273] Although the majority of subjects experienced non-epileptic seizure events (dominant motor stiffening or jerking on video-EEG), pseudosyncope (sudden collapse with little motor movements) was also identified. Many of the subjects of the report described significant social and psychological consequences stemming from the events.[273] Mass hysteria has been described in two main categories: mass motor hysteria and mass anxiety hysteria. Motor movements and dissociation, lasting weeks to months, precipitated by social circumstances or stress characterize mass motor hysteria. Mass anxiety hysteria arises from a perceived danger, albeit false, and is generally short-lived (hours to a day), with a predominance of somatic complaints expressed or exhibited.[274] In all cases studied and reported to date, there is no concurrent alteration in blood pressure or heart rate during the event. In those subjects in whom simultaneous cerebral blood flow monitoring and EEG was obtained, these remained normal during the period of lost consciousness as would be expected. Psychiatric or psychological counseling has been effective as an intervention.

There appears to be good data to support the notion of a familial tendency for syncope. This had first been suggested in a study of thirty consecutive children evaluated for syncope by the Camfields.[275] They compared family history data of syncope from these consecutive subjects to that of their best friends (controls). None of the best friends had syncope, and cardiac causes for syncope were excluded; however, 27/30 subjects compared to only 8/24 best friend controls had at least one first degree relative with syncope ($p < 0.01$).[275] Furthermore, 11/30 subjects had both a sibling and a parent with syncope, whereas only 1/24 best friend control families did ($p < 0.01$).[275] Although a recall bias could affect these results, the mutifactorial nature of syncope lends credence to the idea that inherited intrinsic autonomic reflex responsiveness may be an important component to the tendency toward experiencing syncope. This familial tendency has been demonstrated in the context of childhood breath-holding spells (infantile syncope) where careful examination of family pedigree data disclosed an autosomal dominant inheritance pattern with incomplete penetrance.[79] In a more recent multinational population-based study of 443/671 adult subjects who had vasovagal syncope identified by positive HUT testing, subjects with syncope had an average age at onset of 13 years.[276] These data reiterate the common presentation of syncope in the pediatric age group with a significant genetic influence and the potential expectation for lifelong occurrences.

In a final note to this section, clinicians must be mindful of "ictal syncope" as a manifestation of autonomic epileptic seizures. These syncopal seizures are sudden attacks of flaccid tone and loss of consciousness with or without concurrent motor convulsions. Ictal syncope is present in 20% of children with Panayiotopoulos syndrome (PS), an age-dependent epilepsy syndrome affecting about 10%–15% of children ages 3–6 years.[277,278] The majority of children have idiopathic epilepsy, but there are associated cerebral pathologies identified in those with additional neurological impairments. This unique epilepsy syndrome presents with often prolonged autonomic seizures lasting 30 minutes to several hours in 45% of affected children.[277,278] These are characterized by an abrupt onset, most often from sleep (65%), with the child complaining of feeling sick and nauseas. Recurrent emesis accompanied by pallor (less often flushing) and retching are the most prominent and consistent clinical features with preservation of consciousness.[277,278] Urinary and fecal incontinence, intestinal cramps, and concurrent fever from thermoregulatory abnormalities are not unusual. However, mydriasis (less often miosis) with hypersalivation and mild apnea with brief periods of asystole are also well recognized, with rare cardiorespiratory arrest appreciated.[277,278] Although consciousness is usually preserved during seizures, the child may become confused, lose consciousness, and develop motor convulsions.[277,278] The EEG demonstrates occipital predominant but multifocal spikes in 90% of records, with accentuation during sleep.[277,278] These spikes may appear in the centro-temporal regions with shifting predominance exactly as in Rolandic epilepsy. The single routine EEG may be normal at various times and should prompt the inclusion of sleep during the recording. The frequency, location, or persistence of spikes does not correlate with ictal manifestations.[277,278] The EEG abnormalities remit by early adolescence. Many children with PS are initially misdiagnosed as having Rolandic epilepsy, nonetheless; about 20% of children do eventually evolve into having Rolandic epilepsy as they age.[277,278] The syndrome has been deemed a benign epilepsy; however, the autonomic events may be considerably unpleasant. Prophylactic anticonvulsants (e.g., carbamazepine) may be considered.[277,278] Although autonomic seizures may be more frequent than currently appreciated, their similarity to non-epileptic syncope is readily apparent. These have also been described in a child with 18q syndrome.[279]

The fact that epileptic seizures may induce syncope in some patients stems from the fact that ictal discharges often incorporate regions of the cortex that are known to trigger autonomic alterations in cardiac rate and rhythm. These regions have been identified as the insula cortex, posterior temporal and parietal lobe cortexes, cingulate cortex, and amygdala.[66–68,280] The most common alteration upon cardiac rate is tachycardia; however, rarely ictal discharges may induce bradycardia or asystole.[281] A variety of rhythm disturbances have been associated with cortical stimulation of autonomic control regions as well. These have most prominently been reported in adult subjects and have included QT prolongation, bundle branch block, R on T phenomenon, ectopy, and asystole.[282–285] The clinical seizure manifestation may initially be generalized convulsive, partial, or complex partial by observation. The recognition of seizure more rarely may be further complicated by the fact that even ictal apnea has been identified.[286–288]

HYPERVENTILATION

The inability to inhale adequately is generally experienced by adolescents but also occasionally by younger children. This perceived inability usually prompts the youth to engage in taking repeated short, shallow breaths (hyperventilate), often to the point of becoming lightheaded, with accompanying chest pain or headache.[289] When the behavior continues, there is the eventual development of acroparesthesia, tinnitus, and carpopedal spasm with loss of consciousness, similar to that seen in syncope.[289,290] Attacks such as these are born out of a sense of anxiety or panic, generally precipitated by emotional stress or fear. The inherent sense of anxiety may not be initially recognized until the sequence of events has started. Re-breathing into a paper bag has been advocated for the acute attack. If these attacks become frequent and unremitting, psychiatric evaluation and treatment will be needed.[290–292] Anxiety disorders occur in 5%–18% of all children and often have co-morbidity with underlying depression. These disorders can have a significant negative impact upon social and academic functioning. When these attacks persist in the context of depression, suicide attempts and substance abuse in adulthood can result. The primary treatment approach is with cognitive behavioral therapy. Adjunctive pharmacologic treatments are often utilized.[291, 292]

PAROXYSMAL EXTREME PAIN DISORDER

Paroxysmal extreme pain disorder (PEPD; formerly familial rectal pain syndrome) was first described in 1959 when a family of four generations were described, who experienced paroxysmal "very brief episodes of excruciating rectal pain associated with flushing of the buttocks and legs, ocular pain, and flushing of the eyelid and periorbital skin, and submaxillary pain" affecting thirty-two members.[293] An international consortium, which compiled data on the known cases reported worldwide, renamed the disorder to PEPD in 2005.[294] A detailed clinical summary of those affected living individuals, totaling seventy-seven members of fifteen different families worldwide, has been recently published by Fertleman et al.[295]

Discrete painful attacks are abrupt in onset and are "centered" in one body area (e.g., rectum, jaw, peri-orbit); however, the pain itself is experienced somewhat diffusely throughout that same region.[295, 296] Upon subsequent attacks, the pain may migrate to different areas without consistency. It is described as having a deep, lancing, and burning quality with a superficial component.[295, 296] Flushing is a constant feature and usually approximates the painful "center" but may vary.[295, 296] Rectal pains may involve the genitalia and legs, with associated constipation and urinary retention. Jaw pains may be accompanied by hypersalivation, whereas ocular pain is accompanied by lacrimation and mydriasis. Precipitants of the attacks usually involve physical action or a mechanical strain.[295, 296] Thus, depending upon the site of involvement, minor trauma, eating, swallowing, defecating, and being buffeted by a cold wind are all examples of triggers. All subjects experience flushing related to the region of pain, but it can occur in body segments distant from it. There is often additional swelling and immobility, particularly of a limb when it is involved. If attendant weakness is observed, it may outlast the pain for many hours or, exceptionally, a whole day.[295]

Virtually unique to infants and children (rarely in adults), with lessening frequency as the subject enters adulthood, are tonic non-epileptic seizures.[295–298] These appear to develop in those individuals with neonatal onset and during the most painful attacks. The infant will assume a tonic arching posture with resultant apnea, bradycardia, flushing, and loss of consciousness (syncope).[295–298] Peculiar to these infant tonic attacks is the fact that despite the excruciating pain reported to be experienced by adults, infants do not cry during a tonic attack.[295–298] Thus, despite a "painful" trigger with resultant flushing, tonic posturing, apnea, and loss of consciousness, these may be distinguished from breath-holding spells on the basis of color and by the absence of an emotional component.[70] However, there is also a resemblance to the tonic attacks in neonatal hyperekplexia, which may be more difficult to distinguish. This can be clinically discerned by their normal tone and tendon stretch reflexes, and by the absence of a positive response to the nose-tap test.[299] Tonic attacks appear to be triggered by a number of activities such as feeding, bathing, sneezing, loud noises, and defecation. The onset is within the first 3–4 months of age with the triad of (1) pain on defecation or perineal cleansing, (2) flushing over the buttocks/genitalia with harlequin appearance over the limbs and trunk, and (3) bradycardia.[296,297] There may be an associated edema and pseudo-paralysis of the affected limbs. The attacks last from 30 seconds to 30 minutes. The attacks seen in PEPD bear similarity to paramyotonia and periodic paralysis, and appear related to a rare, dominantly inherited form of dysautonomia erythromelalgia.[300–304] As the attacks persist into early childhood, toddlers begin to exhibit inconsolable screaming during the episodes. In adulthood, the attacks are not accompanied by bradycardia despite this being present in infancy.[295] A long-term complication for individuals affected with PEPD is chronic constipation.[295] This undoubtedly is a direct result of fear of attack precipitation with defecation that promotes compensatory stool holding as an avoidance behavior. Fortunately, rectal attacks precipitated by passing stool appear to decrease and stop in adulthood. Many individuals, however, will experience an increase of attacks involving the orbit and jaw in later childhood and into adulthood.

Etiopathological investigations have been unrevealing with essentially normal histopathology of biopsies from rectum, colon, small bowel, skin, muscle, and sural nerves.[295] Routine laboratory evaluations have also been normal. Interictal EEG and EKG recordings, cardiac function testing, brain MRI and CT scanning, EMG, and nerve conduction studies have all been essentially normal.[295] Detailed sensory and autonomic testing in two subjects have also been normal. EKG during painful attacks in older individuals demonstrates sinus tachycardia; however, only during infantile tonic seizures is there a profound bradycardia or asystole associated with an amplitude-attenuated EEG ("slow-flat-slow" pattern). In one child treated with cardiac pacing, there was no remission in attacks.[295]

Genetic studies performed in a number of affected families have now revealed both autosomal dominant inheritance and linkage to chromosome 2q at the SCN9A gene. Mutations in SCN9A have been identified in eleven PEPD families and two sporadic subjects.[305,306] The SCN9A gene encodes for the $Na_v1.7$ family of voltage-gated sodium channel α-subunits.[305,306] These are expressed in dorsal root and sympathetic ganglion neurons.[307,308] This sodium channel serves to modulate pain signal afferents such that most mutations cause a gain in function and result in increased channel activity.[309,310] Conversely, losses of function mutations in the $Nav1.7$ α-subunit domain have been identified in congenital absence of pain.[311] Carbamazepine selectively blocks slow inactivating channel current and effectively ameliorates the clinical condition, eliminating or reducing the severity of pain in nearly all treated patients.[296,297,312,313] A beneficial response from the application of ice water to the trigger zone and treatment with mexiletine has also been reported in erythromelalgia, but neither has been helpful for PEPD.[296, 304] There has been no benefit from gabapentin, amitriptyline, clonidine, and opioids.[296] The institution of CPR or pacemaker insertion appears ineffective in ablating bradycardia-induced tonic attacks of neonates.[296] Whether PEPD could represent a reflex epilepsy has been debated, because ictal pain is a very rare manifestation of epilepsy.[314, 315] This hypothesis seems unlikely, given the identification of the channel defect.

REFERENCES

1. Stephenson JBP. *Fits and Faints*. MacKieth Press: London, UK, 1990.
2. Brignole M, Alboni P, Benditt D, et al. Guidelines on management (diagnosis and treatment) of syncope. Task Force on Syncope, European Society of Cardiology. Eur Heart J 2001; 22; 1256–1306.
3. Strickberger SA, Benson W, Biaggioni I, et al. AHC/ACCF Scientific statement on the evaluation of syncope. Circulation 2006; 113; 316–327.
4. Lempert T, Bauer M, Schmidt D. Syncope: a videometric analysis of 56 episodes of transient cerebral hypoxia. Ann Neurol 1994; 36; 233–237.
5. Lempert T. Recognizing syncope: pitfalls and surprises. J R Soc Med 1996; 89; 372–375.
6. Farel K. Generalized tonic and atonic seizures. In *The Treatment of Epilepsy: Principles and Practice*. Ed. Elaine Wyllie. 2nd edition. Williams and Wilkins, Baltimore, MD, 1996; 522–529.
7. Lempert T, von Brevern M. The eye movements of syncope. Neurology 1996; 46; 1086–1088.
8. Benbadis SR, Wolgamuth BR, Goren H, et al. Value of tongue biting in the diagnosis of seizures. Arch Int Med 1995; 155; 2346–2349.
9. Gastaut H, Fischer-Williams M. Electroencephalographic study of syncope. Its differentiation from epilepsy. Lancet 1957; 2 (November 23); 1018–1025.
10. Rossen R, Kabat H, Anderson JP. Acute arrest of cerebral circulation in man. Arch Neurol Psychiatry 1943; 50; 510–528.
11. Brenner RP. Electroencephalography in syncope. J Clin Neurophysiol 1997; 14(3); 197–209.
12. Stephenson JBP. Anoxic seizures: self-terminating syncopes. Epilep Dis 2003; 3; 3–6.
13. Gastaut H, Fishgold H, Meyer JS. Conclusions of the international colloquium on anoxia and the EEG. In *Cerebral Anoxia and the Electroencephalogram*. Eds: H Gastaut, JS Meyer. Charles C Thomas Publishers, Springfield, IL, 1961.
14. Stephenson JBP. Febrile convulsions and reflex anoxic seizures. In *Research Progress in Epilepsy*. Ed: FC Rose. Pitman Publishers, London, UK, 1983.
15. Aicardi J. Epileptic syndromes in childhood. Epilepsia 1988; 29(suppl 3); S1–S5.
16. Battaglia A, Guerrini R, Gastaut H. Epileptic seizures induced by syncopal attacks. J Epilepsy 1989; 2; 137–146.
17. Stephenson JBP, Breningstall G, Steer C, et al. Anoxic-epileptic seizures: home video recordings of epileptic seizures induced by syncopes. Epilep Dis 2004; 6(1); 15–19.

18. Horrocks IA, Nechay A, Stephenson JBP, et al. Anoxic-epileptic seizures: observational study of epileptic seizures induced by syncopes. Epilep Dis 2005; 90; 1283–1287.

19. DiMario FJ. Breath-holding spells in childhood. Current Problems in Pediatrics 1999; 29(10); 277–308.

20. Lewis DA, Dhala A. Syncope in the pediatric patient. Pediatr Clin North Am 1999; 46; 205–219.

21. Driscoll DJ, Jacobsen SJ, Porter CJ, Wollan PC. Syncope in children and adolescents. J Am Coll Cardiol 1997; 29; 1039–1045.

22. Ganzeboom KS, Colman N, Reitsma JB, et al. Prevalence and triggers for syncope in medical students. Am J Cardiol 2003; 91; 1006–1008.

23. Willis J. Syncope. Pediatr Rev 2000; 21; 201–203.

24. McLeod KA. Syncope in childhood. Arch Dis Child 2003; 88; 350–353.

25. Rossiter EJR. The Geelong study. Acta Paediatr 1993; Suppl 392; 1–56.

26. Kapoor W, Peterson J, Wieand HS, et al. Diagnostic and prognostic implications of recurrences in patients with syncope. Am J Med 1987; 83; 700–708.

27. Kroger AT, Atkinson WL, Marcuse EK, et al. Centers for Disease Control and Prevention. General recommendations on immunization: Recommendations of the Advisory Committee on Immunization Practices (ACIP). MMWR 2006; 55(RR-15); 1–56.

28. Braun MM, Patriarca PA, Ellenberg SS. Arch Pediatr Adol Med 1997; 151(3); 255–259.

29. Woo EJ, Ball R, Braun MM. The VAERS Working Group. Fatal syncope-related fall after immunization. Arch Pediatr Adol Med 2005; 159; 1083.

30. Younkin DP, Reivich M, Jaggi J, et al. Non-invasive method of estimating human newborn regional bloodflow. J Cerebral Blood Flow Metab 1982; 2; 415–420.

31. Kennedy C, Sokoloff L. An adaptation of the nitrous oxide method to the study of the cerebral circulation in children; normal values for cerebral blood flow and cerebral metabolic rate in childhood. J Clin Invest 1957; 36(7):1130–1137.

32. Mosqueda-Garcia R, Furlan R, Tank J, et al. The elusive pathophysiology of neurally mediated syncope. Circulation 2000; 102; 2898–2906.

33. Sealey B, Lui K. Diagnosis and management of vasovagal syncope and Dysautonomia. AACN Clin Issues 2004; 15(3); 462–477.

34. Grubb B. Neurocardiogenic syncope. N Engl J Med 2005; 352(10); 1004–1010.

35. Wieling W, Ganzeboom KS, Saul JP. Reflex syncope in children and adolescents. Heart 2004; 90; 1094–1100.

36. Gastaut H, Broughton R, De Leo G. Syncopal attacks compulsively self-induced by the valsalva manoeuvre in children with mental retardation. EEG 1982; (Suppl35); 323–329.

37. Stewart J. Orthostatic intolerance in pediatrics. J Pediatr 2002; 140(4); 404–411.

38. Grubb BP, Kanjwal Y, Kosinski DJ. The postural tachycardia syndrome: a concise guide to diagnosis and management. J Cardiovasc Electrophysiol 2006; 17; 108–112.

39. Goldschlager N, Epstein AE, Grubb BP. Scheinman MM. Practice guidelines subcommittee, North American Society of Pacing and Electrophysiology: etiologic considerations in the patient with syncope and an apparently normal heart. Arch Int Med 2003; 163; 151–162.

40. Goldstein DS, Eldadah B, Holmes C, et al. Neurocirculatory abnormalities in chronic orthostatic intolerance. Circulation 2005; 111; 839–845.

41. Bergfeldt L. Differential diagnosis of cardiogenic syncope and seizure disorders. Heart 2003; 89; 353–358.
42. DiVasta AD, Alexander ME. Fainting freshman and sinking sophomores: cardiovascular issues of the adolescent. Curr Opin Pediatr 2004; 16; 350–356.
43. Prengler M, Pavlakis SG, Boyd S, et al. Sickle cell disease: Ischemia and seizures. Ann Neurol 2005; 58; 290–302.
44. Millchap JG. Electroencephalography hyperventilation and stroke in children with sickle cell disease. Clin EEG Neurosci 2006; 37(3); 190–192.
45. Bitzer M, Topka H. Progressive cerebral occlusive disease after radiation. Stroke 1995; 26(1); 131–136.
46. Lerman-Sagie T, Lerman P, Mukamel M, et al. A prospective evaluation of pediatric patients with syncope. Clin Pediatr 1994; 33; 66–70.
47. Massin M, Bourguignont A, Coremans C, et al. Syncope in pediatric patients presenting to an emergency department. J Pediatr 2004; 145; 223–228.
48. Steinberg LA, Knilans TK. Syncope in children: diagnostic tests have a high cost and low yield. J Pediatr 2005; 146; 355–358.
49. Ritter S, Tani LY, Etheridge SP, et al. What is the yield of screening echocardiography in pediatric syncope? Pediatrics 2000; 105(5); e58–e60. URL: http://www.pediatrics.org/cgi/content/full/105/5/e58.
50. Ayabakan C, Ozer S, Celiker A, et al. Analysis of 2017 Holter records in pediatrics. Turk J Pediatr 2000; 42(4); 286–293.
51. Kapoor WN, Smith MA, Miller NL. Upright tilt testing in evaluating syncope: comprehensive literature review. Am J Cardiol 1994; 97; 78–88.
52. Passman R, Horvath G, Thomas J, et al. Clinical spectrum and prevalence of neurologic events provoked by tilt table testing. Arch Int Mrd 2003; 163; 1945–1948.
53. Sabri MR, Mahmodian T, Sadri H. Usefulness of the head-up tilt testing distinguishing neurally mediated syncope and epilepsy in children aged 5–20 years old. Pediatr Cardiol 2006; 27; 600–603.
54. Cohen GA, Lewis DA, Berger S. Reproducibility of head-up tilt–table testing in pediatric patients with neurocardiogenic syncope. Pediatr Cardiol 2005; 26; 772–774.
55. Grubb BP, Temesy-Armos P, Moore J, et al. The use of head-upright tilt testing in the evaluation and management of syncope in children and adolescents. Pacing Clin Electrophysiol 1992; 15; 742–748.
56. Levine MM. Neurally mediated syncope in children: results of tilt testing, treatment, and long-term follow-up. Pediatr Cardiol 1999; 20; 331–335.
57. Lewis DA, Zlotocha J, Henke L, et al. Specificity of head-up tilt testing in adolescents: Effect of various degrees of tilt challenge in normal control subjects. J Am Coll Cardiol 1997; 30; 1057–1060.
58. Matsushima R, Tanaka H, Tamai H. Comparison of the active standing test and head-up tilt test for the diagnosis of syncope in childhood and adolescence. Clin Auton Res 2004; 14; 376–384.
59. Kula S, Olgunturk R, Tunaoglu FS, et al. Distribution of syncopal episodes in children and adolescents with neurally mediated cardiac syncope through the day. Europace 2005; 7; 634–637.
60. Lemmer B. Temporal aspects of the effects of cardiovascular active drugs in humans. In *Chronopharmacology*. Ed: B Lemmer. New York, Marcel Decker Inc., 1989; 525–541.

61. Kula S, Olgunturk R, Tunaoglu FS, et al. Circadian variation of QTc dispersion in children with vasovagal syncope. Int J Cardiol 2004; 97; 407–410.

62. DiMario FJ. Increased QT dispersion in breath-holding spells. Acta Paediatrica 2004; 93; 728–730.

63. Kazemi B, Haghjoo M, Arya A, et al. Predictors of response to head-up tilt test in patients with unexplained syncope or pre-syncope. PACE 2006; 29; 846–851.

64. Chen L, Yang Y, Wang C, et al. A multi-center study of hemodynamic characteristics exhibited by children with unexplained syncope. Chin Med J 2006; 119(24); 2062–2068.

65. Ilgin N, Olgunturk R, Kula S, et al. Brain perfusion assessed by 99mTc-ECD SPECT imaging in pediatric patients with neurally mediated reflex syncope. PACE 2005; 28; 534–539.

66. Colivicchi F, Bassi A, Santini M, et al. Cardiac autonomic derangement and arrhythmias in right-sided stroke with insular involvement. Stroke 2004; 35(9); 2094–2098.

67. Tokgozoglu SL, Batur MK, Topcuoglu MA, et al. Effects of stroke on cardiac autonomic balance and sudden death. Stroke 1999; 30(7); 1307–1311.

68. Oppenheimer SM, Gelb AW, Girvin JP, et al. Cardiovascular effects of human insular stimulation. Neurol 1992; 42; 1727–1732.

69. Szufladowicz E, Maniewski R, Kozluk Ezbiec A, et al. Near-infrared spectroscopy in evaluation of cerebral oxygenation during vasovagal syncope. Physiol Meas 2004; 25; 823–836.

70. DiMario FJ. Breath-holding spells in childhood. Am J Dis Child 1992; 146; 125–131.

71. DiMario FJ. Prospective study of children with cyanotic and pallid breath-holding spells. Pediatrics 2001; 107; 265–269.

72. Low NL, Gibbs EL, Gibbs FA. Electroencephalographic findings in breath-holding spells. Pediatrics 1955; 15; 595–599.

73. Lombroso C, Lerman P. Breath-holding spells (cyanotic and pallid infantile syncope). Pediatrics 1967; 39; 563–581.

74. Emery ES. Status epilepticus secondary to breath-holding and pallid syncopal spells. Neurology 1990; 40; 859.

75. Nirale S, Bharucha NE. Breath-holding and status epilepticus. Neurology 1991; 41; 159.

76. Guerrini R, Battaglia A, Gastaut H. Absence status triggered by pallid syncopal spells. Neurology 1991; 41; 1528–1529.

77. Kuhle S, Tiefenthaler M, Seidl R, et al. Prolonged generalized epileptic seizures triggered by breath-holding spells. Pediatr Neurol 2000; 23(3); 271–273.

78. Goroya JS, Virdi VS. Persistence of breath-holding spells into late childhood. J Child Neurol 2001; 16; 697–698.

79. DiMario FJ, Sarfarazi M. Family pedigree analysis of children with severe breath-holding spells. J Pediatr 1997; 130; 646–651.

80. Southall DP, Shinebourne EA. Sudden and unexpected death between 1 and 5 years. Arch Dis Child 1987; 62; 700–705.

81. Paulson G. Breath-holding spells: a fatal case. Dev Med Child Neurol 1963; 5; 246–251.

82. Taiwo B, Hamilton AH. Cardiac arrest: a rare complication of pallid syncope? Postrad Med J 1993; 69; 738–739.

83. Stephenson JBP. Blue breath-holding is benign. Arch Dis Child 1991; 66; 255–258.

84. Bridge EM, Livingston S, Tietze C. Breath-holding spells: their relationship to syncope, convulsions, and other phenomena. J Pediatr 1943; 23; 539–561.
85. Laxdal T, Gomez MR, Reiher J. Cyanotic and pallid syncopal attacks in children (breath-holding spells). Dev Med Child Neurol 1969; 11; 755–763.
86. Moorjani BI, Rothner AD, Kotagal P. Breath-holding spells and prolonged seizures. Ann Neurol 1995; 38; 512–513.
87. Livingston S. Breath-holding spells in children: differentiation from epileptic attacks. JAMA 1970; 212; 2231–2235.
88. Stephenson JBP. Reflex anoxic seizures and ocular compression. Dev Med Child Neurol 1980; 22; 380–386.
89. DiMario FJ, Chee CM, Berman PH. The evaluation of the autonomic nervous system in children with pallid breath-holding spells. Clin Pediatr 1990; 29; 17–24.
90. Haller JS, Duchowny MS, Jaykar P. Ocular compression reapplied. Ann Neurol 1989; 26; 471A.
91. Stephenson JBP. Two types of febrile seizure: anoxic (syncopal) and epileptic mechanisms differentiated by oculocardiac reflex. BMJ 1978; 2; 726–728.
92. Khura DS, Valencia I, Kruthiventi S, et al. Usefulness of ocular compression during electroencephalography in distinguishing breath-holding spells and syncope from epileptic seizures. J Child Neurol 2006; 21(10); 907–910.
93. Maulsby R, Kellaway P. Transient hypoxic crisis in children. In *Neurological and electroencephalographic correlative studies in infancy*. Ed: P Kellaway. New York, Grune and Stratton, 1964; 349–360.
94. Gastaut H, Gastaut Y. Electroencephalographic and clinical study of anoxic convulsions in children. Electroencephalogr Clin Neurophysiol 1958; 10; 607–620.
95. Stephenson JBP. Reflex anoxic seizures ("white breath-holding"): non-epileptic vagal attacks. Arch Dis Child 1978; 53; 193–200.
96. Gauk EW, Kidd L, Pritchard JS. Mechanism of seizures associated with breath-holding spells. N Engl J Med 1963; 268; 1436–1441.
97. Southall DP, Talbert DG, Johnson P, et al. Prolonged expiratory apnoea: a disorder resulting in episodes of severe arterial hypoxaemia in infants and young children. Lancet 1985; 2(8455); 571–577.
98. Gauk EW, Kidd L, Pritchard JS. Aglottic breath-holding spells. N Eng J Med 1966; 275; 1361–1362.
99. Southall DP, Samuels MP, Talbert DG. Recurrent cyanotic episodes with severe arterial hypoxemia and intrapulmonary shunting: a mechanism for sudden death. Arch Dis Child 1990; 65; 953–961.
100. Hills BA, Masters IB, O'Duffy JF. Abnormalities of surfactant in children with recurrent cyanotic episodes. Lancet 1992; 339; 9(May 30); 1323–1324.
101. DiMario FJ, Chee C, Berman PH. Pallid breath-holding spells: Evaluation of the autonomic nervous system. Clin Pediatr 1990; 29(1); 17–24.
102. DiMario FJ, Burleson JA. Autonomic nervous system function in severe breath-holding spells. Pediatr Neurol 1993; 9; 268–274.
103. Malik M, Bigger JT, Camm AJ, et al. Heart rate variability: Standards of measurement, physiological interpretation, and clinical use. Task force of the European Society of Cardiology and the North American Society of Pacing and Electrophysiology. Circulation 1996; 93(5); 1043–1065.
104. Jasson S, Medigue C, Maison-Blanche P, et al. Instant power spectrum analysis of heart rate variability during orthostatic tilt using a time-/frequency-domain method. Circulation 1997; 96(10); 3521–3526.

105. DiMario FJ, Bauer L, Volpe J, et al. Respiratory sinus arrhythmia in children with severe cyanotic breath-holding spells. J Child Neurol 1997; 12; 260–262.

106. DiMario FJ, Bauer L, Baxter D. Respiratory sinus arrhythmia in children with severe cyanotic and pallid breath-holding spells. J Child Neurol 1998; 13; 440–442.

107. Kolkiran A, Tutar E, Atalay S, et al. Autonomic nervous system functions in children with breath-holding spells and iron deficiency. Acta Paediatr 2005; 94; 1227–1231.

108. Orii KE, Kato Z, Osamu F, et al. Changes in autonomic nervous system function in patients with breath-holding spells treated with iron. J Child Neurol 2002; 17(5); 337–340.

109. Holowach J, Thurston DL. Breath-holding spells and anemia. N Eng J Med 1963; 268; 21–23.

110. Bhatia MS, Singshal PR, Dhar NK, et al. Breath-holding spells: an analysis of 50 cases. Indian Pediatr 1990; 27; 1073–1079.

111. Daoud A, Batieha A, Al-Sheyyab M, et al. Effectiveness of iron therapy on breath-holding spells. J Pediatr 1997; 130; 547–550.

112. Mocan H, Alisan Y, Othan F, et al. Breath-hold spells in 91 children and response to treatment with iron. Arch Dis Child 1999; 81; 261–262.

113. Tam DA, Rash FC. Breath-holding spells in a patient with transient erythro-blastopenia of childhood. J Pediatr 1997; 130; 651–653.

114. Colina KF, Abelson HT. Resolution of breath-holding spells with treatment of concomitant anemia. J Pediatr 1995; 126; 395–397.

115. Mackler B, Person R, Miller LR, et al, Finch CA. Iron deficiency in the rat: biochemical studies of brain metabolism. Pediatr Res 1978; 12; 217–220.

116. Voorhees ML, Stuart MJ, Stockman JA, et al. Iron deficiency anemia and increased urinary norepinephrine excretion. J Pediatr 1975; 86; 542–547.

117. Oski FA. The nonhematologic manifestations of iron deficiency. Am J Dis Child 1979; 133; 315–322.

118. Segal S, Lavie P. Sleep and breathing in sleep in children with breath-holding spells. Neuropsychobiology 1984; 12(4); 209–210.

119. Kahn A, Rebuffat E, Sottiaux M, et al. Brief airway obstructions during sleep in infants with breath-holding spells. J Pediatr 1990; 117(2 pt 1); 188–193.

120. Hunt CE. Relationship between breath-holding spells and cardiorespiratory control: a new perspective. J Pediatr 1990; 117(2 pt 1); 245–247.

121. Anas NG, McBride JT, Boettrich C, et al. Ventilatory chemosensitivity in subjects with a history of cyanotic breath-holding spells. Pediatrics 1985; 75; 76–79.

122. Anas NG, McBride JT, Brooks JG. Childhood cyanotic breath-holding spells and cardiorespiratory control. J Pediatr 1991; 118; 656.

123. Cintra F, Poyares D, Do Amaral A, et al. Heart rate variability during sleep in patients with vasovagal syncope. Pace 2005; 28; 1310–1316.

124. Mattie-Luksic M, Javornisky G, DiMario FJ. Assessment of stress in mothers of children with severe breath-holding spells. Pediatr 2000; 106(1):1–5.

125. Hudaoglu O, Dirik E, Yis U, et al. Parental attitude of mothers, iron deficiency anemia, and breath-holding spells. Pediatr Neurol 2006; 35; 18–20.

126. Stephenson JBP. Prolonged expiratory apnoea in children. Lancet 1985; 2(8461); 953.

127. McWilliam RC, Stephenson JBP. Atropine treatment of reflex anoxic seizures. Arch Dis Child 1984; 59; 473–475.

128. Palm L, Blennow G. Transdermal Anticholinergic treatment of reflex anoxic seizures. Acta Paediatr Scand 1985; 74; 804–805.
129. Benditt DG, Benson DW, Kreitt J, et al. Electrophysiologic effects of theophylline in young patients with recurrent symptomatic bradyarrhythmias. Am J Cardiol 1983; 52; 1223–1229.
130. Sapire DW, Casta A, Safely W, et al. Vasovagal syncope in children requiring pacemaker implantation. Am Heart J 1983; 106(6); 1406–1411.
131. Sreeram H, Whitehouse W. Permanent cardiac pacing for reflex anoxic seizures. Arch Dis Child 1996; 75; 462–463.
132. McCleod KA, Wilson N, Hewitt J, et al. Cardiac pacing for severe childhood neurally mediated syncope with reflex anoxic seizures. Heart 1999; 82; 721–725.
133. Kelly AM, Porter CJ, McGoon MD, et al. Breath-holding spells associated with significant bradycardia: successful treatment with permanent pacemaker implantation. Pediatrics 2001; 108(3); 698–702.
134. Wilson D, Moore P, Finucane AK, et al. Cardiac pacing in the management of severe pallid breath-holding attacks. J Paediatr Child Health 2005; 41; 228–230.
135. Sra JS, Jazayeri MR, Avitall B, et al. Comparison of cardiac pacing with drug therapy in the treatment of neurocardiogenic syncope with bradycardia or asystole. N Eng J Med 1993; 328; 1085–1090.
136. DiMario FJ. Breath-holding spells and pacemaker implantation. Pediatr 2001; 108(3); 765–766.
137. Donma MM. Clincal efficacy of piracetam in the treatment of breath-holding spells. Pediatr Neurol 1998; 18; 41–45.
138. Woody RC, Kiel EA. Swallowing syncope in a child. Pediatrics 1986; 78(3); 507–509.
139. Engelhardt W, Kotlarek F, Von Bernuth G. Deglutition syncope in childhood with complete atrioventricular block. Am J Cardiol 1986; 58; 1113–1114.
140. Kenigsberg K. Deglutition syncope in childhood with complete atrioventricular block (letter). Am J Cardiol 1988; 62; 170.
141. Kenigsberg K, Boris M, Joseph P, et al. Reflex bradycardia after tracheoesophageal fistula repair. Surgery 1972; 71; 125–129.
142. Kalloor GJ, Singh SP, Collis JL. Cardiac arrhythmias on swallowing. Am Heart J 1977; 93; 235–238.
143. Levin B, Posner JB. Swallow syncope. Neurol 1972; 22; 1086–1093.
144. Kunis RL, Garfein OB, Pepe AJ, et al. Deglutition syncope and atrioventricular block selectively induced by hot food and liquid. Am J Cardiol 1985; 55; 613.
145. Golf S. Swallowing syncope. Acta Med Scand 1977; 201; 585–586.
146. Stern R, Horwitz SJ, Doershuk CF. Neurologic symptoms during coughing paroxysms in cystic fibrosis. J Pediatr 1988; 112(6); 909–912.
147. Katz RM. Cough syncope in children with asthma. J Pediatr 1970; 77; 48–51.
148. Charcot JM. {Untitled}. Gaz Med Paris 1876; 5; 588–589.
149. Kerr A Jr, Derbes VJ. The syndrome of cough syncope. Ann Intern Med 1953; 39; 1240–1253.
150. Sharpey-Schafer EP. The mechanism of syncope after coughing. BMJ 1953; 2; 860–863.
151. McIntosh HD, Estes EH, Warren JV. The mechanism of cough syncope. Am Heart J 1956; 52; 70–82.
152. Kerr A Jr, Eich RH. Cerebral concussion as a cause of cough syncope. Arch Int Med 1961; 108; 138–142.

153. Wenger TL, Dohrman ML, Strauss HC, et al. Hypersensitive carotid sinus syndrome manifested as cough syncope. Pacing Clin Electrophysiol 1980; 3; 332–339.

154. McCorry DJP, Chadwick DW. Cough syncope in heavy goods vehicle drivers. Q J Med 2004; 97; 631–632.

155. Mattle HP, Nirkko AC, Baumgartner Sturzenegger M. Transient cerebral circulatory arrest coincides with fainting in cough syncope. Neurology 1995; 45; 498–501.

156. Hart G, Oldershaw PJ, Cull RE, et al. Syncope caused by cough-induced complete atrioventricular block. Pacing Clin Electrophysiol 1982; 5; 564–566.

157. SaitoD, Matsuno S, Matsushita K, et al. Cough syncope due to atrioventricular conduction block. Jpn Heart J 1982; 23; 1015–1020.

158. Benditt DG, Samniah N, Pham S, et al. Effect of cough on heart rate and blood pressure in patients with cough syncope. Heart Rhythm 2005; 2; 807–813.

159. Chao A-C, Lin R-T, Liu C-K, et al. Mechanisms of cough syncope as evaluated by valsalva maneuver. Kaohsiung J Med Sci 2007; 23;(2); 55–61.

160. DeMaria AA, Westmoreland BF, Sharbrough FW. EEG in cough syncope. Neurology 1984; 34; 371–374.

161. Puetz TR, Vakil N. Gastroesophageal reflux-induced cough syncope. Am J Gastroent 1995; 90(12); 2204–2206.

162. Lewis DW, Frank LM. Hair-grooming syncope seizures. Pediatrics 1993; 91(4); 836–838.

163. Igarashi M, Boehm RM, May WN, et al. Syncope associated with hair-grooming. Brain Devel 1988; 10(4); 249–251.

164. Pelekanos JT, Dooley JM, Camfield JR, et al. Stretch syncope in adolescence. Neurology 1990; 40; 705–707.

165. Sturtzenegger M. Transcranial Doppler and angiographic findings in adolescent stretch syncope. J Neurol Neurosurg Psychiatr 1995; 58(3); 367–370.

166. Huycke EC, Card HG, Sobol SM, et al. Postexersional cardiac asystole in a young man without organic heart disease. Ann Int Med 1987; 106; 844–845.

167. Arad M, Solomon A, Roth A, et al. Postexercise syncope: evidence for increased activity of the sympathetic nervous system. Cardiology 1993; 83; 121–123.

168. Smith GPD, Mathias CJ. Postural hypotension enhanced by exercise in patients with chronic autonomic failure. Q J Med 1995; 88; 251–256.

169. Sakakibara R, Hattori T, Kita K, et al. Urodynamic and cardiovascular measurements in patients with micturition syncope. Clin Auton Res 1997; 7(5); 219–221.

170. Schiavone A, Biasi MT, Buonomo C, et al. Micturition syncopes. Functional Neurol 1991; 6(3); 305–308.

171. Bednarek N, Arbues AS, Motte J, et al. Familial rectal pain: a familial autonomic disorder as a cause of paroxysmal attacks in the newborn baby. Epileptic Disord 2005; 7(4):360–362.

172. Lin JT-Y, Ziegler DK, Lai C-W, et al. Convulsive syncope in blood donors. Ann Neurol 1982; 11; 525–528.

173. Roddy SM, Ashwal S, Scheider S. Venipuncture fits: a form of reflex anoxic seizure. Pediatr 1983; 72; 715–718.

174. Duvernoy WFC, Nair MRS, Zobl EG. Convulsive disorder mimicked by prolonged asystole and cured by permanent pacing. Heart Lung 1980; 9; 711–714.

175. Cole M, Shen J, Hommer D. Convulsive syncope associated with acupuncture. Am J Med Sci 2002; 324(5); 288–289.

176. Olatunji BO, Williams NL, Sawchuk CN, et al. Disgust, anxiety and fainting symptoms associated with blood-injection-injury fears: a structural model. Anxiety Dis 2006; 20; 23–41.

177. Seri S, Cerquiglini A, Harding GFA. Visually induced syncope: a non-epileptic manifestation of visual sensitivity. Neurology 2006; 67(2); 359–360.

178. Stephenson JBP. Non-epileptic television syncope. BMJ 1978; 1; 1622.

179. Hall DM. Non-epileptic television syncope. BMJ 1978; 2; 205.

180. Clayton-Smith J, Laan L. Angelman syndrome: a review of the clinical and genetic aspects. J Med Genet 2003; 40; 87–95.

181. Vanagt WY, Pulles-Heintzberger CF, Vernooy K, et al. Asystole during outbursts of laughing in a child with Angelman syndrome. Pediatr Cardiol 2005; 26; 866–868.

182. Douchin S, Do-Ngoc D, Rossignol AM, et al. Angelman syndrome and severe vagal hypertonia. Three pediatric case reports. Arch Mal Coeur Vaiss 2000; 93; 559–563.

183. Lai CW, Ziegler DK. Repeated self-induced syncope and subsequent seizures. Arch Neurol 1983; 40; 820–823.

184. Britton JW. Benarroch, E. Seizures and syncope: anatomic basis and diagnostic considerations. Clin Auton Res 2006; 16(1); 18–28.

185. Naritoku DK, Casebeer DJ, Darbin O. Effects of seizure repetition on postictal and interictal neurocardiac regulation in the rat. Epilepsia 2003; 44(7); 912–916.

186. Devinsky O, Price BH, Cohen SI. Cardiac manifestations of complex partial seizures. Am J Med 1986; 80; 195–202.

187. Grubb B. Neurocardiogenic syncope and related disorders of orthostatic intolerance. Circulation 2005; 111; 2997–3006.

188. McLeod KA. Dysautonomia and neurocardiogenic syncope. Curr Opin Cardiol 2001; 16; 92–96.

189. McCleod KA. Dizziness and syncope in adolescence. Heart 2001; 86; 350–354.

190. Stewart J, Weldon A, Arlievsky N, et al. Neurally mediated hypotension and autonomic dysfunction measured by heart rate variability during head-up tilt testing in children with chronic fatigue syndrome. Clin Auton Res 1998; 8; 221–230.

191. Tanaka H, Yamaguchi H, Matushima R, et al. Instantaneous orthostatic hypotension in children and adolescents: A new entity of orthostatic intolerance. Pediatr Res 1999; 46(6); 691–696.

192. Gastaut H, Zifkin B, Rufo M. Compulsive respiratory stereotypies in children with autistic features: Polygraphic recording and treatment with fenfluramine. J Autis Devel Dis 1987; 17(3); 391–406.

193. Aicardi J, Gastaut H, Mises J. Syncopal attacks compulsively self-induced by valsalva's maneuver associated with typical absence seizures. Arch Neurol 1988; 45; 923–925.

194. Murphy JV, Wilkinson IA, Pollack NH. Death following breath holding in an adolescent. Am J Dis Child 1981; 135; 180–181.

195. Howard P, Leathart G, Dornhorst AC, et al. The "mess trick" and the "fainting lark". BMJ 1951; 2; 524–528.

196. Kanjawal Y, Kosinski D, Grubb BP. The postural tachycardia syndrome: definitions, diagnosis, and management. Pacing Clin Electrophysiol 2003; 26; 1747–1757.

197. Grubb BP, Kosinski D, Boehm K, et al. The postural tachycardia syndrome: a neurocardiogenic variant identified during head upright tilt table testing. Pacing Clin Electrophysiol 1997; 20; 2205–2212.
198. Low P, Novak Y, Novak P, et al. Postural tachycardia syndrome. In *Clinical Autonomic Disorders*. Ed: P Low. Philadelphia PA, Lippincott-Raven, 1997; 681–698.
199. Grubb BP, Calkins H, Rowe P. Postural tachycardia, orthostatic intolerance and chronic fatigue syndrome. In *Syncope: Mechanisms and Management*, Eds: BP Grubb, B Olshansky. Malden MA, Blackwell-Futura Press; 2005; 225–244.
200. Grubb BP, Kanjwal Y, Kosinski DJ. The postural tachycardia syndrome: a concise guide to diagnosis and management. J Cardiovasc Electrophysiol 2006; 17; 108–112.
201. Shannon J, Flatten NL, Jordan T, et al. Orthostatic intolerance and tachycardia associated with norepinepherine-transporter deficiency. N Engl J Med 2000; 342; 541–549.
202. Bonyhay I, Freeman R. Sympathetic neural activity, sex dimorphism, and postural tachycardia syndrome. Ann Neurol 2007; 61; 332–339.
203. Singer W, Opfer-Gehrking TL, McPhee BR, et al. Acetylcholinesterase inhibition: a novel approach in the treatment of neurogenic orthostatic hypotension. J Neurol Neurosurg Psychiat 2003; 74; 1294–1298.
204. Satish RR, Black BK, Biaggioni I, et al. Acetylcholinesterase inhibition improves tachycardia in postural tachycardia syndrome. Circulation 2005; 111; 2734–2740.
205. Singer W, Opfer-Gehrking TL, Nikander KK, et al. Acetylcholinesterase inhibition in a patient with orthostatic intolerance. J Clin Neurophysiol 2006; 23(5); 477–482.
206. Filler G, Gow RM, Nadarajah R, et al. Pharmacokinetics of pyridostigmine in a child with postural tachycardia syndrome. Pediatrics 2006; 118(5); e1563–e1568. URL:http://www.pediatrics.org/cgi/content/full/118/5/e1563.
207. DiGirolamo E, DiIorio C, Leonzio L, et al. Usefulness of a tilt training program for the prevention of refractory neurocardiogenic syncope in adolescents: A controlled study. Circulation 1999; 100; 1798–1801.
208. Krediet CTP, deBruin IGJM, Ganzeboom KS, et al. Leg crossing, muscle tensing, squatting, and the crash position are effective against vasovagal reactions soley through increases in cardiac output. J Appl Physiol 2005; 99; 1697–1703.
209. van Dijk N, Quartieri F, Blanc JJ, et al. Effectiveness of physical counterpressure maneuvers in preventing vasovagal syncope: Physical Counterpressure Manoeuvres Trial (PC-Trial). J Am Coll Cardiol 2006; 48; 1652–1657.
210. Salim MA, DiSessa TG. Effectiveness of fludrocortisone and salt in preventing syncope recurrence in children; A double-blind, placebo-controlled, randomized-trial. J Am Coll Cardiol 2005; 45; 484–488.
211. Balaji S, Oszlok PC, Aleen MC, et al. Neurocardiogenic syncope in children with normal hearts. J Am Coll Cardiol 1994; 23; 779–785.
212. Scott WA, Pongiglione G, Bromberg BI, et al. Randomized comparison of atenolol and fludrocortisone acetate in the treatment of pediatric neurally mediated syncope. Am J Cardiol 1995; 76; 400–402.

213. Madrid AH, Ortega J, Rebollo JG, et al. Lack of efficacy of atenolol for the prevention of neurally mediated syncope in a highly symptomatic population: a prospective, double-blind, randomized and placebo controlled study. J Am Coll Cardiol 2001; 37; 554–559.

214. Connolly SJ, Sheldon R, Thorpe KE, et al. Pacemaker therapy for prevention of syncope in patients with recurrent severe vasovagal syncope: Second Vasovagal Pacemaker Study (VPS II): a randomized trial. JAMA 2003; 289; 2224–2229.

215. Biffi M, Boriani G, Brozetti G, et al. Neurocardiogenic syncope in selected pediatric patients-natural history during long-term follow-up and effect of prophylactic pharmacological therapy. Cardiovasc Drugs Thera 2001; 15; 161–167.

216. Stewart-Williams S. The placebo puzzle: putting together the pieces. Health Psychol 2004; 23; 198–206.

217. Buckalew LW, Ross S. Relationship of perceptual characteristics to efficacy of placebos. Psychol Reports 1981; 49; 955–961.

218. Grubb BP, Kosinski D, Kip K. Utility of methylphenidate in the therapy of refractory neurocardiogenic syncope. Pace 1996; 19; 836–840.

219. Grubb BP, Samoil D, Kosinski D, et al. The use of sertraline hydrochloride in the treatment of refractory neurocardiogenic syncope in children and adolescents J Am Coll Cardiol 1994; 24; 490–494.

220. Axelrod FB, Chelimsky GG, Weese-Mayer DE. Pediatric autonomic disorders. Pediatrics 2007; 118 (1); 309–321.

221. Axelrod FB. Hereditary sensory and autonomic neuropathies: familial dysautonomia and other HSANs. Clin Auton Res 2002;12(Suppl 1); 2–14.

222. Anderson SL, Coli R, Daly IW, et al. Familial dysautonomia is caused by mutations of the IKAP gene. Am J Hum Genet 2001; 68; 753–758.

223. Bernardi L, HiltzM, Stemper B, et al. Respiratory and cardiovascular responses to hypoxia and hypercapnia in familial dysautonomia. Am J Respir Crit Care Med 2002; 167; 141–149.

224. Lewis DA, Dhala A. Syncope in the pediatric patient. The cardiologist's view. Ped Clin North Am 1999; 46(2); 205–219.

225. Greeley WJ, Stanley TE, Ungerleider RM, et al. Intraoperative hypoxemic spells in Tetralogy of Fallot. An echocardiographic analysis of diagnosis and treatment. Anesth Analg 1989; 68; 815–819.

226. Farnie, DE, Storrow A, Whitley H. Syncope in a 2-year-old: ED presentation of primary pulmonary hypertension. Ann Emer Med 1997; 30(3); 337–342.

227. Linzer M, Yang EH, Estes NAM, et al. Clinical Guideline: Diagnosing syncope: Part 1: Value of history, physical examination, and electrocardiography. Ann Int Med 1997; 126(12); 989–996.

228. Gospe SM, Campfield P. Cardiac causes of sudden death: virtual panel discussion of posed questions. Sem Pediatr Neurol 2005; 12(1); 67–69.

229. Lai CW, Ziegler DK. Syncope problem solved by continuous ambulatory simultaneous EEG/EKG recording. Neurology 1981; 31; 1152–1154.

230. Khan I. Long QT syndrome: diagnosis and management. Am Heart J 2002; 143(1); 7–14.

231. Khositseth A, Martinez M, Driscoll D, et al. Syncope in children and adolescents and the congenital long QT syndrome. Am J Cardiol 2003; 92; 746–749.

232. Moss A. Long QT syndrome. JAMA 2003; 289(16); 2041–2044.

233. Wilde A, Roden D. Predicting the long-QT genotype from clinical data: from sense to science. Circulation 2000; 102(23); 2796–2798.

234. Schwartz PJ, Priori SG, Spazzolini C, et al. Genotype-phenotype correlation in the long QT syndrome. Gene-specific triggers for life-threatening arrhythmias. Circulation 2001; 103; 89–95.

235. Nemec J, Hejlik JB, Shen W-K, et al. Catecholamine-induced T-wave lability in congenital long QT syndrome: a novel phenomenon associated with syncope and cardiac arrest. Mayo Clin 2003; 78; 40–50.

236. Villain E, Denjoy I, Lupoglazoff JM, et al. Low incidence of cardiac events with B-blocking therapy in children with long QT syndrome. Eur Heart J 2004; 25; 1405–1411.

237. Goldenberg I, Mathew J, Moss AJ, et al. Corrected QT variability in serial electrocardiograms in long QT syndrome. J Am Coll Cardiol 2006; 48(5); 1047–1052.

238. Guistetto C, DiMonte F, Wolpert C, et al. Short QT syndrome: clinical findings and diagnostic-therapeutic implications. Eur Heart J 2006; 27; 2440–2447.

239. Priori SG, Napolitano C, Gasparini M, et al. Natural history of Brugada syndrome. Insights for risk stratification and management. Circulation 2002; 105; 1342–1347.

240. Becker AE, Becker MJ, Edwards JE. Congenital anatomic potentials for subclavian steal. Chest 1971; 60; 4.

241. Gosselin C, Walker PM. Subclavian steal syndrome. Existence, clinical features, diagnosis, management. Semin Vasc Surg 1996; 9; 93–97.

242. Baravelli M, Borghi A, Rogiani S, et al. Clinical, anatomopathological and genetic pattern of 10 pateints with cervical aortic arch. Int J Cardiol 2007; 114; 236–240.

243. Pearson GD, Kan JS, Neill CA, et al. Cervical aortic arch with aneurysm formation. Am J Cardiol 1997; 79; 112–114.

244. Ikonimidis JS, Robbins RC. Cervical aortic arch with pseudocoarctation. Presentation with spontaneous rupture. Ann Thorac Surg 1999; 67; 248–260.

245. Helebrand WE, Kelley MJ, Talner NS, et al. Cervical aortic arch with retro-esophageal aortic obstruction. Report of a case with successful surgical intervention. Ann Thorac Surg 1978; 26; 86–92.

246. Kumar S, Mandalam R, Unni M, et al. Left cervical aortic arch with associated abnormalities. Cardiovasc Intervent Radiol 1989; 12; 88–91.

247. Patel KR, Hurwitz JL, Clauss RH. Cervical aortic arch associated with Tetralogy of Fallot. Cardiovasc Surg 1993; 1; 602–604.

248. Weiberg PM. Aortic arch anomilies. In *Moss and Adams Heart Disease in Infants, Children and Adolescents*. Eds: GC Emmanouiles, TA Riemenscheider, HD Allen, and HP Gutgessel. 5th edition. Baltimore, MD, Williams and Wilkins, 1995; 810–837.

249. Neilsen K, Stewart F, Van Essen T, et al. Spectrum of clinical features associated with interstitial chromosome 22q11 deletions: a European collaborative study. J Med Genet 1997; 34; 798–804.

250. DiMario FJ, Rorke LB. Transient oculomotor nerve palsy in a ten-month-old child with a distal basilar artery aneurysm. Pediatr Neurol 1992: 8; 303–306.

251. Southall DP, Lewis GM, Buchanan R, et al. Prolonged expiratory apnea (cyanotic "breath-holding") in association with a medullary tumor. Dev Med Child Neurol 1987; 29; 784–804.

252. Cochrane DD, Adderley R, White CP, et al. Apnea in patients with myelomeningo-cele. Pediatr Neurosurg 1990–1991; 16; 232–239.

253. Woelfe J, Haverkamp F, Kreft B. Repeated syncopes and extended paediatric hydrosyringomyelia / Chiari I malformation: relation or coincidence? J Neurol Neurosurg Psychiatr 1998; 64(2); 278–279.
254. Nogues M. Repeated syncopes and extended paediatric hydrosyringomyelia/ Chiari I malformation. J Neurol Neurosurg Psychiatr 1998; 65(5); 805.
255. Ireland PD, Mickelsen D, Rodenhouse TG, et al. Evaluation of the autonomic cardiovascular response in Arnold-Chiari deformities and cough syncope syndrome. Arch Neurol 1996; 53(6); 526–531.
256. DiMario FJ, Bauer L, Baxter DP: Respiratory sinus arrhythmia of brainstem lesions. J Child Neurol 1999; 14; 229–232.
257. Plum F, Alvord EC. Apneustic breathing in man. Arch Neurol 1964; 10; 101–112.
258. Wilken B, Lalley P, Bischoff AM, et al. Treatment of apneustic respiratory disturbance with a serotonin-receptor agonist. J Pediatr 1997; 130; 89–94.
259. Southall DP, Stebbens VA, Rees SV, et al. Apnoeic episodes induced by smothering: two cases identified by covert video surveillance. BMJ 1987; 294; 1637–1641.
260. Rosen CL, Frost JD, Bricker T, et al. Two siblings with cardiorespiratory arrest: Munchausen syndrome by proxy or child abuse? Pediatrics 1983; 71; 715–720.
261. Shaffer HC, Parsons DJ, Peden DB, et al. Recurrent syncope and anaphylaxis as a presentation of systemic mastocytosis in a pediatric patient: case report and literature review. J Am Acad Derm 2006; 54(Suppl 5); S210–S213.
262. Mouterde O, Mallet E, Spriet J. Syncope during bathing in infants, a pediatric form of water-induced urticaria? Arch de Pediatrie 1997; 4(11); 1111–1115.
263. Mofenson HC, Weymuller CA, Greensher J. Epilepsy due to water immersion. An unusual case of reflex sensory epilepsy. JAMA 1965; 191; 600–601.
264. Keipert JA. Epilepsy precipitated by bathing: water-immersion epilepsy. Austral Paediatr J 1969; 5; 244–247.
265. Stensman R, Ursing B. Epilepsy precipitated by hot water immersion. Neurology 1971; 21; 559–562.
266. Shaw NJ, Livingston JH, Minns RA, et al. Epilepsy precipitated by bathing. Dev Med Child Neurol 1988; 30; 108–111.
267. Wood BL, Haque S, Weinstock A, et al. Pediatric stress-related seizures: conceptualization, evaluation, and treatment of nonepileptic seizures in children and adolescents. Curr Opin Pediatr 2004; 16(5): 523–531.
268. Luzza F, Pugliatti P, DiRosa S, et al. Tilt-induced pseudosyncope. Int J Clin Pract 2003; 57(5); 373–375.
269. Grubb BP, Gerard G, Wolf DA, et al. Syncope and seizures of psychogenic origin: identification with head-upright tilt table testing. Clin Cardiol 1992; 15; 839–842.
270. Petersen MEV, Williams T, Sutton R. Psychogenic syncope diagnosed by prolonged head–up tilt testing. Q J Med 1995; 88; 209–213.
271. Mathias CJ, Deguchi K, Bleasdale-Barr K, et al. Familial vasovagal syncope and pseudosyncope: observations in a case with both natural and adopted siblings. Clin Auton Res 2000; 10; 43–45.
272. Mathias CJ, Deguchi K, Schatz I. Observations on recurrent syncope and presyncope in 641 patients. Lancet 2001; 357; 348–353.
273. Roach ES, Langley RL. Episodic neurological dysfunction due to mass hysteria. Arch Neurol 2004; 61; 1269–1272.
274. Wessley S. Mass hysteria: two syndromes? Psychol Med 1987; 17; 109–120.
275. Camfield PR, Camfield CS. Syncope in childhood: a case control clinical study of the familial tendency to faint. Can J Neurol Sci 1990; 17; 306–308.

276. Sheldo RS, Sheldo AG, Connolly SJ, et al. Investigators of the syncope symptom study and the prevention of syncope trial. J Cardiovasc Electrophysiol 2006; 17; 49–54.

277. Panayiotopoulos CP. Autonomic seizures and autonomic status epilepticus peculiar to childhood: diagnosis and management. Epilep Behav 2004; 5; 286–295.

278. Covanis A. Panayiotopoulos syndrome: a benign childhood autonomic epilepsy frequently imitating encephalitis, syncope, migraine, sleep disorder or gastro-enteritis. Pediatrics 2006; 118(4); e1237–e1243. URL:http://www.pediatrics. org/cgi/content/full/118/4/e1237.

279. Stephenson JBP. Autonomic seizures in 18q-syndrome. Brain Dev 2005; 27(2); 125–126.

280. Britton JW, Benarroch E. Seizures and syncope: anatomic basis and diagnostic considerations. Clin Auton Res 2006; 16; 18–28.

281. Tinuper P, Bisulli F, Cerullo A, et al. Ictal bradycardia in partial epileptic seizures: Autonomic investigation in three cases and literature review. Brain 2001; 124; 2361–2371.

282. Keilson MJ, Hauser WA, Magrill JP, et al. ECG abnormalities in patients with epilepsy. Neurology 1987; 37; 1624–1626.

283. Opherk C, Coromilas J, Hirsch LJ. Heart rate and EKG changes in 102 seizures; analysis of influencing factors. Epilepsy Res 2002; 52; 117–127.

284. Tavernor SJ, Brown SW, Tavernor RM, et al. Electrocardiograph QT lengthening associated with epileptiform EEG discharges—a role in sudden unexplained death in epilepsy? Seizure 1996; 5; 79–83.

285. Fenichel GM, Olson BJ, Fitzpatrick JR. Heart rate changes in convulsive and nonconvulsive neonatal apnea. Ann Neurol 1980; 7; 577–582.

286. Watanabe K, Hara K, Miyazaki S, et al. Apneic seizures in the newborn. Am J Dis Child 1982; 136(11); 980–984.

287. Andrade EO, Arain A, Malow BA. Partial epilepsy presenting as apneic seizures without posturing. Pediatr Neurol 2006; 35(5); 359–362.

288. Hosain S, La Vega-Talbott M, Solomon G, et al. Apneic seizures in infants: role of continuous EEG monitoring. Clin Electroencephal 2003; 34(4); 197–200.

289. Kanton WJ. Panic disorder. N Engl J Med 2006; 354; 22; 2360–2366.

290. Kendall PC, Pimentel SS. On the physiological symptom constellation in youth with generalized anxiety disorder. J Anxiety Dis 2003; 17; 211–221.

291. James A, Soler A, Weatherall R. Cognitive behavioural therapy for anxiety disorders in children and adolescents. Cochrane Database of Syst Rev 2005; (4); CD004690.

292. Clark DB, Birmaher B, Axelson D, et al. Fluoxetine for the treatment of childhood anxiety disorders: open-label, long-term extension to a controlled trial. J Am Acad Child Adol Psychiatry 2005; 44(12):1263–1270.

293. Hayden R, Grossman M. Rectal, ocular, and submaxillary pain. Am J Dis Child 1959; 97; 479–482.

294. Fertleman CR, Ferrie CD. What's in a name-familial rectal pain syndrome becomes paroxysmal extreme pain disorder. J Neurol Neurosurg Psychiatr 2006; 77; 1294–1295.

295. Fertleman CR, Ferrie CD, Aicardi J, et al. Paroxysmal extreme pain disorder (previously familial rectal pain syndrome). Neurology 2007; 69; 586–595.

296. Bednarek N, Arbues AS, Motte J, et al. Familial rectal pain: a familial autonomic disorder as a cause of paroxysmal attacks in the newborn baby. Epileptic Disord 2005; 7; 360–362.

297. Schubert R, Cracco JB. Familial rectal pain: a type of reflex epilepsy? Ann Neurol 1992; 32; 824–826.

298. Griesemer DA, Talwar D, Hadden RO, et al. Reflex apnea with autonomic dysynergy (RAAD): a case report. Epilepsia 1993; 34(Suppl 6); 43. Abstract.

299. Gordon N. Startle disease or hyperekplexia. Dev Med Child Neurol 1993; 35(11); 1015–1018.

300. Yang Y, Wang Y, Li S, et al. Mutations in SCN9A, encoding a sodium channel alpha subunit, in patients with primary erythermalgia. J Med Genet 2004; 41; 171–174.

301. Drenth JP, Te Morsche RH, Guillet G, et al. SCN9A mutations define primary erythermalgia as a neuropathic disorder of voltage gated sodium channels. J Invest Dermatol 2005; 124; 1333–1338.

302. Michiels JJ, te Morsche RH, Jansen JB, et al. Autosomal dominant erythermalgia associated with a novel mutation in the voltage-gated sodium channel alpha subunit Nav1.7. Arch Neurol 2005; 62; 1587–1590.

303. Waxman SG, Dib-Hajj SD. Erythromelalgia: a hereditary pain syndrome enters the molecular era. Ann Neurol 2005; 57; 785–788.

304. Nathan A, Rose JB, Guite JW, et al. Primary erythromelalgia in a child responding to intravenous lidocaine and oral mexiletine treatment. Pediatrics 2005; 115; e504–e507.

305. Fertleman CR, Baker MD, Parker KA, et al. SCN9A mutations in paroxysmal extreme pain disorder: allelic variants underlie distinct channel defects and phenotypes. Neuron 2006; 52(5); 767–774.

306. Drenth JPH, Waxman SG. Mutations in sodium-channel gene SCN9A cause a spectrum of human genetic pain disorders. J Clin Invest 2007; 117(12); 3603–3609.

307. Sangameswaran L, Fish LM, Koch BD, et al. A novel tetrodotoxin–sensitive, voltage-gated sodium channel expressed in rat and human dorsal root ganglia. J Biol Chem 1997; 272; 14805–14809.

308. Toledo-Aral JJ, Moss BL, He ZJ, et al. Identification of PN1, a predominant voltage-dependent sodium channel expressed principally in peripheral neurons. Proc Natl Acad Sci USA 1997; 94; 1527–1532.

309. Catterall WA, Yu FH. Painful channels. Neuron 2006; 52; 743–744.

310. Rush AM, Dib-Hajj SD, Liu S, et al. A single sodium channel mutation produces hyper- or hypoexcitability in different types of neurons. Proc Natl Acad Sci USA 2006; 103; 8245–8250.

311. Cox JJ, Reimann F, Nicholas AK, et al. An SCN9A channelopathy causes congenital inability to experience pain. Nature 2006; 444; 894–898.

312. Waxman SG. Neurobiology: a channel sets the gain on pain. Nature 2006; 444; 831–832.

313. Benarroch EE. Sodium channels and pain. Neurology 2007; 68(3); 233–236.

314. Sahota PK, Stacy MA. Pain as a manifestation of seizure disorder. Clin Electroencephalogr 1993; 24; 63–66.

315. Lancman ME, Asconape JJ, Penry KT, et al. Paroxysmal pain as sole manifestation of seizures. Pediatr Neurol 1993; 9(5); 404–406.

4

Sleep-Related Phenomena

INTRODUCTION TO SLEEP-RELATED PHENOMENA

Epileptic seizures may manifest a host of behavioral, motor, and perceptual alterations due to abnormal cortical electrical discharges. All epileptic seizure types can be electrically evident and often clinically manifest during sleep. In fact, sleep may serve as an activator of both epileptic discharges and epileptic seizures through the induction of brain-activated electrographic changes. Sleep itself, however, is a state where an orderly evolution of electrical brain wave patterns induces and reflect the clinical stages and physiologic responses we observe as sleep. It is important to further recognize that many complex physiological as well as pathological behaviors, individual perceptions, and motor activities may be a direct consequence of sleep itself. Many of these clinical features bear resemblance to epileptic events but can be differentiated from them if the clinician has an appreciation for their existence and knowledge of their manifestations.

THE CLINICAL PROBLEM AND EPIDEMIOLOGY

Sleep is a neurobehavioral activity that all mammalian species engage in. It is a complex, cyclical, and neurally regulated state with precise and sequential series of neurally mediated humoral responses that induce and maintain it. Sleep is not merely a passive activity but rather an active brain-initiated function that has a homeostatic purpose, which may consequently produce significant detrimental impacts when not efficiently performed.

The role of sleep in evolution has been the subject of intense study.[1-6] Biologists have attempted to identify the physiologic requirements across species and its relationship to human sleep need. Various theories have been put forward to explain the benefits and functions of sleep.[2-6] These theories have championed a number of physiologic activities that are enhanced during the sleep process. The theories cover the enhancement of tissue growth and restoration, an instinctive behavior designed to prevent maladaptive activity and promote survival, a means to conserve energy, a time to consolidate memory and learned information as well as the time to remove unneeded learning and disengage undesirable cell circuits.[1-6] Mammalian sleep would appear to have specific relevance here.[1] In this context, sleep is divided into two main fractions: rapid-eye-movement (REM) sleep and non-REM sleep. This division is

99

further stratified into stages 1–4 of NREM, where the "light sleep" of stage 1 NREM "deepens" through stages 2, 3, and 4 NREM, followed by the first brief episode of REM sleep approximately 90 minutes thereafter. There is a continual cycling through the stages of NREM and REM every 90–120 minutes in older children and adults.[7] Importantly, there is an age-dependent maturation of this so-called sleep architecture. Prior comparisons of sleep architecture among various mammals suggested that those mammals with bigger brains and higher basal metabolic rates (BMR) had less deep and REM sleep. Species that were also at more risk from predators similarly exhibited less deep and REM sleep.[1] Lesku and colleagues, using path analysis techniques to examine current hypotheses more critically, found that although species with a higher BMR do engage in less deep sleep, species that also had a greater brain mass preferentially engaged in more REM sleep behavior.[1] But again, those mammals experiencing the greatest risk from predators engaged in less REM despite bigger brain mass.[1] This suggests that although multiple factors influence sleep architecture, in support of prior theories, REM sleep is implicated in the maintenance of brain function and possibly cognition, whereas the effect of predatory risk shifts sleep from "deeper" and REM sleep to "lighter" and safer states from the point of view of arousability.[1,8–10] This complements prior hypotheses suggesting a role for sleep in brain plasticity, neural ontogenesis, increased CNS protein synthesis, consolidation of memory, and host immunological defenses.[1,8–11]

Thus, it is important for us humans to obtain both adequate amounts of and appropriately staged sleep for its effectiveness to be felt. Within the United States, recent polls taken from parents about their children's sleep report that almost 75% of parents would like to change something about their children's sleep.[12,13] Almost 15% of these parents report seeking advice from their primary care physician about the adequacy of their child's sleep.[12,13] Data from those surveys identified that children across all age groups were consistently getting less sleep, amounting to only 76%–86% of the amount recommended (Table 4-1).[12–14] In a national random sample of 68,418 participants from the 2003 national survey of children's health of elementary school-aged children (6–11 years) and adolescents (12–17 years), results were analyzed by using

Table 4-1 Typical Amounts of Sleep Needed and Obtained

Age Group	Recommended Amounts	Typically Obtained Amounts
Infants (3–11 months)	14–15 hours	12.7 hours
Toddlers (12–35 months)	12–14 hours	11.7 hours
Preschoolers (3–6 years)	11–13 hours	10.3 hours
School aged (1st–5th grades)	10–11 hours	9.5 hours
Adolescents (6th–12th grades)	9.25 hours	7 hours

Source: Modified from References.[1,2] Data at http://www.sleepfoundation.org.

weighted bivariate and multivariate regression models with a report of "not getting enough sleep one or more times within the week prior to survey" as the dependent variable.[15] Elementary school-aged children with reported inadequate sleep were more likely to have problems in school reported. Adolescents with reported inadequate sleep were more likely to report that they had frequent or severe headaches or experienced frequent parental anger among other findings.[15] These same children with reported inadequate sleep were also described by their parents as appearing depressed, engaged in frequent parental arguments, and were felt to be less safe at home, school, or in the neighborhood.[15] The survey results would extrapolate to potentially impacting upon approximately 15 million similar aged children nationwide and provided solid ground for exploring the family, school, and related health factors contributing to inadequate sleep in children.[15] Clearly, sleep adequacy plays an important role in the prevention of disease and injury, stability of mood, and behavior, and allows for a better ability to learn.[16–19] Importantly, however, teachers' reports may neither be sensitive nor adequate enough to identify the true scope of the problem.[20] An important factor negatively impacting upon the sleep health of children is their use of media such as TV and video games. The negative consequences of these activities seem universal. In a recent study of sleep onset, sleep-wake patterns, and media use in 9718 junior high school children in Japan, a total of 9199 questionnaires were available for analysis.[21] Overall, 27.9% of the subjects reported long sleep onset latency (>20 minutes).[21] This was significantly associated with disturbed sleep: more frequent night awakenings, disturbed sleep depth, and poor overall sleep quality. These difficulties were in turn associated with daytime sleepiness, difficulties in falling asleep, and a "bad morning feeling."[21] Body mass index adjustments revealed no significant results.[21] Both prolonged TV viewing and videogame playing were independently and significantly correlated with long sleep onset latency.[21] Poor sleep hygiene and insufficient sleep time significantly increases sleep onset latency, which itself promotes more disturbed sleep.[21] The appropriate intervention seems obvious: limit TV viewing and videogame playing especially prior to sleep.

Sleep problems in childhood are recognized worldwide. However, the most appropriate ascertainment tool awaits development. There is an ongoing national survey of Australian children aged 4–5 years old. The primary caregiver's reports from 4983 of the 10,596 children (47%) within the families participating in the Longitudinal Study of Australian Children have been studied thus far.[22] The validated study instruments used are the Strengths and Difficulty Questionnaire (SDQ), a measure of behavior and emotional problems; the Pediatric Quality of Life Questionnaire (PedsQL), an assessment of total physical and psychosocial health; the Peabody Picture Vocabulary Test (PPVT-III), a screening test of verbal ability; and the Who Am I (WAI) test to assess the child's developmental vocabulary and preliteracy and numeracy skills.[22] Each measure was correlated with the primary responses to reported sleep problems and their degree of severity. The estimated national prevalence of mild sleep problems was 19.8% and moderate/severe sleep problems were 13.8%.[22] Awakening during the night (18.1%), difficulty getting to bed (12.8%), difficulty breathing (9.7%), and morning fatigue (9.1%) were the most frequently identified national sleep problems.[17] The overall prevalence of 33.6% of mild-to-severe sleep problems was similar to the 27% identified in a study of 1844 Swedish 5- to 7-year-old preschoolers whose parents agreed to participate in a survey from an initial sample of 2215 children.[22, 23] These figures compared similarly as well to the 15.5% with night awakening, 9% difficulty getting to bed, and 5.6% difficulty falling asleep in the Swedish sample.[23] Importantly, there were strong correlations with greater sleep problems and the higher total score on the SDQ in both the Australian and Swedish studies and a strong correlation with attention deficit hyperactivity disorder (ADHD) in both studies on the PedsQL.[22, 23] Children with sleep problems when compared to those without sleep problems had poorer child-health-related quality of life, more behavior problems, and higher rates of ADHD. There was, however, little association between sleep problems and receptive vocabulary, early literacy, or numeracy skills.[22]

The prevalence of other specific disorders of sleep is dependent upon age with particular patterns of problems much more common in one age group over another. In a parental survey of unselected patients seen at a general pediatric clinic, 1038 children ages 2–13.9 years old had sleep problems assessed by means of a validated Pediatric Sleep Questionnaire (PSQ).[24] This tool comprised seventy closed-ended and several open-ended questions that elicit a medical history, which includes sleep disturbances. Habitual snoring was noted in 17%, insomnia in 41%, excessive daytime sleepiness in 14%, and sleepwalking, sleep terrors, or bruxism in another 38%.[24] Two symptoms were present in 18% of the sample.[24] These results suggest that clinicians are faced with vast numbers of children with potential sleep problems. When confronted with a child who has a potential sleep disorder, the evaluation should start by abstracting an accurate history of the behaviors in question as well as obtaining an in-depth sleep history and sleep diary (Table 4-2). These will be the first steps in sorting out the specific sleep problem at hand.[25] The use of one of the aforementioned validated sleep questionnaires can be additionally helpful, especially for small cohorts and population sampling.

We can generally identify an individual at sleep by the observation of their behavior. However, there are more intricate and measurable physiologic parameters, which allow for a precise definition of the underlying properties of sleep. The typical constellation of behaviors associated with sleep includes recumbency, closed eyes, decreased motion, and apparent diminished awareness and level of alertness. The preservation of arousal to a level of normal alertness minimally distinguishes this state behaviorally from coma. Some stimuli may be more effective in producing arousal than others depending upon what level of sleep (light or deep) the individual is encountered in. More familiar sounds such as the cry of a mother's infant or one's own name may be a more potent stimulus than other nonmeaningful sounds.[26] More

Table 4-2 Sleep History

Of Sleep Problem Relative to Age, Associated Illness, Medication,
Home and Life Changes.

- Specify routine for weekdays, weekends, school days, vacation & holidays.
- Sleep environment: Describe where the child sleeps, physical layout of the home, and who sleeps where. Are they alone or in a shared bed or room? Is there access to TV, computers, or other electronic game devices? Is there excessive light or noise immediately apparent? What is the sleep routine of other members of the family? Does the child need a transitional object? Is the bedroom door opened?
- Bedtime behavior: Is there a bedtime ritual or routine? Are there multiple routines? Is the child taking medicine prior to sleep? What happens with each one? Do different routines result in different behavioral outcomes? Does the child engage in refusal, stalling, or complain of fear? Do they have difficulty falling asleep independently? Do they suck their thumb or engage in some type of rhythmic movement (rocking, head banging, leg kicking)?
- Nocturnal behaviors: What is the child's sleep like? Is there snoring or pauses in breathing? Are there frequent night awakenings? What are their timing and duration? Is it due to enuresis, sleep-talking, sleep-walking, agitation/terror, bad dreams, pain, or discomfort? Are there associated movements or motor behaviors? Does the child grind their teeth or have jerking movements? How does the child return to sleep, alone or need other intervention?
- Diurnal behaviors: What hour does the child awaken? Is awakening spontaneous? Does the hour of awakening vary in relation to school or activities? Does the child take naps? When, where, and how long are naps? Is the child sleepy during the day? Are there any anxieties voiced by the child? Are there school or family stresses evident?
- Concurrent medical history and review of systems
- Family history of sleep problems
- Psychosocial history
- Sleep Diary over 2–4 weeks

objective measures of sleep include the use of an actigraph recording and the polysomnogram.

An actigraph is a small watch-like device worn by the child during a multiple-day recording segment. The devise records body activity and converts this into a bar graph over several days, with time plotted in hours. By viewing the graphs of activity and the converse, quiet times, the exact times of sleep onset and termination can be seen. The recording can only identify the appearance of gross body movement and not more specific types. The benefit, however, is that it is an easily obtained sleep diary over extended time frames within the individual's home sleep environment. Polysomnography allows for an in-depth exact physiological monitoring of sleep and thus a more accurate definition of sleep states and accompanying activity. The polysomnogram allows for the simultaneous monitoring of muscle activity by electromyogram (EMG), extraocular eye movements via electro-oculogram (EOG), and brain electrical activity with concurrent electroencephalogram

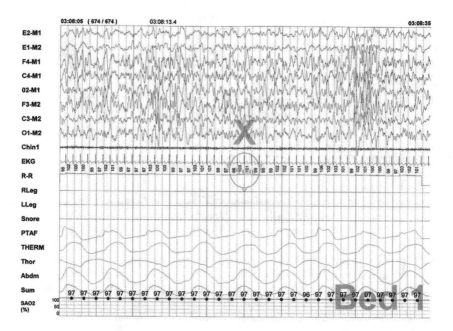

Figure 4-1. Pictured is a single page of a normal segment from a typical polysomnographic tracing. Electrode placements are identified on the y-axis and elapsed time along the bottom (x-axis). Numeric subscripts locate left side of head with odd numbers and right side of head with even numbers. $E_{1,2}$ = ears, $M_{1,2}$ = middline, $F_{1,2}$ = frontal location, $C_{1,2}$ = central location, $O_{1,2}$ = occipital location.

(EEG) (see Figure 4-1). With the recording of these three parameters, the identification of the specific sleep stages through which an individual descends and ascends during segments of recorded sleep can be made (Table 4-3). Concomitant recording of other physiological parameters allow for the identification of respiratory rate and effort, nasal and mouth airflow, heart rate and rhythm, transcutaneous blood oxygen saturation, and exhaled gas constituents (pCO_2, pO_2). All these parameters along with a video recorded observation of the patient in sleep allow for detection of the specific characteristics of recognized sleep disorders.[7]

When examining the EEG tracing during sleep, specific sleep stages are defined by the associated waveform amplitude and frequency in conjunction with the other two aforementioned physiological measures, EMG and EOG.[7] The EEG background is described with the subject at rest with eyes closed. The resting wakeful state is characterized by low-voltage rhythmic alpha activity (8–13 cycles per second [Hz]) in children at or older than 3 years. As sleep develops the alpha waves of wakefulness give way to low-voltage mixed frequencies of alpha- and theta-dominant (4–8 Hz) rhythms in stage-1 NREM with the evolution of sharp waves over the vertex region. The EEG of NREM is considered synchronized because of its regularity and uninterrupted wave

Table 4-3 Sleep Components in Mature Sleep

Sleep State	Eye Movements	Respirations (R) Heart Rate (HR) Blood Pressure (BP)	Muscle Activity	EEG Background	Behaviors
Awake	Variable & conjugate	Variable R & BP Sinus rhythm	Active	Low voltage α	Alert
NREM					
Stage-1	Slow & dysconjugate	Regular R & BP Sinus rhythm	Active Rest	Synchronized Low voltage mixed α & τ	Drowsy rest with easy arousability
Stage-2	No movement conjugate	Regular R & BP Sinus rhythm	Quiet	Sleep spindles K-complexes	Sleep with harder arousability
Stage-3	No movement conjugate	Slow Regular R Slow sinus rhythm Lower BP	Quiet	High voltage slow δ: <50%	Deeper sleep with difficult arousability
Stage-4	No movement conjugate	Slow Regular R Slow sinus rhythm Lower BP	Quiet	High voltage slow δ: >50%	Deep sleep with difficult arousability
REM					
Tonic	Rapid conjugate eye movements	Irregular R, Lower BP& slow HR	Atonia	Desynchronized Low voltage α	Dream
Phasic	Bursts of REM	Bursts of Irregular elevated R, BP, & HR	Atonia		

Notes: NREM = nonrapid eye movement, REM = rapid eye movement, α = (8–13 Hz), τ = (4–8 Hz), sleep spindles = (12–14 Hz), δ = (0.5–4 Hz).

patterns. There are slow, dysconjugate eye movements noted at this time on EOG with regular respiratory and heart rates. As the subject relaxes, there is diminishing although persistent muscle activity. At this stage, subjects may be aroused promptly and not feel as though they were actually asleep unless they are briefly aroused by their own sleep starts (hypnic jerks). The hallmark of stage-2 NREM sleep is the development of sleep spindles and K-complexes. The sleep spindle arises from synchronous bursts of thalamic pacemaker neurons, which produce bursts of synchronized 12–14 Hz activity. When these bursts are coupled with vertex sharp and after following slow wave, a K-complex is noted. The eye movements disappear and muscle activity quietens. There is more difficulty arousing the subject at this time and stage. The subject will continue to sleep and a gradual evolution of a higher-amplitude ($>75 \mu V$) slow-wave predominant pattern emerges. There are an ever-increasing percentage of synchronized delta waves (0.5–2 Hz). By definition, stage-3 sleep has <50% delta wave activity, and with the acquisition of >50% delta wave activity present stage 4 is reached. Slow-wave sleep, or deep sleep, is associated with a higher arousal threshold than the other stages of NREM sleep. There are no eye movements, and the muscle tone continues to decline as the subject descends into deeper sleep. REM sleep is characterized by the reemergence of low voltage and faster frequencies in the alpha range. At this time there is the appearance of characteristic rapid eye movements and muscle paralysis (atonia). Although the EEG at this time is considered activated (dreaming) as if in wakefulness, the individual is difficult to arouse. The EEG in REM sleep is desynchronized as there is irregularity and randomly appearing wave bursts. REM sleep has been further divided into tonic and phasic stages, referring to the primary continuous muscle atonia and desynchronized EEG (tonic stage) and the superimposed intermittent bursts of rapid eye movements, rapid irregular respirations, and heart rate periods (phasic stages).[27]

The effect of age is paramount in the interpretation of normal sleep behavior and sleep architecture. Between 24 weeks gestation and about 2 months post-term the infant evolves from a near continual intermittent atypical sleep state to a pattern of cycling from wakefulness into a well-defined two-staged sleep state.[28,29] Before 30 weeks gestation there is atypical sleep with a discontinuous background that oscillates between that of early REM and NREM. Recent studies in preterm infants have identified cycling between continuous and discontinuous sleep states for a majority of neonates 25–30 weeks gestation with durations of cycles lasting 37–100 minutes (mean 68 ± 19 minutes).[30] Intermittent and sudden, brief, fragmentary motor activity with little eye movement, absent chin EMG activity, and irregular respirations can be identified. There are bursts of high-voltage polymorphic slow waves alternating with long periods of suppressed activity (trace' discontinu'). At about 30 weeks gestation more identifiable markers of REM sleep (active sleep) emerge with more eye movements, increased irregular respirations and heart rate, intermittent twitching behavior, and more prolonged EEG activity. NREM (quiet sleep) becomes more identifiable by 28–32 weeks gestation with the suppression of associated body and eye movement activity, more regular respirations and heart rate patterns, and an alternating but more continuous EEG pattern. The corresponding more mature EEG pattern demonstrates 2- to 5-second bursts of high-amplitude slow waves with intervening 6–8 seconds of low-voltage mixed activity (trace' alternans) by 36 weeks gestation at which time chin EMG also becomes evident. There is a shift from active sleep predominance in the preterm to about equal proportions of active and quiet sleep states at 40 weeks gestation (term). Further maturation rapidly occurs over the first 3 months post-term with a decreasing frequency of startling behavior and the development of sleep spindle activity. Trace' alternans becomes replaced by NREM sleep stages in the first 3 months post-term with K-complexes becoming apparent by 6 months post-term. Sleep cycles last about 50 minutes at term with an ever-increasing duration to the adult 90-minute duration by early adolescence.[29,31] Over the latter half of the first year of life REM sleep periods are all about equivalent in length and take up nearly 30%–40% of the total sleep time despite daytime naps. As the child approaches 2–3 years of age, the sleep cycle has lengthened to about 60 minutes, with an initial very short REM sleep period and progressively longer ones ensuing later in sleep. It is not until 4–5 years of age that the sleep cycle lengthens to about 60–90 minutes, with concomitant decreases in REM sleep time from 30% to 20%–25%. Sleep latency over these early years of childhood is initially shorter than 15 minutes and begins to lengthen up to 30 minutes by age 5 years, with the majority of early-night sleep in NREM. Over the 5- to 10-year age range there continues to be a gradual lengthening of sleep cycles and more regularly placed and progressively longer periods of REM sleep appreciated in the later segments of sleep. By early adolescence, sleep fractions and total sleep time approximate adult values.[22,29,31]

Normative data for various sleep parameters throughout childhood are scant. In a large meta-analysis of peer reviewed journals published over the years 1960–2003, some 65 articles concerning polysomnographic studies of 3577 subjects between the ages of 5 and 102 years were published by Ohayon et al.[32] The analysis included only "nonclinical" participants who underwent all-night recordings where data were presented and published numerically. There were 1186 children aged 5–19 years included in the analysis. Important conclusions were found within the body of literature reviewed. Those conclusions were as follows: (1) Sleep latency increases with age, defined as the time after lying recumbent to the emergence of three consecutive epochs of stage-1 or entry into any other sleep stage.[32] However, the overall increase in sleep latency between ages 20 and 80 years was only 10 minutes. The majority of change occurred in childhood and accounted for the significant differences noted over time. (2) The percentage of stage 1 sleep increases with age.[32] Although there was an increase in childhood compared to middle-aged adults, there was a greater change after middle age to the elderly, implying that the greatest changes occur in adulthood. (3) The percentage of stage 2 sleep increases with age and occurs across all ages consistently, whereas the percentage of stages 3 and 4 (slow-wave sleep) decreased.[32] (4) The percentage of REM sleep increases throughout childhood until adolescence and then decreases between young adulthood and age 60 years before remaining stable.[32] (5) The total sleep time decreased with age in childhood through adolescence only when related to environmental factors and when recordings were performed on school days.[32] The analysis pointed out that both sleep latency and sleep efficiency (the ratio of total sleep time to time in bed) each remained unchanged throughout childhood and adolescence.[32] There were no gender differences appreciated for any parameter throughout childhood.[32]

In the older child and adolescent extending into adulthood, the sleep cycle progressively lengthens from 50–60 minutes to about 90–120-minute intervals.[22,29,31,33,34] During these intervals, alternating segments of NREM and REM sleep occur 4–7 times over the course of a night's sleep. Stage-1 NREM typically lasts a few minutes and accounts for only 2%–5% of total sleep time.[33–35] Entry into deeper stages of sleep proceeds in a sequential order such that stage-2 NREM will last about 10–20 minutes and the sum of each cycle will ultimately constitute approximately 45%–55% of total sleep time each night.[33–35] Sleep stage 3 ($\leq$5 minutes duration each cycle) and stage 4 (30–40 minutes duration each cycle) will comprise 5%–10% and 30%–40% of total sleep, respectively, and will be predominant within the first third of a night's sleep.[33–35] REM periods are initially brief during the first sleep cycles, but as sleep cycles recur and become progressively longer, the REM periods that occur progressively later in the cycles also lengthen.[33–35] An initial 90-minute cycle length increases to about 120 minutes in cycle length in the later phases of an adolescent's night sleep. The longest REM periods, therefore, are found in the last third of a night's sleep. NREM sleep accounts for about 75%–80% of total sleep time and REM accounts for the remainder (20%–25%).[22,29,31,33–35] These fractions of NREM and REM sleep are drastically different from those in infancy where the fractions of each are more even in duration.

With this basic knowledge of sleep cycling and sleep stage durations it becomes immediately obvious that particular stage-related sleep behaviors and disorders are more prominent at particular ages because of the inherent architecture of that age's sleep. Because REM percentage is greatest in over the first year of life and REM sleep is associated with arousals, difficulties with maintaining sleep and arousal from sleep are prominent clinical problems of this age group. In preschool and school-aged children there is a progressive lengthening of the NREM fraction of sleep and an increased number of transitions between NREM and REM. This cycling behavior promotes more opportunity for disorders of arousal related to this age. The adolescent age group presents with a greater demand for sleep, yet with an ever-decreased time allowed for sleep with social and academic demands. The resulting irregularity in schedule promotes a high risk for circadian rhythm disorders. The International Classification of Sleep Disorders (2nd edition, 2005) identifies eight general categories of sleep disorders and enumerates several specific subcategorized entities within each category (Table 4-4).[36] Not all categories and entities are likely to be confused with epileptic phenomenon; however, many are paroxysmal and potentially

Table 4-4 The International Classification of Sleep Disorders

- Insomnia
- Sleep-related breathing disorders
- Hypersomnias of central origin; not due to a circadian rhythm sleep disorder, sleep-related breathing disorder, or other cause of disturbed nocturnal sleep
- Circadian rhythm sleep disorder
- Parasomnias
- Sleep-related movement disorders
- Isolated symptoms, apparently normal variants, unresolved issues
- Other sleep disorders

Source: Modified from Reference.[36]

the source of neurological evaluation. Subsequent sections will focus on those clinical entities with direct relevance to and considered in the evaluation of children with paroxysmal non-epileptic disorders.

OVERVIEW: PATHOPHYSIOLOGY AND MECHANISMS

An understanding of the basic mechanisms of sleep onset and of sleep-wake regulation is fundamental to the understanding of childhood paroxysmal sleep disorders. Clearly, disturbances in the underlying physiological mechanisms will impact greatly on normal sleep regulation and potentially manifest in a number of clinical paroxysmal symptoms, which must be differentiated as non-epileptic events. Current theory, derived from human and animal sleep experimentation, describes the two-process model to account for our understanding and prediction of sleep-wake patterns.[26, 37] This model explains two complementary intrinsic biological drives: a *homeostatic process*, which depends upon the accumulated sleep time and period of wakefulness over a 24-hour segment, and a *circadian process*, which is driven by endogenous pacemakers.[37, 38] The net balance of these complementary processes results in a near 24-hour sleep-wake cycle. Within this cycle is structured an *ultradian process* whereby there is a regular oscillation and cycling between NREM and REM periods.[38, 39]

An individual's homeostatic drive to sleep will increase over periods of wakefulness. The pressure to sleep maximizes over longer waking periods until reaching the individual's "sleep time." This pressure can be augmented further under circumstances of sleep deprivation. The pressure is reduced when sleep is obtained only to rebuild over the subsequent period of prolonged wakefulness.[26, 39] Sleepiness needs to be differentiated from fatigue, where sleep is not inevitable even when allowed to do so. The human circadian rhythm is derived from endogenous neurohumoral pacemakers located within the suprachiasmatic nuclei (SCN) of the hypothalamus.[40, 41] These nuclei insert an intrinsic nearly 24-hour biological timing clock upon the human sleep-wake cycle. There are other circadian rhythms encountered, which are much less obvious (e.g., cortisol and growth hormone secretion). The circadian rhythm is unaffected by prior amounts of wakefulness and sleep but is influenced by and synchronized to environmental factors and cues (zeitgebers). These cues help to encode the physiologic responses within the SCN to produce the cyclical sleep-wake rhythm through the process of entrainment. There is glutamate release and activation of N-methyl-D-aspartate receptors in the cells of the SCN, which is triggered by light stimulus reaching the retina.[40,41] This activation occurs via projections through the retinohypothalamic tract and are in turn transmitted throughout the body by humoral and autonomic changes (Table 4-5).[42] Light exposure is the most potent entraining stimulus of the circadian rhythm, but its effect is dependent upon the time it is presented. Exposure to light at night shifts the clock forward and exposure to light in the early morning shifts it backward.[26,34,39] Melatonin secretion is linked to the circadian rhythm, with peak excretion at both dusk and dawn, then remaining elevated throughout the hours between these peak secretion times only to decline during daylight.[26,34,39] Because the SCN also has melatonin receptors, it can be influenced (reset) by melatonin exposure endogenously or exogenously. The intrinsic and genetically programmed pacemaker function of the SCN will continue even in the absence of environmental dark-light cues.[43] However, when the genes coding for this intrinsic pacemaker function are mutated, the timing may be inordinately lengthened or truncated.[43]

There are a number of identified neurotransmitters and peptides involved in the induction and cycling of sleep-wake states. Many of these substances

Table 4-5 Physiological Changes During Sleep Compared to Quiet Rest

Function	NREM	REM (Tonic/phasic)
Parasympathetic Activity	Increased	Increased/decreased
Sympathetic Activity	Unchanged	Decreased/increased
Body Temperature	Decreased	Increased (absent sweating & shivering)
Respirations	Regular	Irregular
Heart Rate	Slowed & regular	Fast & irregular
Pupil Size	Miotic	Miotic/mydriatic
PenileTumescence/Clitoral Engorgement	Infrequent	Frequent
Gastric Acid Secretion	Increased	Increased (peaks at 2 AM)
Gastric & Duodenal Motility	Increased	Decreased
Swallowing	Decreased (maximal S-W-S)	Decreased
Plantar Responses	Extensor	Mute
Cytokines	Increased IL-1, IL-6, TNF	No changes

Source: Modified from References.[11,26,41]
Notes: REM = rapid eye movement, NREM = non-REM, S-W-S = slow wave sleep, IL-1, IL-6 = interleukins 1,6, TNF = tumor necrosis factor.

are secreted specifically by neuronal projections emanating from, targeting to, and traversing through the hypothalamus to lower brainstem regions and upper cortical areas (Table 4-6).[34,44–47] There exist reciprocal projections whose activations are orchestrated in an orderly response to SCN-initiated rhythms. Knowledge and understanding of the circuits involved and the roles of specific neurotransmitters in modulating sleep-wake states allow for greater precision in diagnosis and targeting drug therapy in specific sleep disorders. The hypothalamus plays a central role in the modulation of the sleep-wake cycle

Table 4-6 Neurotransmitters of Sleep

Neurotransmitter	Action & Sites of Activity
Adenosine[33]	Promotes sleep transition from awake to NREM • Accumulates within active neurons of basal forebrain
Acetylcholine[42,43]	Promotes sleep transition from awake to REM • Projections from midbrain RAF to cortex through thalamus/hypothalamus to (a) induce cortical activation in REM and quiet rest via "wake/REM-on" cells, (b) induce REM activation of the PRF via "REM-on" neurons
γ-aminobutyric acid[49] (GABA)	Promotes sleep transitions in and out of REM • Reciprocal projections to and from "REM-off" and "REM-on" areas within the mesopontine tegmentum
Glutamine[49]	Promotes REM sleep behavior and cortical EEG correlates • Projections from "REM-on" area to descending medulla and spinal cord and to basal forebrain
Serotonin[43]	Promotes wakefulness by suppression of REM • Projections from dorsal raphe nuclei inhibitory to PRF and anterior hypothalamus via "REM-off" cells
Norepinepherine[43]	Promotes wakefulness by suppression of REM • Projections from locus ceruleus inhibitory to PRF and anterior hypothalamus via "REM-off" cells
Hypocretins[44] (Orexins 1,2)	Promotes wakefulness • With activation from the SCN, projections from the dorsolateral hypothalamus to basal forebrain, thalamus, locus ceruleus, dorsal raphe nucleus, and midbrain RAF are inhibited via *Hcrt1/Hcrt2* receptor-mediated inhibition of "REM-on" cells
Histamine[45]	Promotes wakefulness • Projections from the posterior hypothalamus throughout the cortex provide excitatory inputs

Notes: NREM = nonrapid eye movement, REM = rapid eye movement, RAF = reticular activating formation, PRF = pontine reticular formation, SCN = supra chiasmatic nucleus, *Hcrt1/Hcrt2* = hypocretin 1 and 2 receptors.

by serving as a key "wake-sleep flip-flop switching" area.[48,49] Specific brainstem sites within the mesopontine tegmentum additionally act as a "REM flip-flop switch."[50] The anterior hypothalamic region (ventrolateral preoptic nucleus [VPN]) is involved with the induction of sleep and the posterior region (tuberomammillary nucleus [TMN]) maintenance of wakefulness.[48,49] GABA(γ-aminobutyric acid)-ergic neurons are found throughout these areas within the hypothalamus such that those neurons locate within the VPN. These are important in the initiation of NREM sleep, and those found within the areas adjacent to the VPN promote REM sleep.[48,49] Each area in turn projects to midbrain serotonergic and noradrenergic nuclei thereby inhibiting REM-off cells and thus reinforce the process of sleep.[48,49] The TMN receives excitatory inputs from brainstem histaminergic neurons and from activated hypocretin receptors simultaneous with inhibitory inputs from these same populations of neurons projecting to the VPN.[48,49] These in sum bolster the maintenance of the wake state. The hypothalamic sleep switch can be on or off and the wake state (sleep-off switch) can be stabilized in position by the influence of circulating hypocretin.[46,48,49] The secretion and circulation of hypocretin is in turn influenced by the circadian and homeostatic rhythms. The REM-off region is found in the lateral pontine tegmentum (LPT), with the REM-on neurons found within the adjacent sublateral dorsal nucleus (SLD) of the pontine tegmentum.[50] There are reciprocal mutually inhibitory GABA(γ-aminobutyric acid)-ergic neurons projecting between the REM-off and adjacent REM-on areas. The REM-on area has two additional populations of glutaminergic cells, one projecting to the basal forebrain affecting EEG correlates of REM sleep and the other projecting to the medulla and spinal cord affecting atonia during REM sleep.[50] These additional cell populations modulating REM sleep allow for rapid, discrete, and independent changes in and out of REM with separate cortical/EEG and muscle affects. This dual switch arrangement for sleep-wake and REM off-on prevent entry into REM when awake. Conversely, reductions in excitatory hypocretin effect would allow slipping of both the wake-sleep switch and REM-off side of the REM flip-flop switch as in narcolepsy. This reduction in hypocretin effect could preferentially allow REM atonia without affect on sleep (cataplexy).[50]

A number of environmental factors will influence sleep.[34] An unfamiliar sleep surrounding will increase sleep latency and latency to REM with reduction of slow-wave and REM sleep amounts.[51] This effect is transient, however, with a gradual adaptation over several nights. There are also wide variations in individual sensitivity to the exposure of environmental noises.[52] The inherent relevance of the noise to the individual has a direct impact on its alerting effects. For example, a mother may be awakened readily with the soft cries of her infant yet undisturbed with other more noxious sounds such as thunder. Nonetheless, the effects of noise are measurable even in the absence of being recognized or remembered by the sleeper.[52] Several studies have demonstrated the effects of noise on sleep integrity. As a consequence, there is a quantifiable increase in the number of body movements, sleep-stage shifts, and awakenings identified.

All of these have resulted in subsequent greater daytime sleepiness.[52,53] Sleep position will likewise affect the quality of sleep realized. A polysomnographic study of healthy subjects who were studied while sleeping in chairs with varied degrees of upright seatback inclination from horizontal found that there were increased awakenings and reduced total sleep time.[54] In contrast, there appears to be no objective findings in support of any beneficial effect from different sleep surfaces on the quality of sleep.[55]

There is the potential of any drug that crosses the blood brain barrier to adversely affect the integrity of sleep. The effects of medications and drugs on sleep are dependent upon the degree and concentration to which the compound reaches the brain. Many compounds, but particularly those with direct impact upon the reduction, increase, or availability of those neurotransmitters involved with the sleep-wake cycle may affect specific sleep stages. Antidepressants, which act to increase serotonin and norepinephrine (e.g., selective serotonin reuptake inhibitors, tricyclic antidepressants, norepinephrine reuptake inhibitors, and monoamine oxidase inhibitors), will effectively suppress REM sleep.[56] Their abrupt withdrawal, conversely, will result in a rebound of excess REM and a propensity for REM-related sleep behaviors to emerge. This particular group of drugs, however, does not produce tolerance when used repeatedly over time. The development of drug tolerance can have an even greater impact upon rebound effects. The degree to which this is experienced is in part dependent upon the amount of drug consumed and duration of time that tolerance evolved. Many sedatives act to induce sleep onset and increase slow-wave sleep such as with barbiturates, alcohol, and benzodiazepines.[56,57] Tolerance does develop over time with repeated use of these drugs and thus their discontinuation may induce significant rebound insomnia much like discontinuation of psychostimulants will produce rebound sleepiness.[56,57]

As many of the features of normal sleep are tied to the orderly sequence of the robust physiological functions within the hypothalamus and integrated regions, so too are the childhood experiences of these processes. A vivid and universal experience of sleep is the perception of one's dreams. Although it has been and continues to be debated as to their meaning and purpose, the developmental evolution of dreams is established (Table 4-7).[58–60] There is an ever increasing recall frequency and content complexity recognized over the pediatric age continuum. Initial fragmentary and static images in preschool children develop into more cinematic and emotionally laden remembrances of early elementary school ages. This dream quality takes on a more lifelike situational and self-participatory content as children proceed into their second decade. At this time, dreams often reflect short scenes from the movies or television. Scenes that are frightening to the child are often avoided as these become increasingly better recognized as possibly causing a bad dream in a later sleep. As children enter into adolescence, peers and social interactions become a more dominant content theme. New theories have continued to relate the process of dreams and the sleep stages associated with them as an important

Table 4-7 Developmental Aspects of Childhood Dreams

Age (years)	Stage Awakened and % Recall	Length of Description	Content
0–2	REM	Limited	Uncertain
3–5	25% REM 10% NREM	Brief (14 words)	Lack emotion, static quality, describes animals and humans as animals, nonnarrative
6–7	50% REM 25% NREM	Moderate (50–70 words)	Emotional, cinematic quality, describes adult male strangers, being chased, ghosts, TV/cartoon characters, inability to move, some troubling, most wish to finish dream
8–10	60%–70% REM 20% NREM	Moderate–long	Emotional, cinematic quality, describes self participation in sports/school, and family emphasis, scenes from TV/movies, anticipates bad dreams
11–13	60%–70% REM 20% NREM	Moderate–long	Emotional, cinematic quality, peer focused with verbal interactions and less physical action, pleasant or strange experience
14–15	60%–80% REM 20% NREM	Moderate–long	Emotional, cinematic quality, peer focused with much symbolic activity, often recalled as confusing, searching for implied meaning

Source: Modified from References.[56–58]

time for cognitive processing and memory consolidation.[1–6] The possibility that dream states represent a biological defense mechanism to rehearse simulated life-threatening events or to reestablish equilibrium from a disruption of homeostasis have been forwarded.[61,62] In an investigation of the dream recall of 122 Kurdish children brought up in a military and traumatizing war environment compared to a non-military non-war-exposed group of Finnish children serving as controls, investigators found that the children exposed to real-life threats reported more dreams with more threats, more dangerous content, and incorporated more aggression than the control children.[62] Interestingly, these

Kurdish children did not react to the threat in their dreams more often than nontraumatized children.[62] These findings complement those of an investigation of another group of 190 nontraumatized children ages 4–12 years, where the percentages of children reporting fears, worries, and scary dreams were 75.8%, 67.4%, and 80.5%, respectively.[63] These were common in 4–6-year olds and increased in prominence at 7–9 years old, then declined thereafter. Younger children voiced anxiety about imaginary creatures whereas worry about test performance dominated the older age groups.[64] It has been suggested there may be a significant socialization effect to dream recall.[64] Dream recall as a learned behavior by children from their mothers was investigated and a positive correlation between frequency of dreams reported by mothers and their children found.[64] Whether dreams are solely for the benefit of the physiological functions occurring during sleep or potentially serve as a homeostasis achieving, anxiety reducing or a social integrating function remains under study. There are important caveats to their therapeutic interpretation, particularly in the latency aged child (6–11 years), which may require the child to further elaborate with drawing, story-telling, and play in order to make them more tangible and less traumatic.[65]

In summary, sleep is an essential and elegantly complex physiological occurrence in daily life. It is required, difficult to avoid, and dramatically effects the individual when it is insufficient, ineffective, or of inadequate quality. Similar to any precision timing instrument, there are many potential means to alter the mechanism, but different from precision instruments, the effect of human biological development and variation must be anticipated and accepted. The study and understanding of those variations of normal and divergences from normal are discussed in the following sections.

THE CLINICAL CONDITIONS AND TREATMENTS

Sleep-related disordered breathing could occur at any age. There is a natural and intrinsic immaturity of autonomic respiratory drive mechanisms, which may lead to a failure of respiration (central apnea) in preterm infants, which gradually declines by term gestation as these mechanisms develop. Other genetic and nongenetically determined disorders of respiratory drive will also become manifest in early childhood. These patients may present with daytime sleepiness or frequent nocturnal awakenings with resultant increased sleep fragmentation. Obstructive sleep apnea may have its beginning at any age. Although obesity and tonsilar hypertrophy are predisposing factors, oropharyngeal anatomic problems, an overly compliant rib cage, and pectus excavatum-producing paradoxical inward rib cage movement may also serve as risk factors in young children.[66] The presentation of obstructive sleep apnea is often with snoring or noisy breathing; however, not all children will arouse from sleep (Table 4-8). Early morning headache and behavioral disturbances may predominate the initial picture. Nonrespiratory pediatric sleep disorders

Table 4-8 Classification of Sleep Disorders with Paroxysmal Quality Seen in Children

II. *Sleep-Related Breathing Disorder*
Sleep apnea of infancy
Obstructive sleep apnea
Congenital central alveolar hypoventilation syndrome

III. *Hypersomnias of Central Origin*
Narcolepsy with or without cataplexy
Recurrent hypersomnia (Klein-Levin syndrome)

V. *Parasomnias*
Associated with Non-REM
    Confusional arousals
    Night terrors (pavor nocturnus)
    Sleepwalking (somnambulism)
Associated with REM sleep
    REM sleep behavior
    Sleep paralysis
    Nightmares
Other Parasomnias
    Enuresis
    Catathrenia
    Sleep-related Dissociative disorders
    Hypnogogic/Hypnopompic hallucinations
    Exploding head syndrome
    Sleep-related eating disorder
    Unspecified

VI. *Sleep-Related Movement Disorders*
Restless legs syndrome
Periodic limb movement
Leg cramps
Bruxism
Rhythmic movement disorder

VII. *Isolated Syndromes, Apparently Normal Variants and Unresolved Phenomenon*
Sleep-talking (somniloquy)
Sleep starts (hypnic jerks)
Benign sleep myoclonus of infancy

Other Considerations
Sleep disturbances with medical conditions
Sleep-related epilepsy
Binkie flutter
Hypnogogic paroxysmal dystonia
Benign familial nocturnal alternating hemiplegia of childhood

Source: Modified from References.[36,378,379]

are much more common (Table 4-9). Several population studies have identified prevalence rates for many specific sleep disorders and age groups.[14,36,67–72] Although the percentages vary slightly, trends have been constant across time. Sleep-onset resistance (behavioral insomnia of childhood) and night awakenings are much more a problem in children younger than 3 years.[73] The development of parasomnias such as rhythmic body movements, sleep terrors, and enuresis are most common in the 3- to 7-year old age group. Sleepwalking, bruxism, and nightmares emerge more frequently in latency age children and hypersomnias, circadian rhythm disturbances, cataplexy, and narcolepsy are identified most frequently in adolescence. These targeted age-predominant disorders are in part related to the natural maturation of the sleep cycle. A progressive lengthening of the NREM fraction of sleep and an increased number

Table 4-9 Prevalence of Selected Childhood Sleep Disorders with Paroxysmal Quality

Childhood Sleep Disorder	Repeatedly[14,36,67–72,222]	At Least Once[14,71,72,228]
Insomnia	6%–10%	
Sleep Resistance/Night Awakenings	10%–30%	30%–60%
Sleep-Related Breathing Disorder	<0.5% full term	2% full term
Sleep Apnea of Infancy	2%	
Obstructive Sleep Apnea	0.02%–0.18%	
Hypersomnias of Central Origin	1.3%–17%	17.7%–39.9%
Narcolepsy	1%–14.7%	14%–40%
Parasomnias	3.3%–17%	
Confusional Arousals	6%–15%	
Night Terrors (pavor nocturnus)	10%–50%	
Sleepwalking (somnambulism)	7%–15.4%–7-year olds	45.6%
Associated With REM Sleep	2.3%–3%–12-year olds	9.2%–28.1%
Sleep Paralysis		17.2%–31.7%
Nightmares	1%–2%–18-year olds	55.5%–84.4%
Enuresis	7%	
	9.3%–38%	
Sleep-Related Movements Disorder	17.2%–60%	
Leg Cramps	29.2%–55%	
Bruxism	60%–70%	
Rhythmic Movement Disorder		
Isolated Syndromes		
Sleep Talking (somniloquy)		
Sleep Starts (hypnic jerks)		

Source: Modified from References.[14,36,67–70,227,232,328,334]

of transitions between NREM and REM promote more awakening behavior and disordered arousals in preschool and schoolage children. Adolescents postpone their normal intrinsic drive for sleep in favor of other social and academic pursuits. This constant sleep rescheduling behavior causes enough irregularity that it engenders the development of circadian rhythm disorders.

The prevalence of sleep problems in primary school children appear to be different depending upon whether the population studied is from a mainstream or special education setting. There may be higher frequencies of dysomnias (inefficient, excessive, or insufficient sleep) such as settling and night waking problems, symptoms of obstructed sleep apnea (snoring, gagging, choking), and enuresis.[73] A number of these problems, particularly night awakening, can be correlated to concurrent medical conditions, maternal stress factors, and maternal responsiveness.[73] Clearly, children's quality of life will be expected to be impacted as a result, whether in special education settings or not. Surprisingly, few data on this topic exist. Most have been studies comparing children with sleep disordered breathing due to adenotonsillar hypertrophy to normative samples.[74–76] These parental reports have consistently observed decreased overall health, increased instances of bodily pain, general poorer physical functioning, and greater physical behavioral/emotional limitations, with improvements noted after adenotonsillectomy.[74–76] The only large-scale pediatric health-related quality of life survey report from a pediatric sleep disorders clinic comprised a sample of eighty caretakers of children 5–18 years old.[77] The instruments used were all validated and included the Health-Related Quality of Life (HRQOL), a widely used fifty-item parent report of children's physical, emotional, social, and functional well-being; the Child Health Questionnaire-Parent Form (CHQ-PF50), a fifty-item scale of children's physical and psychosocial health; and the Children's Sleep Habits Questionnaire (CSHQ), a forty-five-item rating scale of child sleep behaviors. Comparisons were made to the data derived from a normative sample. Caretakers of children with a sleep disorder reported poorer scores on the CHQ-PF50.[77] Importantly, however, scores on the HRQOL did not differ across diagnostic sleep groups. CSHQ scores were not associated with scores on the CHQ-PF50.[77] The results are important because a wide range of sleep diagnoses affect children's health-related quality of life, as reported by their parents. Furthermore, the effects do not simply impact upon physical health but rather across a broad range of functioning: emotional, social, and physical.

SLEEP-DISORDERED BREATHING

Primary Sleep Apnea of Infancy

This disorder has been identified by a host of alternative names including, apnea of prematurity, apparent life-threatening events (ALTE), idiopathic apnea, infant sleep apnea, and near-SIDS. This later terminology, near-SIDS, should be abandoned because there is no data in support of a relation-ship between apnea and SIDS.[78,79] Sleep apnea can be defined as central, obstructive, and mixed. Central apnea results from inadequate or immature respiratory drive. Obstructive apnea is due to airway collapse or glottic clo-sure in the presence of centrally stimulated respiratory efforts. Mixed patterns involve the combination of these two types. The clinical characterization of sleep apnea of infancy is of prolonged central, mixed, or obstructive apnea of sufficient duration to cause physiologic compromise (bradycardia, hypox-emia, cyanosis/pallor) or a need for intervention.[36] Apneic periods are often ≥ 20 seconds and without other predisposing cause. The underlying prob-lem is the developmentally immature brainstem respiratory control mecha-nism. Although concurrent medical conditions and treatments may also be predisposing or contributory factors, these may not be the primary causes. Physiologic disturbances in the respiratory drive centers, oversensitivity to reflex respiratory inhibition, and aberrant chemoreceptor and mechanorecep-tor reflex mechanisms may all or in part result in the production of apnea. Although nearly all preterm infants weighing less than 1000 grams will expe-rience apnea, the vast majority, 92% of preterm infants, have it resolved by 37 weeks, and by 40 weeks postconceptual age, 98% have it resolved. Most infants beyond 44–46 weeks postconception will be apnea free.[79,80] Those infants who continue to experience apnea at ages as late as 50 weeks postcon-ception are those who had been born at the most extreme premature ages and who often have additional problems such as bronchopulmonary dysplasia.[80] When apnea does not resolve beyond this age, then the exclusion of underly-ing medical conditions will generally need to be undertaken. This will involve evaluations for infectious causes, cardiac diseases, pulmonary causes, cen-tral nervous system structural lesions, neuromuscular conditions, anemia and metabolic disturbances, gastroesophageal reflux, thermal dysregulation, and iatrogenic conditions.[81] However, the diagnostic yield of extensive investiga-tions has been generally very poor. A recent review of over 3776 tests performed on 243 infants younger than 12 months of age admitted to a tertiary care cen-ter for apparent life-threatening events (ALTE) over a 3-year period found that 17.7% of tests were positive but only 5.9% contributed to the diagnosis.[82] In the absence of an important element in the history or finding on physical examination to direct investigations, some specific tests may have greater utility than others such as gastroesophageal reflux screening, chest radiograph, urine analysis and culture, pneumogram, brain imaging, and white blood count.[82] A contemporary meta-analysis of eight studies involving 646 subjects identi-fied 728 diagnoses in ALTE investigations, which found that metabolic studies in addition to a consideration of child abuse also be considered as part of an initial screening evaluation.[83] An important study concerning the effect of gastroesophageal reflux (GER) on the duration of apnea in premature infants found no evidence of a temporal relationship between the two.[84] In a study of 119 infants who were monitored with concurrent cardiorespiratory monitor-ing, O_2 saturation, and esophageal pH probe, there were 6255 episodes of GER recorded. Only 1% of GER episodes were associated with apnea ≥15 seconds, with no difference in apnea rate before, during, or after GER events.[84] Thus, although there are a number of potential associations with infantile apnea, the true cause of apnea may relate most often to an underlying immaturity of the respiratory drive mechanisms and not to an additional underlying etiology.

Bonkowsky and colleagues reviewed their experience of 1148 infants evaluated in their health care system for ALTE.[85] The study focused upon the longitudinal outcomes with an average length of follow-up for the study cohort of 5.1 years (range 2.6–7.6 years). An ALTE is defined by the perception of the observer. The commonly utilized definition was provided by the NIH Consensus Development Conference on infantile apnea and home monitoring from October of 1986, which defined an ALTE in a child less than 1 year of age as an episode that is "frightening to the observer and that is characterized by some combination of apnea . . . , color change . . . , marked change in muscle tone . . . , choking, or gagging . . . . The observer fears that the infant has died."[86] These same manifestations could be exhibited by a multitude of clinical phenomena recognized as abnormal infant behavior and evoke extreme observer anxiety. Of the 1148 initially screened subjects, there was a cohort of 471 subjects (22% premature infants) evaluated.[85]

Three main outcomes characterized were deaths, child abuse, and adverse neurological outcomes (chronic epilepsy and/or developmental delays). Only two subjects died, the first at 18 months and the second 5.5 years after the initial ALTE evaluation. Each had concurrent chronic epilepsy and static encephalopathy described as severe with chronic respiratory and bulbar insufficiency.[85] These are known risk factors for survival even in the absence of ALTE.[87]

Adverse neurological outcomes were identified in twenty-three (4.9%) of the cohort, which included chronic epilepsy in seventeen subjects.[85] Each of these subjects shared in common a family history of epilepsy. Approximately three-quarters of the cohort were diagnosed with epilepsy at the time of a second event, all within 1 month of initial presentation. It is important to acknowledge that a diagnosis of epilepsy is neither an imperative nor always possible at initial presentation. The institution of therapy after the first epileptic event does not appear to alter the prognosis for long-term seizure remission and natural history of epilepsy.[88,89] Despite the fact that many of these infants underwent inpatient neurological evaluation, few of these infants were prospectively identified as having either chronic epilepsy or an identifiable neurological cause for their presentation.

A more compelling finding of the study was that 11% (fifty-four subjects) were ultimately found to be victims of child abuse (physical or sexual abuse), either directly or via exposure within their environments.[85] Two subjects were diagnosed as victims of physical abuse during their initial evaluation and seventeen others were identified within 1 year.[1] Thus, there may still be value in CNS imaging even though it is a low yield procedure. A consideration for Munchausen by proxy abuse is an additional important consideration in this context and should be more seriously pursued if prior siblings have suffered a similar presentation or death.[90,91] When there is a high index of suspicion for potential child abuse, protective measures augmented by the utilization of diagnostic testing are warranted.

Infant apnea may combine an additional element of respiratory obstruction especially if the infant is allowed to sleep in the prone position. Safe sleep position for infants is in the supine position or on their sides. When a complete investigation of possible medical causes is indicated and these as well as body postural contributions have been excluded yet recurrent apnea persists, healthcare providers must be mindful of the possibility of Munchausen by proxy.[83,89,90] This should be suspected when repeated apneic episodes occur only in the presence of parents or primary caretakers, no recognizable cardiorespiratory abnormalities exist, resuscitation is begun only in the presence of parents, and a sibling has a similar illness history.[90]

The most commonly employed treatment strategies for infant apnea have included nasal continuous positive airway pressure (NCPAP), mechanical stimulation devices, the use of respiratory stimulant drugs (e.g., caffeine, theophylline, doxapram), and enhancement of CO_2 sensitivity with acetazolamide.[91–97] When compared to NCPAP the relative efficacy of methylxanthines in reducing central apneas is greater. There are studies, however, that demonstrate a reduction in cerebral blood flow with aminophylline use.[98] Each of the methylxanthines enhances inspiratory drive with a concomitant increase in ventilatory rate and tidal volume. Doxapram given as an intravenous infusion has been beneficial in cases where theophylline has been ineffective.[96] The use of acetazolamide in twelve infants with a median age of 42 weeks gestation has been demonstrated to improve respiratory patterns and basal oxygen saturation, and reduce central apneas when comparison polysomnograms were obtained pre- and post-treatment at 6 weeks.[97]

OBSTRUCTIVE SLEEP APNEA

Obstructive sleep apnea (OSA) is characterized by prolonged partial upper airway obstruction, intermittent complete or partial obstruction, or both prolonged and intermittent obstruction, which disrupts normal ventilation during sleep, normal sleep patterns, or both.[36] Infants and young children may have prolonged periods of partial obstruction leading to isolated hypercarbia or oxygen desaturation, or a combination of both (see Figure 4-2).[99–101] Older children present with a history of snoring or noisy breathing as seen in adults.[101,102] However, children do not typically manifest cortical arousals in response to these obstructions, which tend to occur during REM sleep, but rather some movement or autonomic arousals.[101,102] As a result, sleep architecture is usually preserved although numerous microarousals (apneas that result in arousals of extremely short duration) over a sleep period can result in significant sleep fragmentation.[101,102] There are few recognized definitions, however, which have resulted in the spectrum of childhood obstructive sleep disordered

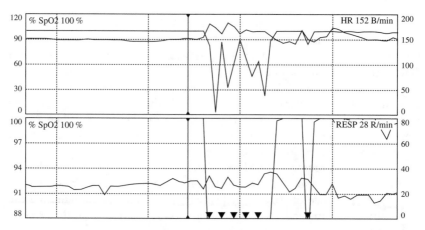

Figure 4-2. A panel from a multichannel vital function trend monitor during the recording of several obstructive apneic spells in a child with previously known typical breath-holding spells and reflex anoxic convulsions. The upper panel displays trends in concurrent % oxygen saturation and heart rates and the lower panel displays abdominal movements and thermistor respiratory rates. The vertical dotted lines demarcate 15 minute intervals. Six separate obstructive spells occur during the recording denoted by the black triangles along the bottom of the lower panel. Line A shows intermittent oxygen desaturation and concurrent increases in heart rate (line B) in upper panel. The correlated drops in thermistor-triggered respiratory rate to zero (triangles) are highlighted in the lower panel along with continued abdominal efforts (line C).

breathing (OSDB). This spectrum recognizes that in children, classical OSA merges with obstructive hypoventilation and may manifest as snoring with daytime symptoms. The new classification of sleep disorders has attempted to offer clearer definition.[36]

OSA may be due to airway collapse, glottic closure, or adenotonsillar hypertrophy in the presence of centrally stimulated respiratory efforts. The size of the tonsil and adenoidal tissue is not predictive of OSA in individual patients. In infants and young children snoring may not be prominent because of a relatively weak inspiratory force and thus paradoxical breathing may be a more obvious sign.[66] Unusual sleeping postures are important features to identify, although not typical. These include neck hyperextension and preference to sleep in a seated position. An important concept to emerge in recent years has been the realization that the diagnosis may be suspected when at least one of the following is observed: paradoxical rib cage motion during inspiration, frequent arousals, diaphoresis, neck extension, excessive daytime sleepiness, hyperactivity and aggressive behavior, slow growth rate, morning headaches, or secondary enuresis, in addition to a positive polysomnographic recording. Although OSDB can occur at any age, preschool children have the highest prevalence.

Certain predisposing features aside from adenotonsillar hypertrophy increase the risk for developing OSA. Craniofacial anatomic anomalies, orthodontic abnormalities, facial dysmorphisms associated with certain underlying genetic syndromes, obesity, and both central and peripheral causes of neuromuscular hypotonia and weakness all predispose to OSA.[102, 103] This is particularly true for children with neurological impairments such as cerebral palsy and neuromuscular diseases.[103] In this population, there is a substantial frequency, up to 75%, who experience recurrent gastroesophageal reflux with attendant aspiration and sleep apnea.[103–105] A familial predisposition also exists, although the mechanism may be mutifactorial, and includes body habitus, skeletal structure, and the heritable factors responsible for respiratory control mechanisms. There have also been several genes found responsible for the embryonic development of the respiratory centers and their interconnections. These include HOX paralogs and the HOX regulating genes, *Kreisler/mafB* and *Krox20*.[106] Furthermore, a number of brainstem structural abnormalities in isolation or in combination with underlying disease syndromes will further accentuate the potential for OSA.[107] As a corollary to these factors, it is important to recognize that OSA tends not to regress spontaneously. Therefore specific etiologic causes need to be defined in order to effectuate an appropriate intervention. Although most children will have anatomic upper airway narrowing, the addition of significant airway and pharyngeal hypotonia contribute additional elements. This contribution will be accentuated during different sleep stages in accordance with their physiological correlates (Tables 4-3 and 4-5). Recent studies of upper airway neuromotor tone in otherwise normal children have demonstrated that children have less collapsible upper airways when compared to adults when exposed to subatmospheric pressure.[108] This was due to greater neuromuscular activity resulting in greater airway patency.[108] However, children who are unable to compensate with increased upper airway neuromotor responses would be at greater risk for collapse and subsequent obstruction. With repeated significant OSA episodes over a long duration (months to years), the child will develop the physiological consequences: growth impairment, neurocognitive and behavioral effects (aggression, inattention, hyperactivity, poor school performance), poorer quality of life, enuresis, cardiovascular complications (cor pulmonale, pulmonary hypertension), and, rarely, seizures and asphyxial brain injury.[36, 101, 109–116] A recent meta-analysis of 66 studies which met inclusion criteria that investigated the relationship of sleep-disordered breathing and blood pressure, surprisingly found no evidence that moderate-to-severe sleep-disordered breathing increases the risk of elevated blood pressure.[117] Methodological issues may mitigate this finding despite individual studies holding a contrary view. Further study is called for. The exact relationship of childhood obesity and OSA may be complex. As noted previously, failure to thrive is a more common association with OSA, identified in as high as 27% in one study.[109] Childhood obesity itself may additionally predispose to OSA.[118] However, the converse may also be true, with OSA predisposing to hyperinsulinemia and relative insulin resistance, hyperlipidemia, and obesity.[119]

The question of who should undergo a sleep study may not always be entirely clear.[120] If reliance is placed on the presence of habitual sleep-related snoring as the key symptom to trigger evaluation, then about 10% (3%–21%) of the worldwide general population of children will be identi-fied.[102] Habitual sleep-related snoring is most often due to primary snoring, a benign disorder not associated with hypoxemia, hypercapnia, sleep dis-ruption, or other symptoms. The reliability to predict severe OSA based upon parental responses to scored sleep questionnaires has been demon-strated; however, these scoring schemas have not been able to identify milder but clinically significant OSA. Therefore, clinical evaluation alone is not sufficient to identify these children.[102, 120–123] Current guidelines from the American Academy of Pediatrics suggest that polysomnography remains the gold standard and that those children with habitual snoring and additional signs or symptoms of OSA should undergo investigation.[123] Complex and high-risk patients with craniofacial abnormalities, neuromuscular disorders, and suspected central hypoventilation should be further investigated.[123] The recognition of the so-called first night effect during polysomnography is an additional important phenomenon.[124] This is when there is a signif-icant (as high as 9%) false negative rate in identifying clinically signifi-cant OSA across age groups when only one night of recording is obtained in comparison to two.[124] The second night of recording may be needed when there is a suggestive history and supportive physical examination findings.

Treatment of OSA depends in part upon whether there exist potentially reversible or correctable causes such as obesity and adenotonsillar hypertrophy. For children who require surgical intervention, tonsillectomy or adenoidec-tomy is the primary intervention for most OSA, with demonstrated efficacy in children with cerebral palsy, Down's syndrome, and obesity.[125–128] Follow-up reassessment will be crucial in determining the effectiveness of any interven-tion utilized. Even in children where only adenotonsillar hypertrophy was the primary indication for surgery, there has been improvement in both symptoms and repeat sleep study parameters.[102, 126, 128, 129] There have been measurable improvements in growth rates in children with growth failure and in both cognitive and behavioral measures where these symptoms were adversely affected prior to treatment. Nonetheless, surgery may be accom-panied by postoperative mortality and morbidity, particularly in high-risk patients. These have been enumerated in the clinical practice guidelines of the American Academy of Pediatrics subcommittee on obstructive sleep apnea and include patients with (1) age younger than 3 years, (2) severe obstruc-tive sleep apnea on polysomnography, (3) cardiac complications, (4) failure to thrive, (5) obesity, (6) prior prematurity, (7) recent respiratory infection, (8) craniofacial anomalies, and (9) neuromuscular disorders.[118]

Continuous positive airway pressure (CPAP) is an effective intervention for a small minority of patients in whom surgery is unsuccessful or contraindicated. These are often children with significant obesity, craniofacial anomalies, bleeding disorders, or neuromuscular disorders.[129] Experience with and demonstrated efficacy from other treatment measures is limited in children. These include weight loss in obese patients, other craniofacial surgical approaches such as uvulopalatopharyngoplasty, mandibular distraction and tongue reduction, oral appliances and orthodontic repair, supplemental oxygen, topical nasal steroids and systemic glucocorticosteroids.[130–132] Tracheostomy is thought to be an effective but last resort intervention, most often utilized in patients with concurrent cerebral palsy or neuromuscular disorders.[130]

CONGENITAL CENTRAL ALVEOLAR HYPOVENTILATION SYNDROME

Congenital central alveolar hypoventilation syndrome (CCHS) is the intrinsic failure of the brainstem autonomic breathing control mechanisms. It is not explained by any underlying neurologic, metabolic, or pulmonary cause.[36] It is worse in sleep, evident at birth, and requires mechanical ventilation for episodes of hypoventilation (not usually apnea) characterized by hypoxemia and hypercapnia due to the absence of a ventilatory response to hypoxia and a negligible sensitivity to hypercarbia. The hypoventilation may be present in wakefulness but often not significant enough to require intervention. Similarly, some children are recognized later in childhood when presenting with ALTE, cyanosis, or cor pulmonale.

The genetic predisposition to central apnea is due to the lack of a CNS chemosensitive response to hypercapnia.[99, 133] In contrast to most sleep-related breathing disorders, hypoventilation and apnea is most marked during non-REM sleep but may happen in other stages of sleep as well as wakefulness. There is a lack of respiratory drive in the face of hypercapnia and hypoxia. The current hypothesis explains this failure on the basis of faulty brainstem integration of chemoreceptor inputs. However, recent evidence of cardiac and respiratory responses with ventilatory challenges to hypercarbia and hypoxia in a group of twelve pediatric subjects with CCHS compared to controls show that there is not a simple failure of either central or peripheral responsiveness.[134] CCHS subjects showed reduced rapid respiratory-related cardiac variation at baseline and after challenge, especially with hypercapnia but also hypoxia in contrast to controls. In response to hypoxia, CCHS subjects did not escalate breathing rate, whereas in response to hypercapnia there was a slow rise in respiratory rate as was seen in controls but much delayed.[134] These findings suggest a degree of sensitivity to hypoxia and some retention of an appropriate cardiovascular response. The major finding was that of a deficiency of the rapid integration of stimuli inputs as distinct from those voluntary and slower integrative components.[134] The culmination of recent work has resulted in at least one homeobox gene identified as causative, *PHOX2B*, on chromosome 4p12.[133,135] This gene encodes a highly conserved homeobox domain transcription factor with an early embryologic role in neuronal differentiation and a later suppressor effect upon neurogenesis inhibitors, thus allowing neurogenesis to proceed.[135] It is needed to allow several noradrenergic hydroxylase enzymes to be expressed and thus has a role in embryologic noradrenergic regulation.[135] The identified gene mutation results in an expansion of the *PHOX2B* allele. The degree of expansion has been correlated with the degree of respiratory deficit, associated symptoms, and age of onset.[135] Inheritance has been demonstrated to be autosomal dominant with reduced penetrance.

The degree of hypoventilation expressed varies individually in part due to the influence from efferent signals from the carotid and aortic peripheral chemoreceptors that maintain some extent of respiratory drive in less severely affected patients.[136–140] There is also a higher incidence of neural crest tumors (e.g., ganglioneuroblastoma, neuroblastoma, ganglioneuroma) in individuals with CCHS.[141] There is an additional widespread autonomic dysfunction (i.e., cardiovascular and blood pressure instability, thermoregulatory abnormalities, sweating disturbances, altered pupillary responses, and aberrant perceptions of pain and anxiety).[140–147] These clinical expressions are not always homogeneous across all children studied, but many individual autonomic function responses form a consistent pattern of deficit. Formal autonomic testing has demonstrated decreased heart rate beat-to-beat variability, increased ratios of low-frequency to high-frequency respiratory power spectra analysis, blunted heart rate response to exercise, constipation, and esophageal dysmotility.[140,147–149] The associated dysautonomia appears to be prominently associated with agenesis of the enteric plexus resulting in Hirschprung disease (16%) and has been referred to as Haddad syndrome.[145] These findings reflect an embryologic affliction of the neural crest. The majority of CCHS-associated neuroblastoma also occurs in combination with Hirsprung's disease.[141] More recent autonomic investigations of nineteen children with CCHS in comparison to thirty-one parents of these children and twenty-four child and fifteen adult controls demonstrated attenuated responses to sympathetic stimulation tests.[150]

There has been a recently published series of forty-five individuals with *PHOX2B*-confirmed CCHS and forty-five matched controls studied with facial digital photography and systematically analyzed for dysmorphologic features.[151] Results of findings on 104 specific measures identified 20 variables that were statistically significant, which were then further subjected to a stepwise logistic regression analysis to identify those features that best discriminated subjects from controls.[151] The results describe a facial appearance that is generally shorter and flatter, with a characteristic "box-shape" and an inferior deflection of the lateral segments of the vermillion borders to the upper lip.[151] Males seemed more strongly affected than females.[151]

Lifetime mechanical ventilatory support is required for sleep and often at other times. This may be accomplished with tracheostomy or facial mask in individual children. Passive lower extremity movement during non-REM sleep has been shown to improve alveolar ventilation perhaps by stimulating mechanoreceptor-afferent pathways.[152] Diaphragmatic pacing may be another treatment option in older children.[153] Cognition and long-term survival can be normal when effective ventilatory support is initiated early; however, there is an extreme heterogeneity to the degree of complicating medical and intellectual impairments.[154] Many children will require gastrostomy tubes for feeding and nutritional issues, educational support for learning disabilities, and experience treatment for associated epilepsy as a sequelae to intermittent hypoxemia.[154]

HYPERSOMNIAS OF CENTRAL ORIGIN

Narcolepsy is a lifelong neurological disorder characterized by excessive daytime sleepiness or brief attacks of sleepiness, and sudden loss of motor tone and muscle control (cataplexy). The cataplectic event, a loss of motor control, is provoked by strong positive emotion (laughter, surprise, pride), resulting in physical collapse.[36, 155] The symptoms may be less well expressed in young children but are more typically manifest by teenage years. The classic tetrad of symptoms expanded to include hypnogogic hallucinations and sleep paralysis with a subsequent suggestion of disturbed nocturnal sleep to be added for a pentad of symptoms of insufficient sleep.[156, 157] The current diagnostic criteria include the following: (1) a complaint of excessive daytime sleepiness occurring almost every day for at least 3 months, (2) a definite history of cataplexy, (3) the diagnosis of narcolepsy with cataplexy confirmed by nocturnal polysomnography, followed by an abnormal multiple sleep latency test (MSLT) of latency ≤ 8 minutes and two or more sleep onset REM periods (SOREMP) after sufficient nocturnal sleep the night prior to testing; alternatively, CSF hypocretin-1 levels $\leq 110 \, pg/mL$ or one-third of mean control values, and (4) hypersomnia not explained by another cause.[36] Narcolepsy without cataplexy can be diagnosed, however, the presence of low hypocretin-1 CSF levels may not be identified.

The exact prevalence of narcolepsy in children is difficult to accurately ascertain. Only about 4% (15) of 400 narcolepsy subjects seen at the Mayo Clinic over a span of 4 years (1957–1960) were younger than 15 years old.[158] Retrospective meta-analysis data on 235 adult subjects with narcolepsy from three studies described by Challamel and colleagues observed that 34% reported symptom onset prior to age 15 years and 16% prior to age 10 years and 4.5% prior to the age of 5 years.[159] Adult population studies have yielded prevalence rates of 0.02%–0.18% in the United States and Europe.[160–164] An Olmstead County, MN, community-based survey yielded a prevalence of 1.37 per 100,000 persons per year with other reports estimating 20–60 per 100,000 persons.[165] The adult population of Japan has been noted to have the highest prevalence, approaching 1 in 600.[166] These variances in epidemiology are in part related to the diagnostic criteria used and the application of current laboratory and neurophysiologic testing. Diagnosis under age 5 years is especially unusual but symptoms suggesting diagnosis at ages 6, 12, and 15 months of age with later confirmation have been reported.[166–169] A 2½-year-old has been reported with cataplexy and hypersomnolence identified at 6 months of age.[164]

Excessive daytime sleepiness can be the most disabling symptom in older children and adolescents. This can be appreciated by the perpetuation of frequent napping behavior, particularly when engaged in passive activities, such as watching television, listening in a classroom, or reading a book. Children are often perceived and described as if they were in a "fog." There may be individual daily fluctuations of sleepiness appreciated with difficulty in maintaining attention. The emergence of behavioral disturbances such as hyperactivity, aggression, irritability, and impulsivity may supersede the appearance of excessive sleepiness.[170] A recent cross-sectional survey of 4–18-year olds included forty-two children with narcolepsy, eighteen children with excessive daytime sleepiness of undetermined cause, and a comparison group of matched controls.[171] Each study group showed significant rates of behavioral problems and depression in comparison to controls.[171] Validated measures included use of the Behavior: Strengths and Difficulties Questionnaire, the Child Depression Inventory for mood assessment, and the fifty-item Child Health Questionnaire for quality of life assessment.[171] Neither subject group could be distinguished from one another, suggesting that excessive sleepiness may be the main cause of these difficulties.[171] Interestingly, although the duration of naps can be extended in children with narcolepsy, the degree of refreshment experienced is generally limited. The actual cumulative amount of sleep obtained is usually not extreme but rather it is the frequency of short sleeps that is excessive.[170, 172] The individuals natural circadian rhythm appears to be intact, however, such that despite the repeated brief sleep intrusions throughout the day, there remains a substantial period of continual and uninterrupted nocturnal sleep.[172]

Cataplexy is a unique and defining characteristic of narcolepsy noted in up to 80% of idiopathic childhood narcolepsy.[159, 173, 174] This symptom can be recognized even in prepubertal children under age 5 years as sudden "drops" and often interpreted as clumsiness.[173] Although the loss of muscle control most usually impacts all four limbs, with preferential effects noted in the legs, both segmental and focal expressions are noted. This can be apparent in the neck, mouth, eyelids, and even in the eyes, with a subjective experience of blurred vision during attacks, although extraocular muscles are not involved.[173] There is a preservation of consciousness with an occasional sense of choking and respiratory irregularity despite the absence of respiratory musculature involvement. This may be a function of abdominal muscular weakness. Subtle drooping of the eyelids, head, jaw, or mouth corners can easily be overlooked. The child can sometimes attempt to "hold it back," which may result in some evident twitching or jerking movements. The attacks may last only a few seconds to at most a few minutes with complete recovery and no residua. Rarely, prolonged repetitive episodes may last several minutes to hours and are described as *status cataplectus*.[36] The underlying pathophysiology incorporates the sudden intrusion of REM sleep into wakefulness with the associated muscle atonia of this stage of sleep exhibited (Table 4-3).[173,175,176] This is explained on the basis of a sudden inappropriate central inhibition of the monosynaptic H-reflex arc and of the multisynaptic tendon reflexes.[175,176] The resultant muscle atonia due to this H-reflex inhibition is only seen in REM sleep, emphasizing the relationship between the cataplectic attacks and the underlying REM sleep behavioral intrusion. The central brainstem regions responsible for the atonia of REM sleep and that of cataplexy may differ, however, with dorsal raphe neurons active in cataplexy and silent in REM sleep.[177] The emotion-activated cataplectic mechanism has been demonstrated by use of ^{99m}Tc-ECD brain SPECT in two adult subjects to incorporate the amygdala, cingulate gyrus, basal ganglia, and brainstem circuits.[177]

The additional symptoms experienced by children with narcolepsy include sleep paralysis, sleep-onset (hynogogic) and sleep-awakening (hypnopompic) hallucinations, and disturbed nocturnal sleep.[158,168,170,174,178,179] Sleep paralysis is experienced either upon entry into sleep or at the time of arousal out of sleep. This is a terrifying experience of complete immobility accompanied by an inability to speak, cry out, or breathe deeply. This occurrence is often accompanied by hallucinations that serve to intensify the anxiety. Hallucinations can be of both visual and auditory quality, and are experienced by 50%–60% of children.[158,168,170,178] The resultant reluctance to return to sleep is a natural and understandable consequence. These are again associated with a sudden entry into REM sleep from wakefulness or an arousal from REM sleep upon awakening. Disturbed nocturnal sleep may be significant and has been noted in approximately 65% of some childhood series.[158,178,179] This disturbance produces frequent night awakenings, which result in sleep fragmentation. Some authors have attributed this to frequent periodic limb movements, particularly during stages 1 and 2 of non-REM sleep but may also be independent of these.[179]

The diagnosis of narcolepsy can be established on clinical grounds when an unequivocal diagnosis of cataplexy is made by observation in the appropriate context of excessive daytime sleepiness.[36,174] Otherwise, ancillary sleep studies and laboratory will be needed to establish the diagnosis. Normative reference values for both nonrespiratory and respiratory sleep parameters in children have been reported and expanded upon.[32,36,180–183] These include some studies of home polysomnographic monitoring as well.[181] The combination of the nocturnal polysomnogram and the MSLT are the gold standards for the assessment of excessive daytime sleepiness. The goal of these investigations is to simply objectify the propensity of sleepy children to fall asleep faster during daytime than those who are not. The MSLT measures sleep latency over five

20-minute scheduled nap intervals 2 hours apart divided over a day. Narcolepsy can be identified when sleep latency (into stage 1) is 8 minutes or less and there are at least two SOREMP (onset within 15 minutes of sleep) during five naps. Debate exists as to the exact duration of sleep latency needed, however, as pre-pubertal children remain very alert during the day and sleep onset even within 12 minutes may be abnormally short.[173]

Human leukocyte antigen testing has been used as an adjunctive test for narcolepsy.[162,164,173,184] The class II antigens of the major histocompatability complex, HLA markers DR15 (formerly DR2), DQw6, and Dw2, have been found positive in a great majority (85%) of Caucasian and Japanese narcoleptic subjects.[162,164,173,184] The DNA-defined subtype of HLA DQ, the DQβ1-0602 gene located on the chromosome 6, is the best marker for narcolepsy overall. This is also identified within the African-American population, where DR15 is not, but it is neither sensitive nor diagnostic for the condition. Further-more, it is neither sufficient nor necessary for its development and therefore determining the HLA haplotypes in children suspected of having narcolepsy is usually not helpful.[173] There are subjects with definite narcolepsy without HLA DQβ1-0602 positivity; conversely, up to 35% of the general population who are positive do not have narcolepsy. Therefore, transmission of narcolepsy even within families is multifactorial and requires at least two genes, one of which is not related to the HLA marker.[184] In a phone survey conducted on 96 narcoleptic probands and 337 of their first-degree relatives compared to 6694 individuals from an unselected general population, investigators found that compared to controls, family members were at a 75-fold increased risk for narcolepsy.[185] Among the narcoleptic probands were childhood onset cataplexy 15.4%, sleep paralysis 8.3%, and hypnogogic hallucinations 22.2%. Twenty of the ninety-six probands had at least one family member with narcolepsy (20.8%) and when compared to the control population all proband family members had increased risks for dysomnias and parasomnias.[185]

The discovery of hypocretin peptides (hcrt-1, hcrt-2), identical to and previously called orexin peptides, is an important link in our understand-ing of the pathophysiology of narcolepsy. These peptides emanate from hypocretin-containing neurons within the dorsolateral hypothalamus that project widely throughout the cerebral cortex, basal forebrain, spinal cord, and brainstem regions.[44,186-189] They have some intrinsic involvement with the control of energy metabolism, neuroendocrine regulation, and in the genesis of narcolepsy/cataplexy.[164,186-189] This system of integrated hypocretin-containing neurons directly innervates and excites noradrenergic, dopamin-ergic, serotonergic, histaminergic, and cholinergic neurons in addition to modulating release of several neurotransmitters including glutamate.[186] At the core of its physiological function is the relationship of its release at ele-vated levels during wakefulness and REM sleep cycling down to be minimized during non-REM sleep. The role of CSF hypocretin measurement in the diagnosis of narcolepsy/cataplexy has been the subject of ongoing study.[190-193] The conclusion of this work definitively establishes hypocretin deficiency as a diagnostic entity.[190–193] From the largest investigative study (798 subjects), the measurement of CSF hypocretin-1 (<110 pg/mL) was useful as a diagnostic test (sensitivity 60%, specificity 98%, positive predictive value 94%, negative predictive value 84%; $n = 570$).[190] This measurement may be most valuable in cases of narcolepsy/cataplexy where the MSLT is equivocal.[190, 191] In a smaller series of 138 subjects (88 neurological controls, 35 narcolepsy, 11 other hypersomnias, 4 Klein-Levin syndrome), similar findings were reported with low CSF hypocretin-1 being highly specific (99.1%) and sensitive (88.5%) for narcolepsy with cataplexy. There exists a positive correlation between the degree of reduction of CSF hypocretin concentration and the severity of narcolepsy/cataplexy, where undetectable levels characterize a homogeneous group of patients with definite cataplexy, severe daytime sleepiness, and frequent SOREMP.[191] This has also been the case in two children reported separately and found to have undetectable levels and children (≤17 years old) included in the larger adult series.[192, 193] The role of hypocretin in other sleep disorders, particularly those characterized by excessive daytime sleepiness, awaits clarification. At this time, however, it appears to be quite specific for narcolepsy/cataplexy. From the previously mentioned studies, only 10 subjects from 570 in the sleep-disordered group and 30 subjects from 228 in the neurological disordered control group were identified with partial deficiencies of hypocretin with intermediate levels detected.[190] This later group included three children with secondary narcolepsy: a 7-year-old with congenital central hypoventilation syndrome, a 16-year-old with Prader-Willi syndrome, and a 14-year-old with Niemann-Pick type-C disease.[190] An important finding from these studies overall was the identification of sixty-five subjects with narcolepsy who had normal hypocretin-1 levels. These individuals tended to be younger and without cataplexy (26%), or with doubtful/atypical cataplexy (35%), and HLA negative (66%). This profile will bear importance for the more widespread application of the test.

The treatment of narcolepsy is aimed at the primary symptoms of excessive daytime sleepiness and the disabling cataplectic attacks (Table 4-10). The forgoing table is modified from that currently used for adolescents and adults in clinical practice at many sleep clinics.[173, 200] The use of stimulants has been a mainstay of treatment for daytime sleepiness; however, a number of common side effects may limit their tolerability in individual children.[195] The development of new agents for use in adults has cautious applicability in younger patients. The use of modafinil, a somnolytic, has been shown to be additionally effective although not as efficacious as amphetamines.[168, 191, 193] It does differ from amphetamines in its mechanism of action, has no intrinsic anti-cataplectic activity, and appears to be less effective in individuals who have had prior amphetamine exposure. Headaches can be an associated side effect, which necessitates a slow titration. The use of sodium oxybate for cataplexy rather than excessive daytime sleepiness has been gaining appeal in adult treatment centers.[173, 197, 198] There is limited published experience with this agent in children. A small series of 8 children 9–16 years

Table 4-10 Medication Treatment for Narcolepsy and Cataplexy

Excessive Daytime Sleepiness
Dextroamphetamine (2.5–40 mg/d)
Methamphetamine (5–40 mg/d)
Methylphenidate hydrochloride(5–60 mg/d)
Modafinil (100–400 mg/d)
Pemoline (37.5–112.5 mg/d)
Mazindol (4–8 mg/d)

*Anticataplexy with Hypnogogic/Hypnopompic Hallucinations and Sleep
Paralysis Effects*
Sodium oxybate (γ-hydroxybutarate) (3–9 g divided in two doses HS)
Clomipramine (25–75 mg/d)
Imipramine (25–100 mg/d)
Protryptyline (2.5–10 mg/d)
Viloxazine (50–200 mg/d)

*Additional Anticataplectics with some Hypnogogic/Hypnopompic Hallucinations
and Sleep Paralysis Effects*
Fluoxetine (20–60 mg/d)
Sertraline (25–100 mg/d)

Periodic Leg Movements
Clonazepam (0.5–1.0 mg HS)
Levodopa-carbidopa (25/100–50/200 HS)
Pramipexol (0.125–0.25 mg HS)

Source: Modified from References.[173, 194–197, 199, 200]
Notes: Mg/d = milligrams per day, HS = at hour of sleep.

of age showed that 7/8 (88%) had objective improvements in both narcoleptic and cataplectic symptoms.[199] The doses used were not described in
detail but one subject took 1.5 g twice nightly. Duration of treatment was
as long as 3–28 months with only three subjects taking the medication for
more than 10 months. Importantly, side effects were similar to that reported
in adults: tremor, insomnia, and an exacerbation (suicidal ideation) of an
underlying psychiatric disorder (oppositional disorder and anxiety) in one
subject.[199] There exists abuse potential with this agent as with the stimulants,
however.

Aside from medications, there are additional sleep hygiene approaches that
may help those with narcolepsy better cope.[198] These include structured nocturnal sleep of a consistent bedtime-duration-arising time, structured regularly
scheduled daytime naps, avoidance of irregular sleep-wake schedules, caution
driving with avoidance of prolonged drives, and counseling.

Lastly, the symptoms of narcolepsy (excessive daytime sleepiness,
hynogogic/hypnopompic hallucinations, sleep paralysis, SOREMP) and
cataplexy can be both a primary genetic condition, as discussed above, and secondary to another underlying cause or other sleep disorder (Table 4-11).[200–209]

Table 4-11 Differential Diagnosis for the Symptoms of Narcolepsy and Cataplexy

Excessive Daytime Sleepiness
Sleep-apnea syndrome
Periodic limb movement disorder
Insufficient sleep disorder
Circadian rhythm disorder
Idiopathic hypersomnias
Recurrent hypersomnias (e.g., Klein-Levin syndrome)
Concurrent sedating drug use/withdrawal from stimulant drug use
Psychiatric disease (e.g., depression)
Fatigue
Organic CNS diseases
    Hypothalamic/thalamic/amygdala region tumor or infarction/precocious
        puberty
    Encephalitis
    Metabolic encephalopathy
    Acute disseminated encephalomyelitis/anti-Ma2 encephalitis
    Closed head injury
    Multiple sclerosis
    CNS sarcoidosis
    Gliomatosis cerebrii
    Parkinson's disease
    CNS lymphoma
    Poliomyelitis
    Suprasellar prolactinoma
    s/p Hypoxic-ischemic encephalopathy
    s/p Surgical resection pituitary adenoma
    s/p Childhood CNS tumor therapy
    s/p CNS radiation to craniopharyngioma, prolactinoma, frontal lobe glioma,
        A.L.L.

Cataplexy
Niemann-Pick disease type C
Prader-Willi syndrome
Norrie disease
Coffin-Lowry syndrome
Autosomal-dominant cerebellar ataxia, deafness, narcolepsy syndrome
Diencephalic tumors
Stiff startle syndromes (hyperekplexia)
Periodic paralysis
Seizures

Hypnogogic/Hypnopompic Hallucinations
Isolated, sporadic events
In association with other sleep disorders
In association with parasomnias
In association with psychiatric disease (e.g., schizophrenia)
In association with peduncular hallucinosis

continued

Table 4-11 continued

Retinal and visual pathway disease
Metabolic encephalopathy
Psychoactive drug use

Sleep Paralysis
Isolated, sporadic events
In association with other sleep disorders
Familial

Source: Modified from References.[36, 164, 200–207]
Notes: s/p = status post, A.L.L. = acute lymphocytic leukemia.

These considerations should be kept in mind when evaluating patients who present with the classic symptoms of narcolepsy/cataplexy but in whom progressive symptoms develop or additional clinical signs and features become more prominent. This is particularly true for patients in whom excessive sleepiness is present in the absence of cataplexy. The recent identification of increased plasma tumor necrosis factor (sTNF-Rp75) suggests a functional alteration of the TNF-α cytokine system and a potential pathogenic role for the immune system in human narcolepsy.[210]

THE KLEIN-LEVIN SYNDROME

The Klein-Levin syndrome is the best characterized of the recurrent hypersomnia syndromes. It is, nonetheless, a rare and infrequently reported clinical entity that affects males more often than females in a ratio of approximately 4:1.[36, 211, 212] The clinical manifestations usually begin in the adolescent age group with recurrent episodes of profound sleepiness, which may last up to several weeks, punctuated by a number of behavioral and mood disturbances. The diagnosis is based upon (1) recurrent episodes of excessive sleepiness lasting 2 days to 4 weeks in duration; (2) recurrence at least once per year; (3) normal behavior, alertness, and cognition between attacks; and (4) the hypersomnia is not better explained by another sleep disorder, medical or neurological disease, mental disorder, medication use, or substance use disorder.[36] The appearance of hyperphagia and hypersexuality is not required for diagnosis. Irritability may be the main behavioral change observed.

   A typical episode may begin with an early prodromal period of mild headache and fatigue. A gradual onset of sleepiness is often observed, although more sudden initiation of sleepiness can also occur. Prolonged periods of sleep are interrupted by an abrupt change in personality, typically manifest by irritability. Hyperphagia or binge eating, acts of hypersexuality, and aggressive behavior are interrupted only by the need to return to sleep.[36, 211, 212] Patients are sometimes described as having a ruddy appearance with diaphoresis during the attacks.[213] The sleep periods may persist for up to 16–18 hours per day only to experience a reemergence to wakefulness and altered behavioral state. The children may describe a sense of unreality, visual and auditory hallucinations, and confusion. Attacks often terminate with a sense of lingering dysphoria, amnesia for the event, and a period of insomnia. Recurrent episodes have durations of 7–30 days and may persist periodically over a period of 4–5 years on average but can continue for up to 20 years. Rare familial cases have been reported. There is a single report of siblings (brother and sister) who experienced extremely prolonged attacks of up to 72–81 days.[214] There is a gradual reduction in symptom severity and frequency over time until termination. Menstruation may serve as a trigger in some girls.

The underlying cause of the syndrome is not known. Although many of the symptoms suggest a hypothalamic origin, neuroimaging have been normal and hypothalamic/pituitary function testing has failed to demonstrate consistent abnormalities.[215,216] Postmortem examinations in a few cases have likewise failed to identify consistent neuropathological findings aside from inflammatory microglia in various locations.[217–219] SPECT studies had demonstrated normal findings overall, with isolated findings of thalamic hypoperfusion in one subject and frontal and temporal lobe hypoperfusion in others, both during and between symptomatic periods.[198,220,221] However, recent studies carried out in seven subjects during asymptomatic periods and in five during symptomatic periods have revealed consistent hypoperfusion in the thalamus during symptomatic periods.[220] Additional hypoperfusion was demonstrated in the basal ganglia (4/5 subjects), and temporal, frontal, and occipital lobe cortices in (3/5 subjects) each.[220] Neuropsychological testing during symptomatic periods showed a marked reduction in verbal memory encoding associated with the temporal lobe hypoperfusion, which persisted some 6 years after resolution of the syndrome when retesting took place.[221] Sleep studies demonstrate SOREMPs and short latencies on MSLTs with slowed backgrounds on routine EEG tracings during attacks. Prolonged total sleep time, decreased sleep efficiency, and frequent awakenings from stage 2 sleep have been objectified as well.[222,223] Blood endocrinologic studies and CSF routine chemistry and neurotransmitter studies have been unremarkable, as have various cultures for viral, fungal, and bacterial causes. An autoimmune hypothesis has emerged from an extensive study of thirty unrelated subjects based upon their results combined with available data concerning the age of onset, commonly identified preceding infections triggering episodes, previously published neuropathological findings, and an association with the HLA DQB1*0201 allele.[224] There have been a few cases studied and found to have normal CSF hypocretin-1 measurements during asymptomatic periods. A single subject was found to have elevated levels, and another subject had a 50% decrease from measurements done when asymptomatic compared to when symptomatic.[192]

The treatment of Kleine-Levin syndrome is symptomatic. Various approaches have been tried, including stimulant drugs (amphetamines, methylphenidate), modafinil, lithium, carbamazepine, valproic acid, melatonin, and light therapy, all with individual responsiveness. No consistently and universally successful intervention has been identified as yet.[198, 219, 224–227] In the largest contemporary literature review on the topic, Arnulf and colleagues reviewed 186 reported cases in the literature.[219] From among seventy-five patients who were reported to have received some drug treatment, somnolence decreased with stimulants (amphetamines > others) in 40%; the use of neuroleptics and antidepressants were of limited overall benefit.[219] Only lithium had a high response rate for preventing relapses (41%). They were able to distinguish that primary Kleine-Levin syndrome (168/186 case reports) occurred mostly in men, lasted 8 years on average, and recurred every 3.5 months but was symptomatically more severe and lasted longer in women.[219]

The co-occurrence of Munchausen and Kleine-Levin syndromes has been reported in a woman who after presenting with acromegaly was initially treated for a pituitary tumor with extension into the hypothalamus by means of multiple transphenoidal resections.[228] The tumor later required bromocriptine and octreotide administration with radiation therapy, which resulted in temporal lobe necrosis. She later engaged in self-induced anemia and the triad of hypersomnia, hyperphagia, and hypersexuality. The authors could not exclude either the pituitary tumor or temporal lobe necrosis as contributing to her behavioral syndromes.[228]

PARASOMNIAS

The parasomnias are defined as unwanted behavioral events that happen during entry into sleep, during sleep, or upon arousal from sleep.[36] They encompass any number of abnormal behaviors, movements, perceptions, dreams, and autonomic functions that accompany sleep. Of the parasomnias categorized under Section 5, Parasomnias of the American Academy of Sleep Medicine, only REM sleep behavior disorder requires polysomnography for diagnosis.[36] In addition to the primary clinical characterization of the specific sleep behavior, each requires the absence of another medical or neurological or mental disorder, sleep disorder, medication use or substance use disorder to better explain the behavior. Therapeutic interventions are listed in Table 4-12.

This group of pathologic sleep events all share some common clinical features. The onset of the behavior typically occurs abruptly during the transition from the first NREM slow-wave (stages 3, 4) cycle into the next NREM slow-wave cycle and before the first REM (dream) sleep.[36] This is typically encountered 60–90 minutes into sleep. Their occurrence is when the child gets stuck in the transition between slow-wave or deep sleep and awakening. The child is observed to be in an apparently elevated state of arousal, unresponsive to and misperceiving the environment, with variable displays of autonomic activity and with a general amnesia for the event.[229, 230] Multiple events will recur at 60–90 minute intervals as the sleep cycles evolve, with the majority during the first third of a night's sleep when slow-wave sleep is most prominent

Table 4-12 Treatment Approach for Parasomnias

General Approaches
Education of parents regards the nature and physiologic causes of the events
Managing the safety of the child within their environment
Reinforcing a consistent bedtime routine and schedule
Eliminate caffeine-containing beverages

Confusional Arousals and Night Terrors
Scheduled awakening 15–30 minutes prior to anticipated arousal
Clonazepam (0.25–1.0 mg/hs) and other benzodiazepines
Lorazepam (0.5–2.0 mg/hs)
Melatonin (3–9 mg/30–60 minutes prior to hs)
Imipramine (25–100 mg/d)
L-5-hydroxytryptophan (2mg/kg/d)
? SSRIs

Sleepwalking
Scheduled awakening 15–30 minutes prior to anticipated arousal
Clonazepam (0.25–1.0 mg/hs) and other benzodiazepines
Imipramine (25–100 mg/d)
? SSRIs

REM Sleep Behavior
Clonazepam (0.25–1.0 mg/hs)
Melatonin (3–9 mg/30–60 minutes prior to hs)

Sleep Paralysis
Clonazepam (0.5–1.0 mg/hs)
Clomipramine (25–75 mg/d)
Imipramine (25–100 mg/d)
Protryptyline (2.5–10 mg/d)
Viloxazine (50–200 mg/d)

Nightmares
Withdrawal of potential causative drugs
Cognitive behavioral therapy for underlying stress & anxiety
Imagery therapy
Use of transitional objects

Enuresis
Enuresis alarm method with positive reinforcement
Desmopressin (20–40 mcg IN/hs: tablets 0.2–0.6 mg/hs)
Imipramine (0.9–1.5 mg/kg/d or 25–100 mg/d)
Oxybutynin (10 mg at dinner)

Catathrenia
? CPAP

Source: Modified from References.[199,248,258,260,269–271,274–279]
Notes: mg/hs = milligrams at hour of sleep, mg/kg/d = milligrams per kilogram per day,
mcg = micrograms, IN = intranasal, SSRIs = selective serotonin reuptake inhibitors,
CPAP = continuous positive airway pressure.

in children. The severities of the events lessen in subsequent recurrences over a single night. Each parasomnic event may last from 1 to 90 minutes in duration and the child returning to sleep marks its termination. In comparison, there have been few normative arousal data available for children across the age spectrum.[231] A recent series of sixty-two volunteer children and adolescents (age 5–16 years) on no medication and with no sleep or medical problems identified no significant age-related differences across the school age range in arousal frequency (mean 8.5–10.8 per night) or arousal durations (mean 10.5–11.8 seconds per arousal) with a single home polysomnographic recording.[231]

The prevalence estimates of the various parasomnias in children are given in Table 4-9. Confusional arousals are more generally observed in infants and toddlers and occur in an estimated prevalence of 1%–17%. They are reported in about 4.2% of adult population surveys with a peak incidence in the 15–24-year-old age range.[232] These are most often described as the child arising to a seated position, moaning for a brief period of time, and then returning to sleep. Some events can be characterized by an evolution from a simple confusion and moaning to an extreme degree of agitation and inconsolability. The children resist parents' attempts to comfort them and may at times appear combative. Their eyes may be open or closed and any attempts to intervene will be resisted. The event usually lasts 5–15 minutes before the child spontaneously returns to sleep. In older children there is a period of disorientation with slowed speech and delayed processing may be more evident. The child may appear sluggish with a blunted affect and simply stare through the parent or observer. At other times the child may be more energized with hyperkinetic behavior but little purpose or goal with a degree of agitation that defies being comforted. These arousals as well as the other parasomnias may be precipitated if the child is awakened out of sleep at the appropriate transition time. Predisposing factors may be recovery from recent insufficient sleep, stress, psychotropic medication, and genetic factors. Positive family histories for disorders of arousal are often present.

Night terrors (sleep terrors, pavor nocturnus) are a more dramatic disorder of arousal. These are much more frequent in early-school-age children with a peak at ages 5–7 years (range 4–12 years) and can be active for individual children into late adolescence and early adulthood but affecting only <1% of adults.[232, 233] Children experiencing these will suddenly arise and begin to scream and act out in a confused and crazed manner. Generally, children do not remain in bed but will get up and run or stamp about in an upset and agitated display. Careful observation will reveal autonomic changes consisting of diaphoresis, pupillary mydriasis, hyperventilation, and tachycardia. There is an intensity and sense of fear exhibited or expressed with an often sudden urge to bolt away. The events typically resolve with the child simply wanting to lie down and sleep. The events usually last a few minutes but may extend over 20–30 minutes.[234] Occasionally, attempts at awakening the child will promote increased intensity of the child's agitation and a more prolonged duration of the night terror.[235] The children generally have no recollection for the activity. Rarely, there is some fragmentary recall of a frightening dream but seldom with any detail. There is a common association with other concurrent parasomnias, sleep disordered breathing, and anxiety.[236–238] Children with an onset age of less than 3.5 years attained a peak frequency of at least one episode per week, whereas those children whose age of onset was between 3.5 and 7 years reached a peak frequency of 1–2 episodes per month.[233] The mean duration of the episodes was nearly 4 years in most children, but a positive history of parasomnias is correlated with a longer duration such that 50% of children terminate by 8 years old and 30% continue having events into adolescence.[233] In a polysomnographic study of 84 children (5 with night terrors, 79 with both night terrors and sleepwalking) compared to 36 controls, children with chronic parasomnias also had an additional sleep disorder (sleep disordered breathing, restless legs syndrome) in 61%.[239] A family history of parasomnias was noted in 29/84 (34.5%).[232] In a large survey in Quebec, Canada, parents of 1353 randomly selected children completed sleep questionnaires concerning their children and associated parasomnias between ages 3 and 13 years.[237] Concurrent parasomnias and underlying anxiety were identified in the same children with the later development of sleepwalking noted after prior confusional arousals in infancy had stopped in 36%.[237] A number of pharmacologic and nonpharmacologic interventions have been helpful in children (Table 4-12).

Sleepwalking (somnambulism) is the parasomnia most often identified in late childhood and early puberty, ages 11–12 years old.[239] Although a sudden burst of activity can be as subtle as the child's crawling in bed, or being found sleeping on the floor or in another part of the home, more complex behaviors such as opening a door and exiting the home, urinating in a closet or corner, climbing out of a window, or attempting to drive a motor vehicle can all be part of the sleepwalking spectrum.[240] The risk of injury is a real one with lacerations from breaking glass, trauma from falling, and hypothermia from outdoor exposure, all possible.[240, 241] The majority of children can be easily led back to their bed to sleep without resistance. They typically have no recall for the evening events just as is the case with the other disorders of arousal. The prevalence of sleepwalking in children has been estimated to be 3%–17% with persistence over 5 years in 33%. However, population studies have also identified that as many as 40% of surveyed children experience it once between the ages of 6 and 16 years.[239] The rate of familial sleepwalking also increases with the number of affected parents: 22% no parent, 45% one parent, 60% both parents affected.[36, 242] There has also been a strong genetic component suggested in population-based studies of twins with over 65% of somnambulists having some genetic component identified.[242] The occurrence of violent and paraphilic behaviors has been well established in adult somnambulists, particularly men.[242] This has not been a comorbid feature of childhood parasomnias, however. Clinical guidelines to assist in the determination of the putative role of a sleep disorder in the commission of a violent act have been suggested.[242]

Psychiatric comorbidities have been features of the adolescent with night terrors or sleepwalking in referred sleep clinic populations.[237,238] This has also been true in a community-based, nonreferred junior high school sample using a case-control study format. The study included twenty-one adolescents with parasomnias identified by self-report on a sleep questionnaire in comparison to thirty control adolescents in Taipei City, Taiwan.[242] All study subjects completed the Junior Eysenck Personality Inventory and underwent an audio-taped psychiatric interview using the Schedule for Affective Disorders and Schizophrenia for Children in addition to a standardized sleep and family history. Results demonstrated a high psychiatric comorbidity, especially anxiety, phobic disorders, and a greater tendency for suicidal ideation.[242] A list of potential interventions helpful in children is given in Table 4-12.

In contrast to the arousal parasomnias associated with transitions of NREM sleep cycles, those associated with REM sleep require polysomnographic confirmation. The physiologic disturbance underlying the behaviors of the REM behavior disorder (RBD) is inappropriate persistence of excessive or intermittent muscle activity during REM sleep as identified on EMG recording. Thus, rather than the normal muscle atonia anticipated during this sleep stage, there is the capacity for intermittent or excessive limb and trunk muscle activity resulting in unwanted and sleep disrupting movements. There must also be documented either abnormal REM sleep behaviors or injurious, potentially injurious, or disruptive behaviors by history. These are in addition to the absence of EEG epileptiform activity and no better alternative explanation.[36] The behaviors themselves occur during the experience of a dream and are often referred to as "the acting out of a dream." These actions most often include facial and limb movements such as punching, kicking, slapping, flailing, and grimacing. Vocalizations such as laughing, shouting, crying, and swearing are commonly identified. These are all accompanied by eye closure. However, in distinction to the arousal parasomnias, arising from bed and walking or running is extraordinarily unusual. There is a high likelihood of injury to oneself or bed partner because the individual's eyes remain closed with little attention to the surrounding environment during a sometimes severe and violent limb-thrashing episode. RBD is typically a disorder of middle-aged men and has been rarely described in adolescents.[243,244] Rarer still are isolated reports of RBD in young children as early as 11 months old.[245–247] There appears to be some association with underlying neurological disorders such as xeroderma pigmentosum, Tourette's syndrome, brainstem tumors, and other degenerative conditions in children as well as additional degenerative conditions in adults.[244–247] These later conditions are typically associated with a chronic form of the condition. Perhaps more importantly, this can also be an acute disorder precipitated by certain drugs (e.g., tricyclic antidepressants, SSRIs, benzodiazepines, or barbiturates).[248] It is also important to note that RBD may overlap with other parasomnias concurrently.

Sleep paralysis or isolated sleep paralysis is characterized by the absence of voluntary movement at the beginning (hypnogogic) or end (hypnopompic) of a sleep period in the absence of a diagnosis of narcolepsy.[36] The event happens with the individual completely aware and with preserved respiration. There is inability to speak or move over a period of seconds to minutes with complete recollection for the event. Hallucinations may be present during the event but not required for the diagnosis. It may be interrupted by applied sensory input, such as by touching or speaking to the individual.[249] Individuals may experience isolated events in a lifetime (15%–40% of general population samples worldwide) or several events per year.[249–251] These occur due to a sudden intrusion of REM sleep into wakefulness at sleep entry or exit. This may begin in childhood but has been typically identified in adolescence and adulthood, often peaking at 16–17 years of age.[249, 250] There may be additional risk factors that increase the likelihood of recurrences, including sleep deprivation, stress, and the use of anxiolytic medications. When the meaning of the event has been studied in different populations, the experience of sleep paralysis holds important transcultural significance by those who have experienced it. Those individuals who have experienced the phenomenon often express an intense spiritual experience.[252, 253]

Nightmare disorder is a much more common and compelling sleep occurrence in children than most any other phenomenon. This is defined as recurrent episodes of awakening from sleep with an intensely disturbing dream recall involving fear, anger, disgust, sadness, or other dysphoric emotions.[36] There must be full alertness upon awakening with full immediate recall of the dream experience and little mental confusion.[36] A hallmark of nightmares is the child's reluctance to return to sleep immediately after the episode and/or their occurrence during the second half of the usual sleep period.[36] The dream content typically involves some element of physical danger, the description of which is dependent upon the maturational age of the child (Table 4-7).[56–58] It is estimated that nightmares are experienced by 10%–50% of children aged 3–5 years old in sufficient severity to awaken their parents (Table 4-9). Nightmares are intrinsic to those individuals who are suffering from posttraumatic stress disorder (PTSD). They may develop within 3 months of the inciting traumatic experience and prior to the identification of PTSD.[62, 254, 255]

A number of drugs clearly have an impact upon the orderly progression of sleep and enhance the production of nightmares.[56, 256–258] These compounds have variable effects upon those neurotransmitters imminently associated with the sequential shifting of sleep stage transition and maintenance. Particularly sensitive to the production of nightmares are those compounds affecting concentrations of noradrenergic transmitters norepinephrine, serotonin, and dopamine, such as with tricyclic and selective serotonin reuptake inhibitor antidepressants, monoamine oxidase inhibitors, and anti-Parkinsonian agents.[56, 256–258] Similar effects are induced upon the abrupt withdrawal of REM-sleep suppressant drugs such as those within the classes of central-acting antihypertensive agents (alpha agonists), beta-blockers, antihistamines, sedative hypnotics (barbiturates, benzodiazepines, ethanol), ketamine, and others.[56, 256–258] Potential interventions would logically include the identification of the nightmare-inducing drugs and withdraw them if feasible. Cognitive behavioral therapy and imagery reversal therapy have proved useful as an adjunctive approach, particularly in the context of PTSD.[259, 260]

As an interesting side light to this discussion, Iranzo and colleagues undertook a systematic viewing of Disney films and were able to identify a broad range of sleep disorders, including nightmares, sleepwalking, sleep-related seizures, disruptive snoring, excessive daytime sleepiness, insomnia, and circadian rhythm sleep disorder in various cartoon characters.[261] Some of the most beloved Disney characters run the gambit of sleep-related symptomatology. As we move through the transition from wakefulness through each sleep cycle disturbance, clear examples of many recognizable entities can be identified. As a takeoff on the fact that many people suffer from not being able to fall asleep, at least two Disney characters experience this problem on film: Donald Duck (in *Early to Bed* and in *Drip Dippy Donald*) and Goofy (in *How to Sleep*). By analogy, excessive daytime sleepiness is portrayed by Sleepy (in *Snow White and the Seven Dwarfs*), Aurora (in *Sleeping Beauty*), and Archimedes, the owl (in *The Sword in the Stone*). There are many Disney characters that are depicted as snoring loudly during sleep. A few of the most prominent examples include Sleepy, Doc, Happy, Sneezy, and Dopey (in *Snow White and the Seven Dwarfs*); Humphrey the Grizzly Bear (in *Bearly Asleep*); and Gepetto (in *Pinocchio*). The symptoms of REM sleep behavior disorder, including twitching, body repositioning, and vocalizing, are exemplified in four Disney dogs, Bruno (in *Cinderella*), Trusty (in *Lady and the Tramp*), Chief (in *The Fox and the Hound*), and Pluto (in *Pluto's Judgment Day*). In several Disney films, nightmares are used as a tool to further the story line. The star of the Disney lineup, Mickey Mouse, is a prime example of our cartoon heroes affected by disturbing dreams, noted in *Mickey's Nightmare*, *The Mad Doctor*, and *Thru the Looking Glass*. Each nightmare experience allows the protagonist to experience a harrowing situation without real physical threat. In a similar vane, extreme danger can be danced around and taunted with by using sleepwalking as a ploy. This is portrayed by Pluto (in *The Sleepwalker*), Monte the Pelican (in *The Pelican and the Snipe*), and Donald Duck (in *Sleepy Time Donald*).[261] While the study revealed that the cartoonists consciously or unconsciously identified and portrayed several sleep disturbances in child-friendly media, the ease at which a child may identify with the expressed feelings of the characters opens a potential therapeutic window. For children who suffer from extreme nightmare disorder, the use of cartoon imagery to affect therapeutic benefit may be another theoretical mode of intervention. Drug therapy for the various parasomnias including nightmare disorder has been reviewed and a summary table presented[262] (Table 4-12).

Other parasomnias encountered in pediatric patients and not infrequently confused with epileptic events include enuresis, and a much less well-known and newly identified entity, catathrenia. **Enuresis** is the involuntary discharge of urine during sleep in a child older than 5 years.[36] It may be primary if occurring at least twice a week in a child not previously consistently dry through a night's sleep or secondary if previously the child had been consistently continent during sleep for a period of 6 months.[36] Secondary enuresis is more often associated with organic or psychological factors than primary enuresis.[263] However, in a recent study of 179 enuretic children who underwent a careful analysis of a number of elements in history, examination and urological studies revealed that only the presence of constipation distinguished the two.[264] Constipation was noted in 74.59% of primary enuretics compared to 57.54% of secondary enuretics.[264] This suggests that the mechanisms underlying each are similar. There is also an important association with concurrent obstructive sleep apnea with each.[265] The vast majority (80%) of children with primary enuresis wet only during sleep, 5% wet only during wakefulness, and 15% are enuretic during wakefulness and sleep.[262] The problem is a common one, with 7%–15.4% of 7-year-olds, 2.3%–3% of 12-year-olds, and 1%–2% of 18-year-olds having primary enuresis. There is an expected gradual decline in prevalence at about 14%–19% per year.[266] The exact mechanism of enuresis is not known, but because there is resolution spontaneously as children mature through childhood, a delay in the contemporaneous maturation of bladder mechanics and central nervous system bladder control function is likely. Factors impacting upon the delay in development of continence include the gradual but slower increase in bladder capacity, decreased nocturnal antidiuretic hormone secretion, more frequent spontaneous detrusor muscle contractions, and a reduced arousal response to bladder fullness.[267] There appear to be an element of genetic influence (autosomal dominant with decreased penetrance) as well as a behavioral component.[268] The purported genetic loci have been disputed, though.[268, 269]

Effective intervention strategies have consistently demonstrated that the enuresis alarm method results in a response rate approaching 80% with sustained effectiveness and lower relapse rates than with medications.[270] Most children relapse after stopping active drug treatment, whereas only half the children relapse after discontinuing alarm treatment.[270] The enuresis alarm method coupled with bladder training, behavioral modification, motivational techniques, and overlearning (giving extra fluids at bedtime after successfully becoming dry while using an alarm) can be the most gratifying.[270] Dry bed training has been shown to be ineffective without an alarm. A number of medications may also be utilized. A Cochrane review of available clinical trials revealed that treatment with most tricyclic antidepressant drugs (such as imipramine, amitriptyline, viloxazine, nortriptyline, clomipramine, and desipramine) was associated with a reduction of about one to two wet nights per week while on treatment compared with placebo.[271] Imipramine is the most-often-studied and prescribed agent. The use of desmopressin has had slightly higher reduction rates of two to three wet nights per week while on treatment when compared with placebo, but it is no longer advocated for treatment.[271] The evidence comparing desmopressin with various tricyclic antidepressants has been unreliable or conflicting. The use of combination medications has been less frequently employed and not clearly superior but may be beneficial for some children. Furthermore, adverse effects from some of these drugs can be significant in addition to their generally higher costs.[272] The reduction of bladder spasms in sleep with smooth muscle-inhibiting agents such as oxybutynin chloride can be effective for children with neurogenic bladders.

Catathrenia is defined clinically as a history of regularly occurring groaning or related monotonous vocalizations during sleep.[36] The polysomnographic recording of catathrenia reveals respiratory dysrhythmia predominantly or exclusively during REM sleep stage.[36] This dysrhythmia is a characteristic deep inspiration with a protracted expiration and an accompanying groaning or moaning sound. This is periodic in nature without a normal vocal speech differentiating from sleep-talking. It may be exhibited with the sleeping individual lying in any position not purely supine. There is a recurring bradypnea accompanying the respirations bearing similarity to sleep apnea, although no inspiratory distress is typically identified and it does not awaken the subject. The disorder has been predominantly identified and reported in adults, although in many of those reports there has been a prior history of the events since adolescence. In a summary of 27 reported patients, 10/27 (37%) had the onset of catathrenia before 18 years of age and 2 had an onset at 8 years old.[273] Another prior report of four patients had onset identified as young as 5 years old.[274] The main complication arising from the disorder seems to be the awakening of others in close proximity. The use of continuous positive airway pressure as a treatment has been suggested in some patients.[275]

Treatment approaches for most parasomnias, both those of NREM and REM sleep origin, have some general approaches applicable to each. Parents need to be educated as to the physiologic changes occurring during sleep that account for the physical changes they encounter with their child. This understanding will aid the parents in accepting and enforcing a regimented sleep routine and to be compliant with proposed drug regimens if warranted. The uses of nonprescription/nonpharmaceutical treatments coupled with behavioral interventions are important and in many instances the mainstay of therapy.[276–279]

The remaining pediatric parasomnia entities, sleep-related dissociative disorders, sleep-related hallucinations, exploding head syndrome, and sleep-related eating disorder are generally identified infrequently and most often in adolescence. The **sleep-related dissociative disorders** emerge during wakefulness at the transition into sleep or upon arousal from sleep. These episodes fulfill the DSM-IV criteria for dissociative disorder, which is a disruption in the normally integrated functions of consciousness, memory, identity, or perception of the environment.[280] These events are confirmed with polysomnographic evidence of wakefulness or by a compelling history if similar to those observed daytime dissociative behaviors not better explained by alternative neurological, medical, or sleep disorder.[36] During these sleep-related behaviors, patients can run, scream, display sexualized behaviors, or reenact previously endured abuse experiences. There is a corresponding daytime dissociative disorder with a typical prior history of physical or sexual abuse. The event may occur with the individual perceiving the actions as happening in a dream, the dissociative state. Concurrent nightmares, PTSD, and borderline personality, major mood, and anxiety disorders are common, as are prior suicidal attempts and self-mutilating behaviors.[36,281,282] The identification of prior childhood traumatic experiences is more likely in those individuals suffering with nightmares.[283]

Sleep-related hallucinations are primarily visual but may be auditory, tactile, or kinetic, and occur primarily at sleep onset (hypnogogic hallucinations) or upon awakening (hypnopompic hallucinations).[36] These are typically complex, vivid, and distorted images of people or animals. They are perceived when the individual is awake, may persist for several minutes, then resolve especially when ambient lighting is increased.[36] The hypnogogic hallucinations are more common (25%–37%) than hypnopompic events (7%–13%) and are reported in a number of disease states other than narcolepsy.[282,283] Anxiety may be a common predisposing factor.[36,282] Three mechanisms underlying complex visual hallucinations have been postulated by Manford and Andremann: (1) epileptic, caused by a direct irritative process acting on cortical centers integrating complex visual information, (2) visual pathway lesions, which cause defective visual input and visual processing or an abnormal cortical release phenomenon, and (3) brainstem lesions affecting ascending cholinergic and serotonergic pathways.[284] Although many hallucinatory experiences related to sleep are likely associated with the intrusion of REM sleep upon wakefulness, alterations in cholinergic and serotonergic pathways may alternatively play a role. These later functional brainstem pathway abnormalities, even in the absence of a structural lesion or underlying disease state, are often associated with disturbances of sleep and may produce defective modulation of thalamocortical connections leading to these release phenomenons.

The exploding head syndrome is a benign yet peculiar and frightening sleep experience. Despite its name, there is no associated head pain but rather the experience of a sudden, intense, painless, momentarily extreme perception of a loud noise, bang, or explosion within the head at the transition into sleep from wakefulness or upon awakening.[36,285] At times there may be an accompanying flash of bright light (10%).[284] There is an immediate arousal from sleep, occasionally with a jerk, and a lingering but transient sense of fright.[36] This has been usually thought of as a syndrome of middle-aged and older patients but may be an underlying phenomenon of younger persons' sleep disruptions as well. At least one report identifies onset at age 18 years.[286] The condition may happen rarely, sporadically, weekly, or multiple times per week.[284–287] The combination of exploding head syndrome with a brief period of sleep paralysis and then later evolving as an aura to migraine has been reported in a young adult.[286] The combination of exploding head syndrome in association with stabbing headaches in an elderly woman has also been noted.[287] The elderly woman had an elimination of exploding head symptoms with nifedipine treatment and no benefit to her stabbing headaches.[287]

The last sleep-related parasomnia to be discussed here is the **sleep-related eating disorder.** Sleep-related eating disorder is a clinical syndrome that combines characteristics of both eating and sleep disorders, is distinct from other daytime eating disorders, and is seen in both genders, with female predominance.[288] There are nocturnal partial arousals followed by food seeking and rapid ingestion of food. The episodes occur 2–3 hours into a typical sleep period, with the vast majority of patients arising to wakefulness out of NREM sleep.[36,288] Reports by patients of partial amnesia for the eating have been encountered, but this is not universal.[289,290] The patients often have a compulsive urge to awaken and eat, sometimes multiple times per nocturnal sleep. Recent sleep laboratory studies of these patients identify normal wakefulness and conversation during the eating episodes.[290] Polysomnographic studies have identified sleepwalking, somniloquy, restless legs syndrome, and periodic limb movements during sleep in these same patients.[290] These associations, coupled with the reported efficacy of dopaminergic medications and the compulsory food-seeking behaviors, have suggested possible dopaminergic dysfunction as pathogenic.[290] Although generally a disorder of adulthood, many patients in retrospect identify the onset in adolescence, with a few before age 10 years.[288,289]

SLEEP-RELATED MOVEMENT DISORDERS

Restless legs syndrome (RLS) and **periodic limb movements of sleep (PLMS)** are distinct clinical phenotypes that often overlap in the same individual and family. RLS is a sensorimotor phenomenon whereby an intensely uncomfortable sensation disturbs quiet wakeful rest necessitating movement of the legs for temporary relief. It occurs mainly at night while settling to sleep but also at quiet rest during the day. The accompanying dysesthesias and powerful urge to move the legs ultimately disrupts sleep and consequently overall well-being.[36,291] In children, the diagnosis requires both the prior elements and either the child relates this discomfort in his or her own words, or two of three additional features occur: a parent/sibling with RLS, an age-related sleep disturbance, or a polysomnographic-recorded PLM index of 5 or more movements per hour.[36]

Most patients (90%) with RLS also have coexistent PLMS, whereas the majority of patients with PLMS do not have waking symptoms of RLS. The prevalence of RLS in the general population is estimated at 5%–10%. There is also a strong familial pattern expressed, with over 50% of affected, particularly younger subjects (<45 years old), identifying other affected relatives.[36,289] Several genetic loci on multiple chromosomes (14q, 12q, 9p, 2q) have been linked to the presence of RLS in family and population studies.[291–293] These confirm the presence of genetic heterogeneity and the likelihood of susceptibility genes and variants for clinical expression.

In a U.S. population study of 16,202 adults (aged ≥18 years) using validated diagnostic questions to determine the presence, frequency, and severity of RLS correlated to health impact, using the Short Form-36 Health Survey (SF-36), symptoms were identified in 7.2% of respondents and had significant impact on sleep and quality of life in 2.7%.[291] European population studies show a similar prevalence. A cross-sectional telephone survey study using the Sleep-EVAL system performed in the United Kingdom, Germany, Italy, Portugal, and Spain of 18,980 subjects aged 15–100 years old found the prevalence of RLS to be 5.5% and PLMS, 3.9%.[291–294]

PLMS is an involuntary movement of the legs during sleep. The polysomnographic recording of PLMS is characterized by stereotyped, repetitive (in a sequence of four or more) movements of the legs lasting ≥0.5 seconds each at intervals greater than 5 seconds but less than 90 seconds, involving extension of the great toe, dorsiflexion of the ankle, and flexion of the knee and sometimes the hip.[36, 291] A diagnosis in children also requires a PLMS index of >5 per hour and a clinical sleep disturbance or complaint of daytime fatigue.[36] These movements may precede, coincide, or follow an arousal from sleep and are associated with transient elevations of systemic blood pressure.[295] In about one quarter of the movement instances, arousal is provoked, which cumulatively may result in a clinical sleep disturbance or daytime sleepiness.[36, 291] When this disruption in sleep is significant enough to cause symptoms, it is referred to as periodic leg movement disorder (PLMD).[36] PLMS has an estimated prevalence of 35% in adults over 60 years of age.[294] It may also be recognized in conjunction with REM sleep behavior disorder, sleep-related behavior disorder, narcolepsy, uremia and provoked by selective serotonin reuptake inhibitors, tricyclic antidepressants, lithium, and dopamine-receptor blocking agents.[36, 296, 297] The potential genetic patterns associated with PLMS are less well-studied and understood than RLS. Nonetheless, there may be similar genetic susceptibility genes operative here as well. A recent multinational population genetic study in distinct Icelandic and American cohorts of subjects with RLS and their families compared to controls identified a genetic variant on chromosome 6p that conferred the population with periodic limb movements with risk for RLS to be 50%. They found an association between the genetic variant and periodic limb movements in sleep without RLS (and the absence of such an association for RLS without periodic limb movements), which identifies a genetic determinant of periodic limb movements in sleep.[298]

Although these syndromes are mainly identified in adults, with increasing frequencies at older ages, children have become ever more recognized.[299–303] Nearly one-third of a sample of 138 adults with RLS identified symptoms beginning in childhood before the age of 10 years old and as young as 18 months.[301, 302] In a most recently concluded population survey conducted on over 10,000 volunteer families from the United States and the United Kingdom, Picchietti and colleagues used a nonvalidated questionnaire and diagnostic algorithm using current diagnostic criteria to estimate the prevalence of RLS in children.[303] Those data found definite RLS in 1.9% of 8- to 11-year-olds and 2% of 12- to 17-year-olds, with at least one biological parent reporting symptoms of RLS in >70% of the families.[303] The relationship of "growing pains" to RLS may be extrapolated as unrelated, because in most instances only 2.5% of 6661 surveyed individuals with growing pains met diagnostic criteria of RLS.[303] Descriptive terms used by children included "boo-boos," "spiders," "oowies," "tickles," "want to run," and "a lot of energy in my legs."[303] In an early study exploring the relationship between PLMS and ADHD as comorbid causes of sleep disruption and daytime inattention, Picchietti and colleagues questioned sixty-nine consecutive parents of children with ADHD about the symptoms of periodic limb movement disorder. Those children with positive responses (27/69) underwent all-night polysomnography. Eighteen children (aged 2–15 years) of the 27 (26% of the 69 children with ADHD) had 5 or more periodic leg movements in sleep per hour of sleep and had complaints of sleep disruption, thus fulfilling the criteria for periodic limb movement disorder.[299] They concluded that the sleep disruption associated with PLMS, RLS, and the motor restlessness of RLS while awake could contribute to the inattention and hyperactivity seen in a subgroup of ADHD-diagnosed children.[299] In a subsequent retrospective review of 129 children and adolescents who were found to have PLMS >5/hour of sleep, 65 had PLMS of 5–10/hour of sleep, 48 had PLMS of 10–25/hour of sleep, and 16 had PLMS >25/hour of sleep; 117 of the original 129 had ADHD.[299] There was no association of PLMS with concurrent stimulant treatment. Importantly, in only 25 (19%) of the 129 children did their parents note the movements.[300] This suggests that survey data and history alone may not be a sensitive enough indicator of an underlying problem.

The prior studies performed on children referred for sleep disturbances, however, and investigations into other comorbid medical diseases such as diabetes mellitus type 1 (a sample of 46 children, 50 siblings, and 76 parents undergoing a similar questionnaire study) failed to demonstrate any association with PLMS, although there has been a high prevalence of severe RLS and PLMD in samples of adult patients with uremia undergoing dialysis.[296,304,305] Nearly all RLS patients had severe PLMD, which resulted in poor sleep quality, insomnia complaints, depression, and emotional distress.[305] Similar associations have been identified in adult patients with iron deficiency, uremia, pregnancy, and polyneuropathy.[306] Furthermore, recent studies show that RLS may be associated also to type 2 diabetes mellitus and to multiple sclerosis.[306] Whether these findings will be applicable to pediatric populations awaits further study and confirmation.

Data obtained in a general pediatric setting concerning associations between hyperactivity and RLS and PLMS have shown positive correlations, however.[306,307] In a cross-sectional survey of two university-affiliated but community-based general pediatrics clinics, 866 children (469 boys), aged 2.0–13.9 years (mean 6.8 ± 3.2 years) were studied with a validated Pediatric Sleep Questionnaire and assessed for PLMS, restless legs, growing pains, and several other pertinent potential associations.[307] Parents also completed the Connors' Parent Rating Scale of inattention/hyperactivity. The authors found restless legs were reported in 17% of all subjects and hyperactivity in 13%. A significant correlation was found between those children with restless legs (18%) and hyperactivity scores compared to those (11%) without ($p < 0.5$). Results were similar for high PLMS and hyperactivity scores.[307] These associations retained significance after statistical adjustment for sleepiness, snoring, restless sleep in general, or stimulant use. The authors concluded that inattention and hyperactivity among general pediatric patients are associated with symptoms of PLMS and RLS.[307] Why these associations exist may be attributed to greater PLMS/RLS-related arousals, reduced REM sleep, and greater overall sleep fragmentation.[308]

The underlying pathophysiology of RLS and PLMS has yet to be clearly elucidated. Studies evaluating iron, ferritin, and transferrin in both serum and CSF in adult patients with RLS were initiated based on the identification that there was a relationship between low serum ferritin levels and severity of subjective and objective symptoms of RLS.[309] This prompted the hypothesis that iron deficiency in the CNS caused the symptoms of RLS as a result of dysfunction of the dopaminergic systems because iron is required in the metabolic generation of dopamine. Studies on CSF ferritin and iron transport, MRI iron imaging, and neuropathological material have now indicated that there is low brain iron concentration caused by a dysfunction of iron transport from serum to CNS in patients with idiopathic RLS.[309–312] Early metabolic imaging studies using [F18]fluorodeoxyglucose (FDG) positron emission tomography (PET) in six patients with RLS and four of these same patients with [F18]fluorodopa (FDOPA) PET compared with those from age-matched healthy control subjects showed no significant differences between the two groups for any regional blood flow values derived from the FDG scans or for any binding constants derived from the FDOPA scans.[313] However, more recent studies in sixteen RLS patients naive to dopaminergic drugs and sixteen matched control subjects examined with PET [^{11}C]raclopride and [^{11}C]FLB 457 used to estimate D2-receptor availability in striatum and extra-striatal regions, respectively, have shown that in striatum, patients had significantly higher [^{11}C]raclopride-binding potential values than controls.[314] In extra-striatal regions, and in subregions of thalamus and the anterior cingulate cortex, [^{11}C]FLB 457 binding potential was also higher in patients than controls.[314] This may correspond to higher receptor densities or lower levels of endogenous dopamine. These brain regions are involved with the regulation of affect, motivation, and sensory processing and may help to explain the behavioral consequences of the syndrome.[314]

The data concerning pathophysiology of RLS have helped further treatment interventions. Dopaminergic agents such as carbidopa/levodopa, pramipexole, ropinirole, transdermal rotigotine, pergolide, and cabergoline all show clear evidence for efficacy in short-term treatment.[315] Multivalvular heart disease and pleuropulmonary fibrosis can be worrisome consequences of ergot-derived dopaminergic agents that need periodic assessment. Gabapentin and the supplementation of iron in iron deficiency states (ferritin levels <50 mcg/L) have also been shown helpful in adults.[315] Exercise programs and caffeine restriction may also be beneficial.[316]

Seven children with RLS/PLMS and ADHD were studied for the long-term effects of monotherapy with levodopa or the dopamine agonist pergolide.[317] Behavioral, motor/sensory, and cognitive variables were investigated. Five of the seven children had previously been treated with stimulants that had either been determined to be ineffective or to have intolerable side effects. Dopaminergic therapy improved the symptoms of RLS and reduced both the number of PLMS per hour of sleep ($p = 0.018$) and associated arousals ($p = 0.042$) for the entire group.[317] After treatment, three children no longer met the criteria for ADHD, three reverted to normal on the Test of Variable Attention, and all seven had improvement in ADHD symptoms as measured by the Connors parent rating scale ($p < 0.04$), the Child Behavior Checklist ($p < 0.05$) and visual memory scores on the Wide Range Assessment of Memory and Learning ($p < 0.001$).[317] Five children were continued on dopaminergic therapy for 3 years with good response.[317] Whether the improvements seen in both RLS/PLMS and ADHD were the result of improved sleep alone or due to an improvement in a shared dopaminergic deficit is unknown. Elemental iron (3 mg/kg/d) over 3 months has been shown to improve symptoms of PLMS in children as well.[318]

Sleep-related leg cramps are a common complaint of all ages, which increases in prevalence with older ages.[319–321] The prevalence approaches 70% in adults older than 50 years of age.[319] In a large ambulatory survey of 2527 children ages 3–18 years old, complaints of leg cramps were only noted after age 8 years with an overall prevalence of 7.3%.[322] Over 70% of the children experienced them in only sleep and 12% had them during wakefulness and sleep.[322] Here too, an increasing frequency of this complaint was noted at successive ages. Sleep-related or nocturnal leg cramps are the most common form of cramps. In individual children a frequency of once per week was reported in 4.3%, and as many as 81.6% reported having them occur up to 1–4 times per year.[322] In a survey of college students in physical training classes, 115/121 (95%) reported having experienced cramps at least once and 16% having had sleep-related cramps severe enough to awaken them from sleep twice per month.[323]

The cramp is a spontaneous, painful contraction of skeletal muscle, which requires voluntary stretching against the contraction itself for relief. This fact allows distinction from dystonias where co-contracting agonist and antagonist muscles are not relieved by this simple stretching maneuver. Sleep is disrupted because of the pain associated with them, which is probably secondary to accumulated metabolites associated with regional ischemia during the contraction. Neurophysiologic studies have identified the spontaneous discharge of anterior horn cells, which result in motor discharges at high rates at high frequencies (300 Hz) during the contraction.[323,324] These are clearly different from PLMS/RLS in that there is visible, palpable, and prominent muscle tightness. The gastrocnemius muscle is the most common muscle involved but the plantar flexors and digital extensors may also occasionally be involved. Most often these are unilateral at onset (98%) and have durations of 1–2 minutes but may persist longer.[322] About one-third of children have residual tenderness in the muscle for 30–40 minutes (range: 2 minutes to 1 day) after the cramp relaxes and the remainder have none.[322] In the vast majority of children who experience sleep-related cramps, there is an idiopathic etiology and thus laboratory investigations are typically not needed. Inadequate stretching has been a prevailing yet unproved theory on causality. The most pertinent elements of history involve the identification of iron deficiency anemia, renal disease, and medications used.[319,321] A primary intervention includes passive muscle stretching.[316] There have been no clinical treatment trials in children, although there is data in adults to support the efficacy of quinine to provide preventative relief.[325] Other interventions are based largely upon anecdote and published clinical experience.

Sleep bruxism, or teeth grinding, consists of grinding and clenching of the teeth during sleep, which is often associated with sleep arousals.[36] It results in abnormal tooth wear, jaw muscle pain or fatigue upon awakening, and masseter muscle hypertrophy upon voluntary forceful jaw clenching.[36] This may occur in a single prolonged tonic contraction of jaw clenching or in a series of brief (250 ms) rhythmic masseter muscle contractions, also known as rhythmic masticatory muscle activity (RMMA). When the muscle contractions are forceful, a grinding sound is produced, which may disrupt sleep of both the subject and others in close proximity. This can be identified in both healthy children as well in children with neurocognitive disabilities. Facio-mandibular myoclonus, a form of sleep-related dyskinesia, is distinct from bruxism in that it is briefer (15 ms) and involves more facial muscles, the orbicularis oculi and oris in addition to the masseters.[326] Both may coexist in the same child. Polysomnography with masseter muscle EMG monitoring can identify the muscle contractions that must occur in a frequency of at least four episodes per hour or twenty-five individual muscle bursts per hour with at least two audible grinding episodes for diagnosis.[326] The EMG pattern may demonstrate rhythmic or more sustained (1 Hz) bursts of masticatory potentials. Bruxism may be present in any sleep stage but is most predominant in stages 1 and 2 of NREM sleep.[327]

Sleep-related bruxism has its highest prevalence in childhood (17%–38%), with a gradually declining prevalence into later adulthood (3%).[36,328] The mean age of onset has been about 10.5 years old.[329] There is a strong familial influence with up to 20%–50% of subjects having first-degree relatives with bruxism. Studies of bruxism in monozygotic (MZ) and dizygotic (DZ) twins have shown a discordant side of preference in MZ twin pairs compared to DZ twin pairs, suggesting a "mirror-image" effect.[330] In children there has been an association noted with habitual snoring but no relationship to gastroesophageal reflux when concomitant pH-probe and polysomnography have been performed.[327] Sleep architecture remains normal when compared to controls, but there is a higher arousal index. This disruption in sleep has been suggested as the cause of an additional association with attention and behavioral problems.[231,327] One survey of 152 children (77 with bruxism, 75 controls) from a private pediatric dental practice assessed for the coexistence of other parasomnias in concert with bruxism. Results from a stepwise logistic regression analysis of the Children's Sleep Behavior Scale, The Pediatric Questionnaire, Teeth Grinding Questionnaire, and Standardized Questionnaire found several night-time behaviors and physical conditions that occurred in association with bruxism: nocturnal leg cramps, enuresis, drooling in sleep, sleep-talking, and colic.[332] Investigators have found anxiety, stress, and teeth anomalies to be provocative.[329] In a case control study of 86 children (43 bruxers, 43 controls) recruited from a dental practice, ages 1–7 years old, scored assessments of dental wear were compiled with results from an anxiety scale reported by their parents. Seventy-two percent of children with bruxism compared to 12% of controls had significant anxiety scores with an odds ratio revealing that bruxers had a sixteen times greater probability to be anxious.[329] Other sleep-related rhythmic movements and sleep-disordered breathing may also be found simultaneously with bruxism.

The main daytime symptoms of sleep bruxism may include dental wear of the crowns of the teeth, jaw pain, craniofacial pain, headaches, painful loosened teeth, and gum bleeding. Inattention and behavioral problems may be exacerbated if significant sleep disruption occurs.[329] The main interventions have been the management of dental complications. Clearly, reducing potential stressful provocative factors may be helpful, but there does not appear to be effective means to eliminate the bruxism itself. Protection of the teeth and minimizing the pain and headache complications can be accomplished to some degree with mouth guards. If other concurrent sleep-related disorders (e.g., sleep-disordered breathing and habitual snoring) are present, then specific management of these other disorders will be additionally beneficial.[333]

Sleep-related rhythmic movement disorder (RMD) is characterized by repetitive, stereotyped, and rhythmic motor behaviors of large muscle groups during drowsiness and sleep. The criteria of a disorder is met when one of the following is also satisfied: (1) there is an interference with normal sleep, (2) they result in an impairment of daytime function, (3) the behavior results in self-inflicted bodily injury that requires treatment or would otherwise result in injury had no preventative interventions been taken.[36] The movements may involve the head and neck, trunk, and/or limbs in combination or in isolation. The movements may persist through sleep stage transitions, most often from wakefulness into sleep. The most common behaviors include head banging into a pillow or headboard (jactacio capitis nocturna), body rocking (jactacio corporis nocturna), leg kicking or slamming, foot wagging, and head rolling side-to-side while supine.[36,334] Many children engage in humming or groaning at the same time the motor movements are active. These have been typically in a rhythm of 0.5–2-Hz frequencies with duration from 4 minutes to about

15–20 minutes at each event.[335] These behaviors are quite common in infants and young children, with population prevalence rates of up to 60% in infancy, which declines thereafter to 6% in early childhood and 3% by early teenage years.[336,337] It is rare for RMD to persist into adulthood or be acquired after early childhood. Similarly, the type of movement noted in infancy is that of body rocking, with head banging and head rolling behaviors more common in preschool children.[336] The behavior is identified predominantly in normal healthy children; however, children with developmental disabilities may demonstrate these as well. It has been hypothesized that there exists a central motor pattern generator, which may play a role in the genesis of and during motor phenomena such as parasomnias and epileptic seizures, and in the occurrence of RMD in both normal and disabled children.[338] There is little evidence to associate RMD to anxiety or stress.

Polysomnographic studies of children engaging in RMD have demonstrated the occurrence primarily during wake-sleep transition; however there are children who manifest the motor behaviors in REM sleep as well. In a review of 33 published polysomnographically studied cases, Kohyama and colleagues noted that 8/33 (24%) experienced RMD exclusively in REM sleep, 15/33 (46%) had no episodes in REM sleep, and the remaining 10/33 (30%) had them in both REM and NREM sleep.[339] This and other studies have noted stages 1 and 2 sleep to be the most common stages for RMD to appear.[335,339]

Serious injury from RMD has been the exception. Rare and isolated accounts of skull, soft tissue, and eye injury along with carotid dissection, subdural hematoma, and occipital gray matter tissue loss in an adult have been reported.[340–346] Treatment would rarely appear to be necessary as most children experience spontaneous remission by school age. Occasional need for protection against injury must be employed. The use of antihistamines, benzodiazepines, SSRIs, and carbamazepine has anecdotal and variable degrees of success reported.

ISOLATED SYNDROMES

Sleep-talking or somniloquy is a highly prevalent benign sleep behavior of childhood. It is a nocturnal vocalization of varying degrees of comprehensibility, with occasional bursts of words, phrases, and sounds. It is a self-limited disorder that has its greatest impact upon other family members in that sleep disruption affects others and not the sleep-talkers themselves.[36,336] It may arise during any stage of sleep (NREM or REM) and is commonly associated with other parasomnias, sleep-related eating disorder, and sleepwalking.[36,336] Studies have identified it in more than 50% of school-age children, with a reduction in prevalence into adulthood, although the exact prevalence in adults is not known.[36] There appears also to be a genetic predisposition to sleep-talking, with the parents of sleep-talkers commonly engaging in both sleep-talking and sleepwalking themselves.[347] A large cohort study of twins in Finland provided questionnaire data from 1298 monozygotic and 2419 dizygotic twin pairs aged 33–60 years.[348] Structural equation modeling was used to estimate genetic and environmental components of variance in the liability to sleep-talk, and registry data on hospitalizations and use of antipsychotic medications were compiled to assess psychiatric comorbidity.[348] The occurrence of child-hood and adult sleep-talking was highly correlated. The liability to sleep-talk attributed to genetic influences in childhood was 54% (95% CI, 44%–62%) in males and 51% (43%–58%) in females.[348] An association with psychiatric comorbidity was found only for adult sleep-talkers, and it was highest in those adults with adult-onset sleep-talking.

Sleep starts, or hypnic jerks (hypnogogic jerks), are another benign sleep phenomenon in childhood. They are in fact a universal component of the process of falling asleep. Sleep starts occur in the transition from wakefulness into sleep and result in the sudden, single (occasionally multiple in succession), and simultaneous contractions of segments of body musculature.[36, 349] These can be commonly identified as a sudden head and neck jolt or upper body and arm jerk as the child begins to fall asleep. Their frequency may escalate with prior physical activity, stress, or caffeine ingestion. There may be the perception of falling or other hallucinatory sensation often associated with them.[350] However, these rarely interfere with sleep but can frequently be misinterpreted as seizures, particularly in neurologically impaired children.[351] Sleep starts bear resemblance to but are differentiated from proprioceptive myoclonus, which are movements that arise in axial muscles (trunk, neck, abdomen) from a trigger postulated to be a spinal generator. This spinal facilitation, character-istic of the wake-sleep transition, undergoes slow sequential multisegmental propriospinal propagation caudally and rostrally resulting in the sequential myoclonic movements observed. This disorder results in insomnia because the phenomenon is produced in quiet rest.[352]

Benign myoclonus of infancy (benign neonatal sleep myoclonus) is char-acterized by a series of repetitive myoclonic jerks during early sleep onset in infants within the first few days of life to several months old.[36] These can be variable in distribution and vigor. They may involve multiple body segments at different times, with clusters of jerks (40–300 ms each), either isolated or in a series of 4–6 jerks per cluster.[353–357] The clusters may repeat in irregular inter-vals for 3–15 minutes on average but as long as 60 minutes as an exception. The majority of jerks encompass the limbs (50%), with arms more often than legs, whole body (30%), or the proximal trunk muscles (20%).[357, 358] These are unassociated with disruption of sleep or arousals. Awakening the infant pro-duces cessation of the jerks.[358] Restraint will not impede their appearance. They are unaccompanied by any abnormality on concurrent EEG recording.[353–358] Employing a simple and gentle rocking maneuver in supine position while the infant is asleep will provoke them at low frequency until a typical series is entrained.[359] The major importance recognizing these is the benign and self-limited nature of the phenomenon. The majority of infants will experience resolution by 6 months of life.[359]

OTHER CONSIDERATIONS

An unusual movement unique to infants is the so-called binkie-flutter.[360] This is observed as a rapid fine tremor of the pacifier when the infant is pausing from the more vigorous sucking motion. There is an accompanying puckering of the lips during the flutter and an irregular pause from all motion. This usually occurs as the infant is wakeful and sucking peacefully. The sequence may repeat itself (vigorous sucking-pause-flutter-pause) several times as the infant drifts into sleep. The flutter is distinguished from the slow 2 Hz deliberate movements by its vibratory quality and 6–18 Hz frequency range.[361]

Recurrent rhythmic nocturnal tongue biting as a result of **hereditary chin trembling** (geniospasm) has been reported in a number of children.[361–366] This typically presents as multiple tongue-biting episodes in sleep to the point of causing a distal tongue amputation. On clinical examination, the recognition of the fine chin trembling is apparent but often overlooked as insignificant. Further questioning may reveal a familial disorder affecting the siblings, parent, and relatives. Hereditary chin trembling is considered a benign autosomal-dominant disorder that can manifest in concurrence with other more significant medical and neurological problems.[361, 363, 365] Nocturnal tongue biting has been reported several times, including in twins and multigenerational families.[361, 362, 365, 366] The tongue biting becomes apparent at 10–18 months of age, with gradual spontaneous remission in later childhood. The tip of the tongue tends to be bitten preferentially with a nightly or multiple-times-per-night frequency. Tongue biting can also be associated with RMD, sleep starts, and sleep myoclonus. Recurrent rhythmic nocturnal tongue biting as a result of hereditary chin trembling has been responsive to benzodiazepine administration. Whether this too represents another form of parasomnias or not is debated.

Another unusual sleep-related rhythmic tongue movement disorder has been reported in children over a spectrum of ages with Costello syndrome.[367] The tongue movements were a licking- or sucking-like tongue motion associated with a loud noise only while asleep. These were recorded on video-polysomnography in 4/10 subjects with Costello syndrome.[367] This syndrome is a rare condition characterized by polyhydramnios due to impaired deglutination and fetal macrosomia prenatally, followed by postnatal failure to thrive because of poor sucking and feeding.[368] There is later identified mental retardation, compounded by several craniofacial, cardiac/cardiac rhythm, and dermatological abnormalities.[368] Some of the reported subjects had additional sleep-related breathing abnormalities, including snoring and obstructive apnea. The tongue movements were not associated with arousals and were observed in NREM sleep. The subjects were 9 months to 29 years of age, with diminished tongue movements noted with later ages.[367] Rhythmic tongue movements in sleep may occur in the absence of any specific syndrome as well.

A number of additional sleep-related behaviors have been associated with sleep disruption or movements in sleep and are described in older ages beyond childhood.[36,249,369] However, gastroesophageal reflux (GER) may be another common phenomenon seen in childhood but not always recognized as interrupting sleep or confused with epilepsy. The finding of emesis around the mouth or on the pillow after a night's sleep is clear, but more subtle complaints of throat and chest discomfort should arouse suspicion, especially if the child frequently awakens from sleep, crying. GER in childhood will often produce delays in initiating sleep due to esophageal irritation and pain.[36,370] Nocturnal wheezing and laryngospasm can develop and reflux-related apnea can occur particularly in infants.[370] GER may be coupled with or confused with abnormal swallowing syndrome, which is more typical in adults, and produces arousals from sleep due to choking on pooled oral and pharyngeal secretions.[249] The symptoms may simulate obstructive sleep apnea, and polysomnography may be needed to differentiate the two.

An important and easily identified movement of sleep is **excessive fragmentary myoclonus in sleep**.[36,369] These are simple, quick, and small-amplitude movements of the fingers, toes, and corners of the mouth. They occur in any and all sleep stages and resemble quick twitches, which helps to differentiate them from the larger hypnic jerks seen only at the wake-sleep transition. They may continue in both wakefulness and sleep with polysomnographic monitoring demonstrating recurrent and persistent very brief (75–150 ms) EMG potentials in various muscles. These muscle contractions occur asynchronously and asymmetrically in a sustained manner without clustering. There must be more than five potentials per minute sustained for at least 20 minutes of NREM sleep stages 2, 3, or, 4 for diagnosis.[36] No treatment is needed for this disorder. Although this is more often identified in older men, all ages can be affected and should be considered as one of the sleep-related movement disorders primarily seen in childhood.

Hypnogogic paroxysmal dystonia is another non-epileptic entity to consider in children who present with stereotyped periods of choreo-athetosis and dystonic posturing during NREM sleep.[371] This rare disorder usually begins in infancy and extends into adulthood. Patients may display variable durations of involuntary movements lasting from a few minutes to several hours and may repeat during a single night's sleep period. The posturing is typically manifest in the distal portions of the limbs but may also involve the face and trunk. As further patients are studied, however, the epileptic etiology of many short attacks is being recognized (autosomal-dominant nocturnal frontal lobe epilepsy, ADNFLE), making telemetry and polysomnography study most important to differentiate the causes.[372] Thus, there are both non-epileptic and epileptic etiologies to consider when evaluating these patients. Similarly, an epileptic etiology for nocturnal laryngospasm and night terrors (pavor nocturnus) in children has been reported as well.[373–375] There appear to be no clearly distinguishable clinical features that would allow differentiation of the epileptic from a non-epileptic etiology in these cases except that non-epileptic events are exceedingly more usual. There is also a number of specific epilepsy syndromes associated predominantly or exclusively with sleep-related epileptic seizures (Table 4-13).[376,377]

Table 4-13 Epilepsy Syndromes with Predominantly or Exclusively Sleep-Related Epileptic Seizures

1. Nocturnal temporal lobe epilepsy
2. Benign epilepsy of childhood with centrotemporal spikes
3. Nocturnal paroxysmal dystonia
4. Supplementary sensorimoter seizures
5. Autosomal-dominant nocturnal frontal lobe epilepsy
6. Continuous spike-waves during slow-wave sleep
7. Juvenile myoclonic epilepsy
8. Generalized tonic-clonic seizures upon awakening
9. Infantile spasms/West syndrome
10. Childhood epilepsy with occipital paroxysms
    Early onset: Panayiotopoulos type
    Late onset: Gastaut type

Source: Modified from References.[376,377]

Benign familial nocturnal alternating hemiplegia of childhood is a rare paroxysmal syndrome constituting a benign and familial form of the progressive disorder.[378,379] Six patients have had full description, all of whom are males, four within the same family, suggesting an autosomal recessive or X-linked dominant inheritance pattern distinct from the sporadic malignant form.[378,379] The events give the appearance of a post-ictal epileptic paralysis (Todd's paralysis). Each child had recurrent attacks of flaccid hemiplegia (arm more than the leg and included the face) develop upon arousal from sleep without apparent concurrent neurological or cognitive impairment.[373,374] There has been associated drooling and breathing difficulty encountered with a positive Babinski sign during attacks.[378,379] These attacks first occur between the ages of 4 months and 3.5 years (median age 18.5 months). The episodes of hemiplegia were transient and relatively mild, lasting from 5–20 minutes.[378,379] Hemiplegia alternated from side-to-side in successive attacks, although two children experienced bilateral plegia of less intensity than isolated hemiplegia.[378,379] These often began 20–30 minutes into drowsiness or sleep, with the onset heralded by crying. Only one child experienced them during wakefulness. The attacks have been variable in frequency, occurring two to twelve times per month and over time evolved dystonic posturing and an associated limb ataxia.[378,379] There is no concurrent headache or visual impairment. Associated precipitants appear to be sleep deprivation, a stressful or a "busy and exciting day." A parental (maternal) family history of migraine with or without aura has been noted in four of the families.[378,379] All biological and neuroradiological investigations, except cerebellar hypometabolism noted on the PET scan of one child, have been reported as normal.[379] Interictal and sleep EEGs have been normal, and ictal EEGs have demonstrated contralateral hemispheric slowing.[379] Long-term follow-up data reported a decreasing frequency of attacks with age, with cessation at 19 months, and 4.5 and 7 years of age in three children.[379] Treatment responses were only modest with flunarizine and clobazam, and negligible with other anticonvulsants.[379]

REFERENCES

1. Lesku JA, Roth TC, Amlaner CJ, et al. A phylogenetic analysis of sleep architecture in mamals: The integration of anatomy, physiology, and ecology. Am Nat 2006; 168(4); 441–453.
2. Adam K, Oswald I. Sleep is for tissue restoration. J RColl Phys 1977; 11; 376.
3. Allison T, Cicchetti DV. Sleep in mammals: ecological and constitutional corre-lates. Science 1976; 194; 732–734.
4. Zeplin H, Rechtschaffen A. Mammilian sleep, longevity, and energy conservation. Brain Behav Evol 1974; 10; 425–470.
5. Smith C, Butler S. Paradoxical sleep at selective times following training is necessary for learning. Physiol Behav 1982; 29; 469.
6. Crick F, Mitchson G. The function of dreamsleep. Nature 1983; 304; 111.
7. Carskadon MA, Rechtschaffen A. Monitoring and staging human sleep. In *Prin-ciples and Practice of Sleep Medicine.* Eds: MH Kryger, T Roth, and WC Dement. Philadelphia PA, Saunders Co., 2005; 1359–1377.
8. Walker MP, Stickgold R. Sleep-dependent learning and memory consolidation. Neuron 2004; 44; 121–133.
9. Marks GA, Shaffery JP, Oksenberg A, et al. A functional role for REM sleep in brain maturation. Behav Brain Res 1995; 69; 1–11.
10. Lima SL, Rattenborg NC, Lesku JA, et al. Sleeping under the risk of predation. Anim Behav 2005; 70; 723–736.
11. Opp MR. Sleep and psychoneuroimmunology. Neurol Clin 2006; 24; 493–506.
12. The National Sleep Foundation. *Sleep in America Poll 2004.* Washington, DC: National Sleep Foundation, 2004; 1–183.
13. The National Sleep Foundation. *Sleep in America Poll 2004.* Washington, DC: National Sleep Foundation, 2006; 1–195. http://www.sleepfoundation.org
14. Moore M, Allison D, Rosen CL. A review of pediatric nonrespiratory sleep disorders. Chest 2006; 130(4); 1252–1262.
15. Smaldone A, Honig JC, Byrne MW. Sleepless in America: inadequate sleep and relationships to health and well being of our nation's children. Pediatrics 2007; 119 (Suppl 1); S29–S37.
16. Karen M, Feldman R, Tanyo S. Diagnoses and interactive patterns of infants referred to a community-based infant mental health clinic. J Am Acad Child Adolesc Psychiatry 2001; 40; 27–35.
17. Gais S, Plihal W, Wagner U, et al. Early sleep triggers memory for early visual discrimination skills. Nat Neurosci 2000; 3; 1335–1339.
18. Lavigne JV, Arend R, Rosenbaum D, et al. Sleep and behavior problems among preschoolers. J Dev Behav Pediatr 1999; 20; 164–169.
19. Sadeh A, Gruber R, Raviv A. Sleep, neurobehavioral functioning, and behavior problems in school-age children. Child Dev 2002; 73; 405–417.
20. Amschler DH, McKenzie JF. Elementary students' sleep habits and teacher obser-vations of sleep-related problems. J Sch Health 2005; 75(2); 50–56.
21. Alexandru G, Michikazu S, Shimako H, et al. Epidemiological aspects of self-reported sleep onset latency in Japanese junior high school children. J Sleep Res 2006; 15(3); 266–275.

22. Hiscock H, Canterford L, Ukoumunne OC, et al. Adverse associations of sleep problems in Australian preschoolers: a national population study. Pediatrics 2007; 119(1); 86–93.

23. Smedge H, Broman JE, Hetta J. Parents' reports of disturbed sleep in 5-7-year-old Sweedish children. Acta Paediatr 1999; 88; 858–865.

24. Archibald KH, Pituich KJ, Panahi P, et al. Symptoms of sleep disturbances among children at two general pediatric clinics. J Pediatr 2002; 140(1); 97–102.

25. Ferber R. Clinical assessment of child and adolescent sleep disorders. Child Adolesc Psychiatr Clin N Am 1996; 5; 569–580.

26. Markov D, Goldman M. Normal sleep and circadian rhythms: Neurobiologic mechanisms underlying sleep and wakefulness. Psychiatr Clin N Am 2006; 29; 841–853.

27. Siegel JM. REM sleep. In *Principles and practice of sleep medicine.* Eds: MH Kryger, T Roth, and WC Dement. Philadelphia PA, Saunders Co., 2005; 120–135.

28. Kahn A, Dan B, Groswasser J, et al. Normal sleep architecture in infants and children. J Clin Neurophysiol 1996; 13(3); 184–197.

29. Sheldon SH, Spire JP, Levy HB. Normal sleep in children and young adults. *Pediatric Sleep Medicine.* Philadelphia, PA: Saunders Co., 1992; 14–27.

30. Scher M, Johnson MW, Holditch-Davis D. Cyclicity of neonatal sleep behaviors at 25 to 30 weeks' postconceptional age. Pediatr Res 2005; 57(6); 879–882.

31. Meltzer LJ, Mindell JA. Sleep and sleep disorders in children and adolescents. Psychiatr Clin N Am 2006; 29; 1059–1076.

32. Ohayon MM, Carskadon MA, Guilleminault C, et al. Meta-analysis of quantitative sleep parameters from childhood to old age in healthy individuals: Developing normative sleep values across the human lifespan. Sleep 2004; 27(7); 1255–1273.

33. Chokroverty S. Physiologic changes in sleep. In *Sleep Disorders Medicine: Basic Science, Technical Considerations, and Clinical Aspects,* Ed: Chokroverty S. Boston, MA: Butterworth Heinemann, 1999; 95–126.

34. Roth T, Roehrs T. Sleep organization and regulation. Neurology 2000; 54 (Suppl 1); S2–S7.

35. Roth T. Characteristics and determinants of normal sleep. J Clin Psychiatr 2004; 65(Suppl 16); 8–11.

36. The American Academy of Sleep Medicine. International classification of sleep disorders, 2nd edition. Diagnostic and coding manual. Westchester, IL: American Academy of Sleep Medicine, 2005.

37. Borbely AA. A two process model of sleep regulation. Hum Neurobiol 1982; 1; 195–204.

38. Van Gelder RN. Recent insights into mammalian circadian rhythms. Sleep 2004; 27; 166–171.

39. Jenni OG, LeBourgeois MK. Understanding sleep-wake behavior and sleep disorders in children: the value of a model. Curr Opin Psychiatr 2006; 19(3); 282–287.

40. Hattar S, Liao HW, Takao M, et al. Melanopsin-containing retinal ganglion cells: architecture, projections, and intrinsic photosensitivity. Science 2002; 295; 1065–1070.

41. Berson DM, Dunn FA, Takao M. Phototransduction by retinal ganglion cells that set the circadian clock. Science 2002; 295; 1070–1073.

42. Sheldon SH, Spire JP, Levy HB. Physiological variations during sleep. *Pediatric Sleep Medicine.* Philadelphia, PA, Saunders Co., 1992; 46–57.

43. Pace-Schott EF, Hobson JA. The neurobiology of sleep: genetics, cellular physiology and subcortical networks. Nat Rev Neurosci 2002; 3; 591–605.

44. Hobson JA. The cellular basis of sleep cycle control. Adv Sleep Res 1974; 1; 217–250.

45. Jones BE. Basic mechanisms of sleep-wake states. In *Principles and Practice of Sleep Medicine*. Eds: Kryger MH, Roth T, and Dement WC. Philadelphia, PA, Saunders Co., 2005; 136–153.

46. Sutcliffe JG, de Lecea L. The hypocretins: setting the arousal threshold. Nat Rev Neurosci 2002; 3; 339–349.

47. Seigel JM. The neurotransmitters of sleep. J Clin Psychiatr 2004; 65(Suppl 16); 4–7.

48. Mignot E, Taheri S, Nishino S. Sleeping with the hypothalamus: emerging therapeutic targets for sleep disorders. Nat Neurosci 2002; 5(Suppl); 1071–1075.

49. Saper CB, Chou TC, Scammell TE. The sleep switch: hypothalamic control of sleep and wakefulness. Trends Neurosci 2001; 24; 726–731.

50. Lu J, Sherman D, Devor M, et al. A putative flip-flop switch for control of REM sleep. Nature 2006; 441; 589–594.

51. Stepanski E, Roehrs T, Saab P, et al. Readaption to the laboratory in long-term sleep studies. Bull Psychonomic Soc 1981; 17; 224–226.

52. Lukas JS. Noise and sleep: a literature review and proposed criteria for assessing effects. J Acoust Soc Am 1975; 58; 1232–1242.

53. Oswald I, Taylor AM, Treisman M. Discriminative responses to stimulation during human sleep. Brain 1960; 83; 440–453.

54. Haskell EH, Palca JW, Walker JM, et al. The effects of high and low ambient temperatures on human sleep stages. Electroencephalog Clin Neurophysiol 1981; 46; 29–32.

55. Nicholson AN, Stone BM. Influence of back angle on the quality of sleep in seats. Ergonomics 1987; 30; 1033–1041.

56. Obemyer WH, Benca RM. Effects of drugs on sleep. Neurol Clin 1996; 14; 827–840.

57. Roehrs T, Merlotti L, Zorick F, et al. Rebound insomnia and hypnotic self-administration. Psychopharmacology 1992; 107; 480–484.

58. Foulkes D, Larson JD, Swanson EM, et al. Two studies of childhood dreaming. Am J Orthopsy 1969; 39; 627–643.

59. Ames LB. Sleep and dreams in children. In *Problems of Sleep and Dreams in Children*. Ed: Harmes E. New York: Macmillan Co., 1964; 6–29.

60. Sheldon SH, Spire JP, Levy HB. Dreams. *Pediatric Sleep Medicine*. Philadelphia, PA: Saunders Co., 1992; 58–68.

61. Schulze G. The dual origins of affect in nightmares: the roles of physiological homeostasis and memory. Medical Hypoth 2006; 66(6); 1082–1084.

62. Valli K, Revonsuo A, Palkas O, et al. The threat simulation theory of the evolutionary function of dreaming: Evidence from dreams of traumatized children. Consciousness Cogn 2005; 14(1); 188–218.

63. Muris P, Merkelbach H, Gadet B, et al. Fears, worries, and scary dreams in 4- to 12-year old children: their content, developmental pattern, and origins. J Clin Child Psychol 2000; 29(1); 43–52.

64. Schredl M, Sartorius H. Frequency of dream recall by children and their mothers. Percept Motor Skills 2006; 103(3); 657–658.

65. Lewis O, O'Brien J. Clinical use of dreams in latency-age children. Am J Psychotherapy 1991; 45(4); 527–543.
66. Kohyama J, Shiiki T, Shimohira M, et al. Asynchronous breathing during sleep. Arch Dis Child 2001; 84; 174–177.
67. Owens J, Mindell J. *Take Charge of your Child's Sleep.* New York: Marlow & Company, 2005.
68. Littner MR, Kushida C, Wise M, et al. Practice parameters for the clinical use of the multiple sleep latency test and the maintenance of wakefulness test. Sleep 2005; 28; 113–121.
69. Hoban TF, Chervin RD. Assessment of sleepiness in children. Semin Ped Neurol 2001; 8; 216–228.
70. Anderson NE. Late complications in childhood central nervous system tumour survivors. Curr Opin Neurol 2003; 16; 677–683.
71. Petit D, Touchette E, Tremblay RE, et al. Dyssomnias and parasomnias in early childhood. Pediatrics 2007; 119; e1016–e1025. http://www.pediatrics.org/cgi/content/full/119/5/e1016.
72. Laberge L, Tremblay RE, Vitaro F, et al. Development of parasomnias from childhood to early adolescence. Pediatrics 2000; 106(1); 67–74.
73. Mindell JA, Kuhn B, Lewin DS, et al. Behavioral treatment of bedtime problems and night awakenings in infants and young children. Sleep 2006; 29(10); 1263–1276.
74. de Serres LM, Derkay C, Sie K, et al. Impact of adenotonsilectomy on quality of life in children with obstructive sleep disorders. Arch Otol Head Neck Surg 2002; 128; 489–496.
75. Rosen CL, Palmero TM, Larkin EK, et al. Health-related quality of life and sleep disordered breathing in children. Sleep 2002; 25; 648–654.
76. Stewart MG, Friedman EM, Sulek M, et al. Quality of life and health status in pediatric tonsil and adenoid disease. Arch Otol Head Neck Surg 2000; 126; 45–48.
77. Hart CN, Palmero TM, Rosen CL. Health-related quality of life among children presenting to a pediatric sleep disorders clinic. Behav Sleep Med 2005; 3(1); 4–17.
78. Committee on Fetus and Newborn. American Academy of Pediatrics. Apnea, sudden infant death syndrome and home monitoring. Pediatrics 2003; 111; 914–917.
79. Ender A, Wennborg M, Alm B, et al. Why do ALTE infants not die of SIDS? Acta Paediatr 2006; 96; 191–194.
80. Naulaers G, Daniels H, Allegaert K, et al. Cardiorespiratory events recorded on home monitors: the effect of prematurity on later serious events. Acta Paediatr 2006; 96; 195–198.
81. Anstead M. Pediatric sleep disorders: new developments and evolving understanding. Curr Opin Pulm Med 2000; 6; 501–506.
82. Brand DA, Altman RL, Purtill K, et al. Yield of diagnostic testing in infants who have had an apparent life-threatening event. Pediatrics 2005; 115(4); 885–893.
83. McGovern MC, Smith MBH. Causes of apparent life-threatening events in infants; a systematic review. Arch Dis Child 2004; 89; 1043–1048.
84. DiFiore JM, Arko M, Whitehouse M, et al. Apnea is not prolonged by acid gastroesophageal reflux in preterm infants. Pediatrics 2005; 116(5); 1059–1063.
85. Bonkowski J, Guenther E, Filoux F, et al. Death, child abuse, and adverse neurological outcome in infants after an apparent life threatening event. Pediatrics 2008; 122(1); 125–131.

86. Hirtz D, Berg A, Bettis D, et al. Practice parameter: treatment of the child with a first unprovoked seizure: Report of the Quality Standards Subcommittee of the American Academy of Neurology and the Practice Committee of the Child Neurology Society. Neurology 2003; 60(2); 166–175.

87. Strauss D, Shavelle R, Reynolds R, et al. Survival in cerebral palsy in the last 20 years: signs of improvement? Dev Med Child Neurol 2007; 49; 86–92.

88. Camfield P, Camfield C, Smith S, et al. Long-term outcome is unchanged by antiepileptic drug treatment after a first seizure: a 15-year follow-up from a randomized trial in childhood. Epilepsia 2002; 43(6); 662–663.

89. Meadow R. Munchausen syndrome by proxy. Arch Dis Child 1982; 57; 92–98.

90. Rosen CL, Frost JD, Glaze DG. Child abuse and recurrent infant apnea. J Pediatr 1986; 109(6); 1065–1067.

91. Kriter KE, Blanchard J. Management of apnea in infants. Clin Pharmacol 1989; 8; 577–587.

92. Kelly DH, Shannon DC. Treatment of apnea and excessive periodic breathing in the full-term infant. Pediatrics 1981; 68; 183–186.

93. Miller MJ, Carlo WA, Martin RJ. Continuous positive airway pressure selectively reduces obstructive apnea in preterm infants. J Pediatr 1985; 106; 91–94.

94. Bairam A, Boutroy MJ, Badonnel Y, et al. Theophylline versus caffeine: Comparative effects in treatment of idiopathic apnea in the preterm infant. J Pediatr 1987; 110; 636–639.

95. Jones RAK. Apnoea of prematurity: I. A controlled trial of theophylline and face mask continuous positive airway pressure. Arch Dis Child 1982; 57; 761–765.

96. Barrington KJ, Finner NN, Peters KL, et al. Physiologic effects of doxapram in idiopathic apnea of prematurity. J Pediatr 1986; 108; 124–129.

97. Philippi H, Bieber I, Reitter B. Acetazolamide treatment for infantile central sleep apnea. J Child Neurol 2001; 16(8); 600–603.

98. Rosenkrantz TS, Oh W. Aminophylline reduces cerebral blood flow velocity in low birth weight infants. Am J Dis Child 1984; 138; 489–491.

99. Gozal, D. New concepts in abnormalities of respiratory control in children. Curr Opin Pediatr 2004; 16(3); 305–308.

100. Kahn A, Groswasser J, Sottiaux M, et al. Mechanisms of obstructive sleep apneas in infants. Biol Neonate 1994; 65; 235–239.

101. Marcus CL. Sleep-disordered breathing in children. Curr Opin Pediatr 2000; 12; 208–212.

102. Carroll JL. Obstructive sleep-disordered breathing in children: new controversies, new directions. Clin Chest Med 2003; 24; 261–282.

103. Seddon PC, Khan Y. Respiratory problems in children with neurological impairment. Arch Dis Child 2003; 88; 75–78.

104. Abrahams P, Burkitt BF. Hiatus hernia and Gastroesophageal reflux in children and adolescents with cerebral palsy. Aust Paediatr J 1970; 6; 41–46.

105. Kortagal S, Gibbons VP, Stith JA. Sleep abnormalities in patients with severe cerebral palsy. Dex Med Child Neurol 1994; 36; 304–311.

106. Chantonnet F, Dominguez del Toro E, Thoby-Brisson M, et al. From hindbrain segmentation to breathing after birth: developmental patterning in rhombomeres 3 and 4. Mol Neurobiol 2003; 28; 277–294.

107. Brazy EB, Kinney HC, Oakes WJ. Central nervous system structural lesions causing apnea at birth. J Pediatr 1987; 111(2); 163–175.

108. Marcus CL, Lutz J, Hamer A, Smith pL, Schwartz A. Developmental changes in response to subatmospheric pressure loading of the upper airway. J Appl Physiol 1999; 87; 626–633.
109. Brouillette RT, Fernbach SK, Hunt CE. Obstructive sleep apnea in infants and children. J Pediatr 1982; 100; 31–40.
110. Gozal D. Sleep-disordered breathing and school performance in children. Pediatrics 1998; 102; 616–620.
111. Gozal D, Pope DW Jr. Snoring during early childhood and academic performance at ages 13–14 years. Pediatrics 2001; 107; 1394–1399.
112. Huang Y-S, Guilleminault C, Li H-Y, et al. Attention-deficit/hyperactivity disorder with obstructive sleep apnea: a treatment outcome study. Sleep Med 2007; 8; 18–30.
113. Ungkanont K, Areyasathidmon S. Factors affecting quality of life of pediatric outpatients with symptoms suggestive of sleep-disordered breathing. Int J Pediatr Otorhinolaringol 2006; 70; 1945–1948.
114. Brooks LJ, Topol HI. Enuresis in children with sleep apnea. J Pediatr 2003; 142; 515–518.
115. Bandla HPR, Gozal D. Dynamic changes in EEG spectra during obstructive sleep apnea in children. Pediatr Pulmonol 2000; 29; 359–365.
116. Row BW, Kheirandish L, Neville JJ, et al. Impaired spatial learning and hyperactivity in developing rats exposed to intermittent hypoxia. Pediatr Res 2002; 52; 449–453.
117. Zintzaras E, Kaditis AG. Sleep-disordered breathing and blood pressure in children. Arch Pediatr Adolesc Med 2007; 161; 172–178.
118. Levers-Landis CE, Redline S. Pediatric sleep apnea: Implications of the epidemic of childhood overweight. Am J Respir Crit Care Med 2007; 175; 436–441.
119. de la Eva RC, Baur LA, Donaghue KC, et al. Metabolic correlates with sleep apnea in obese subjects. J Pediatr 2002; 140; 654–659.
120. Carrol J, McColley S, Marcus C, et al. Inability of clinical history to distinguish primary snoring from obstructive sleep apnea syndrome in children. Chest 1995; 108; 610–618.
121. Rosen CL. Clinical features of obstructive sleep apnea hypoventilation syndrome in otherwise healthy children. Pediatr Pulmonol 1999; 27; 403–409.
122. Broulliette R, Hanson D, David R, et al. A diagnostic approach to suspected obstructed sleep apnea in children. J Pediatr 1984; 105; 10–14.
123. American Acadaemy of Pediatrics, Section on Pediatric Pulmonology, Subcommittee on Obstructive Sleep Apnea: Clinical practice guideline: Diagnosis and management of childhood obstructive sleep apnea syndrome. Pediatrics 2002; 109; 704–712.
124. Verhulst SL, Schrauwen N, De Backer WA, et al. First night effect for polysomnographic data in children and adolescents with suspected sleep disordered breathing. Arch Dis Child 2006; 91; 233–237.
125. Kudoh F, Sani A. Effect of tonsillectomy and adenoidectomy on obese children with sleep-associated breathing disorders. Acta Otolaryngol Suppl 1996; 523; 216–218.
126. Wiet GJ, Bower C, Seibert R, et al. Surgical correction of obstructive sleep apnea in the complicated pediatric patient documented by polysomnography. Int J Pediatr Otorhinolaryngol 1997; 41; 133–143.
127. Marcus CL, Keens TG, Bautista DB, et al. Obstructive sleep apnea in children with Down syndrome. Pediatrics 1991; 88; 132–139.

128. Grundfast K, Berkowitz R, Fox L. Outcome and complications following surgery for obstructive adenotonsillar hypertrophy in children with neuromuscular disorders. Ear Nose Throat J 1990; 69; 756, 759–760.

129. Schecter MS. Technical report: Diagnosis and management of childhood obstructive sleep apnea syndrome. Pediatrics 2002; 109; e69. http://www.pediatrics.org/cgi/content/full/109/4/e69.

130. Marcus CL. Treatment of obstructive sleep apnea syndrome in children. In *Principles and Practice of Pediatric Sleep Medicine*. Eds: SH Sheldon, R Ferber, MH Kryger, Elsevier/Saunders 2005, 235–247.

131. Gulleminault C, Lee JH, Chan A. Pediatric obstructive sleep apnea syndrome. Arch Pediatr Adolesc Med 2005; 159(8); 775–785.

132. Davis CL, Tkacz J, Gregoski M, et al. Aerobic exercise and snoring in overweight children: a randomized controlled trial. Obesity 2006; 14(11); 1985–1991.

133. Gaultier C, Amiel J, Dauger S, et al. Genetics and early disturbances of breathing control. Pediat Res 2004; 55(5); 729–733.

134. Macey PM, Valderama C, Kim AH, et al. Temporal trends of cardiac and respiratory responses to ventilatory challenges in congenital central hypoventilation syndrome. Pediatr Res 2004; 55(6); 953–959.

135. Matera I, Bachetti T, Puppo F, et al. PHOX2B mutations and polyalanine expansions correlate with the severity of the respiratory phenotype and associated symptoms in both congenital and late onset Central Hypoventilation syndrome. J Med Genet 2004; 41; 373–380.

136. Deonna T, Arczynska W, Torrado A. Congenital failure of automatic ventilation (Ondine's curse). A case report. J Pediatr 1974; 84; 710–714.

137. Fleming PJ, Cade D, Bryan MH, et al. Congenital central hypoventilation and sleep state. Pediatrics 1980; 66; 425–428.

138. Guilleminault C, McQuitty J, Ariagno RL, et al. Congenital central hypoventilation syndrome in six infants. Pediatrics 1982; 70; 684–694.

139. Paton JY, Swaminathan S, Sargent CW, et al. Hypoxic and hypercapnic ventilatory responses in awake children with congenital central hypoventilation syndrome. Am Rev Respir Dis 1989; 140; 368–372.

140. Weese-Mayer DE, Sylvestri JM, Menzies LJ, et al. Congenital central hypoventilation syndrome: diagnosis, management, and long term outcome in thirty-two children. J Pediatr 1992; 120; 381–387.

141. Rohrer T, Trachsel D, Engelcke G, et al. Congenital central hypoventilation syndrome associated with Hirsprung's disease and neuroblastoma: Case of multiple neurocristopathies. Pediatr Pulm 2002; 33; 71–76.

142. Woo MS, Woo MA, Gozal D, et al. Heart rate variability in congenital central hypoventilation syndrome. Pediatr Res 1992; 31; 291–296.

143. Ogawa T, Kojo M, Fukushima N, et al. Cardio-respiratory control in an infant with Ondine's curse: a multivariate autoregressive modeling approach. J Auton Nrv Syst 1993; 42; 41–52.

144. Silvestri JM, Hanna BD, Volgman AS, et al. Cardiac rhythm disturbances among children with idiopathic congenital central hypoventilation syndrome. Pediatr Pulmonol 2000; 29; 351–358.

145. Silvestri JM, Weese-Mayer DE, Flanagan EA. Congenital central hypoventilation syndrome: cardiorespiratory responses to moderate exercise, simulating daily activity. Pediatr Pulmonol 1995; 20; 89–93.

146. Haddad GG, Mazza NM, Defendini R, et al. Cogenital failure of automatic control of ventilation, gastrointestinal motility and heart rate. Medicine 1978; 57; 517–526.

147. Pine DS, Weese-Mayer DE, Sylvestri JM, et al. Anxiety and congenital central hypoventilation syndrome. Am J Psychiatr 1994; 151; 864–870.

148. Weese-Mayer DE, Sylvestri JM, Huffman AD, et al. Case/control family study of autonomic nervous system dysfunction in idiopathic congenital central hypoventilation syndrome. Am J Med Genet 2001; 100; 237–245.

149. Weese-Mayer DE, Shannon DC, Keens TG, et al. American Thoracic Society Statement. Idiopathic congenital central hypoventilation syndrome. Am J Crit Care Med 1999; 160; 368–373.

150. O'Brien LM, Holbrook CR, Vanderlaan M, et al. Autonomic function in children with congenital central hypoventilation syndrome and their families. Chest 2005; 128; 2478–2484.

151. Todd ES, Weinberg SM, Berry-Kravis EM, et al. Facial phenotype in children and young adults with PHOX2B-determined congenital central hypoventilation syndrome: Quantitative pattern of dysmorphology. Pediatr Res 2006; 59(1); 39–45.

152. Gozal D, Simakajornboon N. Passive motion of the extremities modifies alveolar ventilation during sleep in patients with congenital central hypoventilation syndrome. Am J Respir Crit Care Med 2000; 162; 1747–1751.

153. Shaul DB, Danielson PD, McComb JG, et al. Thoracoscopic placement of phrenic nerve electrodes for diaphragmatic pacing in children. J Pediatr Surg 2002; 37; 974–978.

154. Chen ML, Keens TG. Congenital central hypoventilation syndrome: not just another rare disorder. Ped Resp Rev 2004; 5; 182–189.

155. Black JE, Brooks SN, Nishino S. Narcolepsy and syndromes of primary excessive daytime somnolence. Seminars in Neurology. Introduction to Sleep and Its Disorders 2004; 24(3); 271–282.

156. Yoss RE, Daly DD. Criteria for the diagnosis of the narcoleptic syndrome. Proc Mayo Clin 1957; 32; 320–328.

157. Guilleminault C, Cataplexy. In Narcolepsy. Eds: C Guilleminault, WC Dement, and P Passouant. New York, Spectrum, 1976; 125–144.

158. Yoss RE, Daly DD. Narcolepsy in children. Pediatrics 1960; 25; 1025–1033.

159. Challamel MJ, Mazzola ME, Nevsimalova S, et al. Narcolepsy in children. Sleep 1994; 17; S17–S20.

160. Aldrich MS. Narcolepsy. Neurology 1992; 42; 34–43.

161. Hublin C, Partinen M, Kaprio J, et al. Epidemiology of narcolepsy. Sleep 1994; 17; S7–S12.

162. Mignot E. Genetic and familial aspects of narcolepsy. Neurology 1998; 50(2 Suppl 1); S16–S22.

163. Roth B. Narcolepsy and Hypersomnia. Ed: S Karger, Basel, Switzerland, 1980.

164. Overeem S, Mignot E, van Dijk GJ, et al. Narcolepsy: Clinical features, new pathophysiologic insights, and future perspectives. J Clin Neurophysiol 2001; 18(2); 78–105.

165. Silber M, Krahn L, Olson E, et al. The epidemiology of narcolepsy in Olmstead County, Minnesota: A population-based study. Sleep 2002; 25; 197–202.

166. Honda Y. Census of narcolepsy, cataplexy, and sleeplife among teenagers in Fujisawa city. Sleep Res 1979; 8; 191.

167. Sharp SJ, D'Cruz OF. Narcolepsy in a 12 month old boy. J Child Neurol 2001; 16; 145–146.
168. Hood BM, Harbord MG. Paediatric narcolepsy: Complexities of diagnosis. J Paediatr Child Health 2002; 38; 618–621.
169. Nevsimalova S, Roth B, Zouhar A, et al. Narkolepsie-Kataplexie a periodicka hypersomnie se zacatkem v kojeneckem veku. Cs Pediatr 1986; 41; 324–327.
170. Wise MS. Childhood narcolepsy. Neurology 1998; 50(Suppl 1); S37–S42.
171. Stores G, Montgomery P, Wiggs L. The psychosocial problems of children with narcolepsy and those with excessive daytime sleepiness of uncertain origin. Pediatrics 2006; 118(4); e1116–e1123. http://www.pediatrics.org/cgi/content/full/118/4/e1116.
172. Pollack CP. The rhythms of narcolepsy. Narcolepsy Network 1995; 8; 171–177.
173. Guilleminault C, Wilson RA, Dement WC. A study of cataplexy. Arch Neurol 1974; 31; 255–261.
174. Guilleminault C, Pelayo R. Narcolepsy in prepubertal children. Ann Neurol 1998; 43; 135–142.
175. Hishikawa Y, Shimizu T. Physiology of REM sleep, cataplexy, and sleep paralysis. Adv Neurol 1995; 67; 245–271.
176. Guilleminault C, Heinzer R, Mignot E, et al. Investigations into the neurological basis of narcolepsy. Neurol 1998; 50(2 Suppl 1); S8–S15.
177. Hong SB, Tae WS, Joo EY. Cerebral perfusion changes during cataplexy in narcolepsy patients. Neurology 2006; 66; 1747–1749.
178. Dahl RE, Holttum J, Trubnick L. A clinical picture of child and adolescent narcolepsy. J Am Acad Child Adolesc Psychiatry 1994; 33; 834–841.
179. Young D, Zorick F, Wittig R, et al. Narcolepsy in a pediatric population. Am J Dis Child 1988; 142; 210–213.
180. Verhulst SL, Schrauwen N, Haentjens D, et al. Reference values for sleep-related respiratory variables in asymptomatic European children and adolescents. Pediatr Pul 2007; 42; 159–167.
181. Moss D, Urschitz MS, Von Bodman A, et al. Reference values for nocturnal home polysomnography in primary schoolchildren. Pediatr Res 2005; 58(5); 958–965.
182. Kotagal S, Goulding PM. The laboratory assessment of daytime sleepiness in childhood. J Clin Neurophysiol 1996; 13(3); 208–218.
183. Carskadon MA. Measuring daytime sleepiness. In Principles and Practice of Sleep Medicine, Eds: MH Kryger, T Roth, and WC Dement. 3rd edition, Philadelphia, PA, Saunders Co., 2005; 99–125.
184. Guilleminault C, Mignot E, Grummet FC. Familial patterns of narcolepsy. Lancet 1989; II (8676); 1376–1379.
185. Ohayon MM, Okun ML. Occurrence of sleep disorders in the families of narcoleptic patients. Neurology 2006; 67; 703–705.
186. Seigel JM. Hypocretin (orexin): role in normal behavior and neuropathology. Annu Rev Psychol 2004; 55; 125–148.
187. Thannickal TC, Moore RY, Nienhuis R, et al. Reduced number of hypocretin neurons in human narcolepsy. Neuron 2000; 27(3); 469–474.
188. Overeem S, Scammell TE, Lammers GJ. Hypocretin/Orexin and sleep: implications for the pathophysiology and diagnosis of narcolepsy. Curr Opin Neurol 2002; 15; 739–745.

189. Nishino S, Ripley B, Overeem S, et al. Hypocretin (orexin) deficiency in human narcolepsy. Lancet 2000; 355; 39–40.
190. Mignot E, Lammers GJ, Ripley B, et al. The role of cerebrospinal fluid hypocretin measurement in the diagnosis of narcolepsy and other hypersomnias. Arch Neurol 2002; 59; 1553–1562.
191. Baumann CR, Khatami R, Werth E, et al. Hypocretin (orexin) deficiency predicts severe objective excessive daytime sleepiness in narcolepsy with cataplexy. J Neurol Neurosurg Psychiatr 2006; 77; 402–404.
192. Dauvilliers Y, Baumann CR, Carlander B, et al. CSF hypocretin-1 levels in nacolepsy, Kleine-Levin syndrome, and other hypersomnias and neurological conditions. J Neurol Neurosurg Psychiatr 2003; 74; 1667–1673.
193. Tsukamoto H, Ishikawa T, Fujii Y, et al. Undetectable levels of CSF hypocretin-1 (orexin-A) in two prepubertal boys with narcolepsy. Neuropediatrics 2002; 33; 51–52.
194. Guilleminault C, Pelayo R. Narcolepsy in children. A practical gude to its diagnosis, treatment and follow-up. Paediatr Drugs 2000; 2(1); 1–9.
195. Mitler MM. Evaluation of treatment with stimulants in narcolepsy. Sleep 1994; 17(8 Suppl); S103–S106.
196. US Modafinil in Narcolepsy Multicenter Study Group: randomized trial of modafinil as a treatment for the excessive daytime somnolence of narcolepsy. Neurology 2000; 54(5); 1166–1175.
197. Brooks SN, Guilleminault C. New insights into the pathogenesis and treatment of narcolepsy. Curr Opin Pul Med 2001; 7; 407–410.
198. Black JE, Brokks SN, Nishino S. Conditions of primary excessive daytime sleepiness. Neurol Clin 2005; 23; 1025–1044.
199. Murali H, Kotagal S. Off-label treatment of severe childhood narcolepsy-cataplexy with sodium oxybate. Sleep 2006; 29(8); 1025–1029.
200. Bassetti C, Aldrich MS. Narcolepsy. Neurol Clin 1996; 14(3); 545–571.
201. Malik S, Boeve BF, Krahn LE, et al. Narcolepsy associated with other central nervous system disorders. Neurology 2001; 57; 539–541.
202. Overeem S, Dalmau J, Bataller L, et al. Hypocretin-1 CSF levels in anti-Ma2 associated encephalitis. Neurology 2004; 62; 138–140.
203. Gledhill RF, Bartel PR, Yoshida Y, et al. Narcoplepsy caused by acute disseminated encephalomyelitis. Arch Neurol 2004; 61; 758–760.
204. Anderson NE. Late complications in childhood central nervous system tumour survivors. Curr Opin Neurol 2003; 16; 677–683.
205. Scammell TE, Nishino S, Mignot E, et al. Narcolepsy and low CSF orexin (hypocretin) concentration after a diencephalic stroke. Neurology 2001; 56; 1751–1753.
206. Plazzi G, Parmeggiani A, Mignot E, et al. Narcolepsy-cataplexy associated with precocious puberty. Neurology 2006; 66; 1577–1579.
207. Kubota H, Kanbayashi T, Tanabe Y, et al. Decreased cerebrospinal fluid hypocretin-1 levels near the onset of narcolepsy in 2 prepubertal children. Sleep 2003; 26(5); 555–557.
208. Marcus CL, Trescher WH, Halbower AC, et al. Secondary narcolepsy in children with brain tumors. Sleep 2002; 25;(4); 435–439.
209. Marcus CL, Mignot E. Letter to the editor regarding our previous publication: "Secondary narcolepsy in children with brain tumors," Sleep 2002; 25; 435–439. Sleep 2003; 26(2); 228.

210. Himmerich H, Beitinger PA, Fulda S, et al. Plasma levels of tumor necrosis factor α and soluable tumor necrosis factor receptors in patients with narcolepsy. Arch Int Med 2006; 166; 1739–1743.

211. Critchley M. Periodic hypersomnia and megaphagia in adolescent males. Brain 1962; 85; 627–656.

212. Takahashi Y. Clinical studies of periodic somnolence. Analysis of 28 personal cases. Psychiatr Neurol Jpn 1965; 67; 853–889.

213. Hegarty A, Merriam AE. Autonomic events in Kleine-Levin syndrome. Am J Psychiatr 1990; 147; 951–952.

214. Katz JD, Ropper AH. Familial Kleine-Levin syndrome. Two siblings with unusually long hypersomnic spells. Arch Neurol 2002; 59; 1959–1961.

215. Chesson AL, Levine SN. Neuroendocrine evaluation in Kleine-Levin syndrome: Evidence of reduced dopaminergic tone during hypersomnolence. Sleep 1991; 14; 226–232.

216. Mayer G, Leonhard E, Kreig J, et al. Endocrinological and polysomnographic findings in Kleine-Levin syndrome: No evidence for hypothalamic and circadian dysfunction. Sleep 1998; 21; 278–284.

217. Carpenter S, Yassa R, Ochs R. A pathologic basis for Kleine-Levin syndrome. Arch Neurol 1982; 39; 25–28.

218. Fenzi F, Simonati A, Crosato F, et al. Clinical features of Kliene-Levin syndrome with localized encephalitis. Neuropediatrics 1993; 24; 292–295.

219. Arnulf I, Zeitzer JM, File J, et al. Kleine-Levin syndrome: a review of 186 cases in the literature. Brain 2005; 128; 2763–2776.

220. Huang YS, Guilleminault C, Kao PF, et al. SPECT findings in the Kleine-Levin syndrome. Sleep 2005; 28; 955–960.

221. Landtblom AM, Dige N, Schwerdt K, et al. A case of Kleine-Levin syndrome examined with SPECT and neuropsychological testing. Acta Neurol Scand 2002; 105; 318–321.

222. Gadoth N, Kesler A, Vainstein G, et al. Clinical and polysomnographic characteristics of 34 patients with Kleine-Levin syndrome. J Sleep Res 2001; 10; 337–341.

223. Rosenow F, Kotagal P, Cohen B, et al. Multiple sleep latency test and polysomnography in diagnosing Kleine-Levin syndrome and periodic hypersomnia. J Clin Neurophysiol 2000; 17(4); 519–522.

224. Dauvilliers Y, Mayer G, Lecendreux M, et al. Kleine-Levin syndrome. An autoimmune hypothesis based upon clinical and genetic analyses. Neurology 2002; 59; 1739–1745.

225. Mukaddes NM, Kora ME, Bilge S. Carbamazepine for Kleine-Levin syndrome. J Am Acad Child Adolesc Psychiatry 1999; 38(7); 791–792.

226. Kornreich C, Fossion P, Hoffman G, et al. Treatment of Kleine-Levin syndrome: Melatonin on the starting block. J Clin Psychiatry 2000; 61(3); 215.

227. Crumley FE. Light therapy for Kleine-Levin syndrome. J Am Acad Child Adolesc Psychiatry 1998; 37(12); 1245.

228. Jungheim K, Badenhoop K, Ottmann OG, et al. Kleine-Levin and Munchausen syndromes in a patient with recurrent acromegaly. Eur J Endo 1999; 140(2); 140–142.

229. Mason TBA, Pack AI. Pediatric parasomnias. Sleep 2007; 30(2); 141–151.

230. Derry CP, Duncan JS, Berkovic SF. Paroxysmal motor disorders of sleep: The clinical spectrum and differentiation from epilepsy. Epilepsia 2006; 47(110); 1775–1791.

231. Stores G, Crawford C. Arousal norms for children age 5–16 years based on home polysomnography. Technol Health Care 2000; 8; 285–290.
232. Ohanyon MM, Guilleminault C, Priest RG. Night terrors, sleepwalking, and confusional arousals in the general population: their frequency and relationship to other sleep and mental disorders. J Clin Psychiatr 1999; 60; 268–276.
233. DiMario FJ, Emery ES. The natural history of night terrors. J Clin Pediatr 1987; 26; 505–511.
234. Pesikoff RB, Davis PC. Treatment of pavor nocturnus and somnambulism in children. Am J Psychiatr 1971; 128; 134–137.
235. Cooper AJ. Treatment of coexisitent night-terrors and somnambulism in adults with imipramine and diazepam. J Clin Psychiatr 1987; 48; 209–210.
236. Guilleminault C, Palombini L, Pelayo R, et al. Sleepwalking and sleep terrors in prepubertal children: What triggers them? Pediatrics 2003; 111; e17–e25. http://www.pediatrics.org/cgi/content/full/111/1/e17.
237. Laberge L, Tremblay RE, Vitaro F, et al. Development of parasomnias from childhood to early adolescence. Pediatrics 2000; 106; 67–74.
238. Mason TBA, Pack AI. Sleep terrors in childhood. J Pediatr 2005; 147; 388–392.
239. Klackenberg G. Somnambulism in childhood-prevalence, course, and behavioral correlates: A prospective longitudinal study. Acta Paediatr Scand 1982; 71; 495–499.
240. Stores G. Dramatic parasomnias. J R Soc Med 2001; 94; 173–176.
241. Hublin C, Kaprio J, Partinen M, et al. Prevelence and genetics of sleepwalking: a population-based twin study. Neurology 1997; 48; 177–181.
242. Bornemann MAC, Mahowald MW, Schenck CH. Parasomnias Clinical features and forensic implications. Chest 2006; 130; 605–610.
243. Gau S-F, Soong W-T. Psychiatric comorbidity of adolescents with sleep terrors or sleepwalking: a case control study. Aust New Zeal J Psychiatr 1999; 33; 734–739.
244. Schenck CH, Mahowald MW. REM sleep behavior disorder: clinical, developmental, and neuroscience perspectives 16 years after its formal identification in sleep. Sleep 2002; 25; 120–138.
245. Sheldon SH, Jacobsen J. REM-sleep motor disorder in children. J Child Neurol 1998; 13; 257–260.
246. Kohyama J, Shimohira M, Kondo S, et al. Motor disturbance during REM sleep in group A xeroderma pigmentosum. Acta Neurol Scand 1995; 92; 91–95.
247. Rye DB, Johnston LH, Watts RL, et al. Juvenile Parkinson's disease with REM sleep behavior disorder, sleepiness, and daytime REM onset. Neurology 1999; 53; 1868–1870.
248. Stores G. Medication for sleep-wake disorders. Arch Dis Child 2003; 88; 899–903.
249. Derry CP, Duncan JS, Berkovic SF. Paroxysmal motor disorders of sleep: The clinical spectrum and differentiation from epilepsy. Epilepsia 2006; 47(11); 1775–1791.
250. Ohayon M, Zulley J, Guilleminault C, et al. Prevalence and pathologic associations of sleep paralysis in the general population. Neurology 1999; 52; 1194–2000.
251. Kotorii T, Kotorii T, Uchimura N, et al. Questionnaire relating to sleep paralysis. Psychiatry Clin Neurosci. 2001; 55(3); 265–266.
252. Hufford DJ. Sleep paralysis as a spiritual experience. Transcult Psychiatr 2005; 42(1); 11–45.
253. Awadalla A, Al-Fayez G, Harville M, et al. Comparative prevalence of isolated sleep paralysis in Kuwaiti, Sudanese, and American college students. Psychol Rep 2004; 95(1); 317–322.

254. Germain A, Nielsen T. Sleep pathophysiology in posttraumatic stress disorder and idiopathic nightmare sufferers. Biol Psychiatr 2003; 54; 1092–1098.

255. Zandra A, Donderi D. Nightmares and bad dreams: their prevalence and relationship to well-being. J Abnorm Psychol 2000; 109; 273–281.

256. Pagel J, Helfter P. Drug induced nightmares – an etiology based review. Hum Psychopharmachol 2003; 18; 59–67.

257. Thompson DF, Pierce DR. Drug-induced nightmares. Ann Pharmacother 1999; 33(1); 93–98.

258. Pagel JF. Nightmares and disorders of dreaming. Am Fam Phys 2000; 61; 2037–2042, 2044.

259. Davis JL, Wright DC. Randomized clinical trial for treatment of chronic nightmares in trauma-exposed adults. J Trauma Stress 2007; 20(2); 123–133.

260. Krakow B, Sandoval D, Schrader R, et al. Treatment of chronic nightmares in adjudicated adolescent girls in a residential facility. J Adol Health 2001; 29; 94–100.

261. Iranzo A, Schenck CH, Font J. REM sleep behavior and other disturbances in Disney animated films. Sleep Med 2007; 8(5); 531–536.

262. Wills L, Garcia J. Parasomnias. Epidemiology and management. CNS Drugs 2002; 16(12); 803–810.

263. Sheldon SH. Sleep-related enuresis. Child Adolesc Psychiatr Clin North Am 1996; 5; 661–672.

264. Robson WLM, Leung AKC, Van Howe R. Primary and secondary nocturnal enuresis: similarities in presentation. Pediatrics 2005; 115; 956–959.

265. Brooks LJ, Topol HI. Enuresis in children with sleep apnea. J Pediatr 2003; 142; 515–518.

266. Forsythe WI, Redmond A. Enuresis and spontaneous cure rate: Study of 1129 enuretics. Arch Dis Child 1974; 49; 259–263.

267. Muellner SR. Development of urinary control in children: Some aspects of the cause and treatment of primary enuresis. JAMA 1960; 172; 1256–1262.

268. von Gontrard A, Schaumburg H, Hollmann E, Eiberg H, Rittig S. The genetics of enuresis: A review. J Urol 2001; 166(6); 2438–2443.

269. Bayoumi RA, Eapen V, AlYahyee S, et al. The genetic basis of primary inherited nocturnal enuresis: A UAE study. J Psychosom Res 2006; 61(3); 317–320.

270. Glazener CM, Evans JH, Peto RE. Alarm interventions for nocturnal enuresis in children. Cochrane Database Syst Rev 2005; 18(2); CD002911. Update of: Cochrane Database Syst Rev 2003; (2); CD002911.

271. Glazener CM, Evans JH, Peto RE. Tricyclic and related drugs for nocturnal enuresis in children. Cochrane Database Syst Rev 2003; (3); CD002117. Update of: Cochrane Database Syst Rev 2000; (3); CD002117.

272. Theidke CC. Nocturnal enuresis. Am Fam Phys 2003; 67(7); 1499–1506.

273. Oldani A, Manconi M, Zucconi M, et al. Nocturnal groaning: just a sound or parasomnia? J Sleep Res 2005; 14; 305–310.

274. Vertrugno R, Provini F, Plazzi G, et al. Catathrenia (nocturnal groaning): a new type of parasomnia. Neurology 2001; 56(5); 681–683.

275. Iriate J, Alegre M, Urrestarazu E, et al. Continuous positive airway pressure as treatment for catathrenia (nocturnal groaning). Neurology 2006; 66(2 of 2); 609.

276. Bruni O, Ferri R, Miano S, et al. L-5-hydroxytryprophan treatment of sleep terrors in children. Eur J Pediatr 2004; 163(7); 402–407.

277. Jan JE, Freeman RD, Wasdell MB, et al. A child with severe night terrors and sleep-walking responds to melatonin. Devel Med Child Neurol 2004; 46; 789.

278. Lask B. Novel and non-toxic treatment for night terrors. BMJ 1988; 297 (September 3); 592.

279. Frank NC, Spirito A, Stark L, et al. The use of scheduled awakenings to eliminate childhood sleepwalking. J Pediatr Psychol 1997; 22(3); 345–353.

280. American Psychiatric Association. *Diagnostic and Statistical Manual of Mental Disorders DSM-IV*, 4th edition. Washington, DC, American Psychiatric Association, 1994.

281. Agargun MY, Kara H, Ozer OA, et al. Clinical importance of nightmare disorder in patients with dissociative disorders. Psychiatr Clin Neurosci 2003; 57(6); 575–579.

282. Agargun MY, Kara H, Ozer OA, et al. Nightmares and dissociative experiences: the key role of childhood traumatic events. Psychiatr Clin Neurosci 2003; 57(2); 139–145.

283. Silber MH, Hansen MR, Girish M. Complex nocturnal visual hallucinations. Sleep Med 2005; 6(4); 363–366.

284. Manford M, Andermann F. Complex visual hallucinations. Clinical and neuro biological insights. Brain 1998; 121(Pt 10); 1819–1840.

285. Evans RW. Exploding head syndrome. Headache 2001; 41; 602–603.

286. Evans RW. Exploding head syndrome followed by sleep paralysis: A rare migraine aura. Headache 2006; 46; 682–683.

287. Jacome DE. Exploding head syndrome and idiopathic stabbing headache relieved by nifedipine. Cephalalgia 2001; 21; 617–618.

288. Manni R, Ratti MT, Tartara A. Nocturnal eating: prevalence and features in 120 insomniac referrals. Sleep 1997; 20(9); 734–738.

289. Winkelman JW. Clinical and polysomnographic features of sleep-related eating disorder. J Clin Psychiatr 1998; 59(1); 14–19.

290. Vetrugno R, Manconi M, Ferini-Strambi L, et al. Nocturnal eating: sleep-related eating disorder or night eating syndrome? A videopolysomnographic study. Sleep 2006; 29(1); 876–877.

291. Allen RP, Walters AS, Montplaisir J, et al. Restless legs syndrome prevalence and impact: REST general population study. Arch Intern Med 2005; 165; 1286–1292.

292. Winklemann J, Ferini-Strambi L. Genetics of restless legs syndrome. Sleep Med Rev 2006 21(1); 28–33.

293. Pichler I, Marrooni F, Volpato CB, et al. Linkage analysis identifies a novel locus for restless legs syndrome on chromosome 2q in a South Tyrolean population isolate. Am J Hum Genet 2006; 79(4); 716–723.

294. Ohayon MM, Roth T. Prevalence of restless legs syndrome and periodic limb movement disorder in the general population. J Psychosom Res 2002; 53(1); 547–554.

295. Pennestri MH, Montplaisir J, Colombo R, et al. Nocturnal blood pressure changes in patients with restless legs syndrome. Neurology 2007; 68; 1213–1218.

296. Rijsman RM, de Weerd AW, Stam CJ, et al. Periodic limb movement disorder and restless legs syndrome in dialysis patients. Nephrology 2004; 9(6); 353–361.

297. Hening WA. Current guidelines and standards of practice for restless legs syndrome. Am J Med 2007; 120(Suppl 1); S22–S27.

298. Stefansson H, Rye DB, Hicks A, et al. A genetic risk factor for periodic limb movements in sleep. A genetic risk factor for periodic limb movements in sleep. N Engl J Med 2007; 357. DOI: 10.1056/NEJMoa072743.

299. Picchietti D, England SJ, Walters A, et al. Periodic limb movement disorder and restless legs syndrome in children with attention-deficit hyperactivity disorder. J Child Neurol 1998; 13(12); 588–594.

300. Picchietti D, Walters A. Moderate to severe periodic limb movement disorder in childhood and adolescence. Sleep 1999; 22; 297–300.

301. Walters AS, Hickey K, Maltzman J, et al. A questionnaire study of 138 patients with restless legs syndrome: The "Night-Walkers" survey. Neurology 1996; 46; 92–95.

302. Walters AS, Picchietti DL, Ehrenberg BL, et al. Restless legs syndrome in childhood and adolescence. Pediatr Neurol 1994; 11; 241–245.

303. Picchietti D, Allen RP, Walters A, et al. Restless legs syndrome: Prevalence and impact in children and adolescence-The Peds REST study. Pediatrics 2007; 120(2); 253–266.

304. Happe S, Treptau N, Ziegler R, et al. Restless legs syndrome and sleep problems in children and adolescents with insulin-dependent diabetes mellitus type 1. Neuropediatrics 2005; 36(2); 98–103.

305. Merlino G, Valente M, Serafini A, et al. Restless legs syndrome: diagnosis, epidemiology, classification and consequences. Neurol Sci 2007; 28(Suppl 1); S37–S46.

306. Chervin RD, Hedger KM. Clinical prediction of periodic leg movements during sleep in children. Sleep Med 2001; 2; 501–510.

307. Chervin RD, Archibold KH, Dillon JE, et al. Associations between symptoms of inattention, hyperactivity, restless legs, and periodic leg movements. Sleep 2002; 25(2); 213–218.

308. Crabtree VM, Ivanenko A, O'Brien LM, et al. Periodic limb movement disorder of sleep in children. J Sleep Res 2003; 12; 73–81.

309. Sun ER, Chen CA, Ho G, et al. Iron and the restless legs syndrome. Sleep 1998; 15; 21(4); 371–377.

310. Mizumo S, Mihara T, Miyoka T, et al. CSF iron, ferritin and transferring levels in restless legs syndrome. J Sleep Res 2005; 14(1); 43–47.

311. Connor JR, Boyer PJ, Menzies SL, et al. Neuropathological examination suggests impaired brain iron acquisition in restless legs syndrome. Neurology 2003; 61(3); 304–309.

312. Earley CJ, Barker P, Horska A, et al. MRI-determined regional brain iron concentrations in early- and late- onset restless legs syndrome. Sleep Med 2006; 7(5); 458–461.

313. Trenkwalder C, Walters AS, Hening WA, et al. Positron emission tomographic studies in restless legs syndrome. Mov Disord 1999; 14(1); 141–145.

314. Cervenka S, Palhagen SE, Comley RA, et al. Support for dopaminergic hypoactivity in restless legs syndrome: a PET study on D2-receptor binding. Brain 2006; 129(Pt 8); 2017–2028.

315. Montagna P. The treatment of restless legs syndrome. Neurol Sci 2007; 28(Suppl1); S61–S66.

316. Aukerman MM, Aukerman D, Bayard M, et al. Exercise and restless legs syndrome: a randomized controlled trial. J Am Board Fam Med 2006; 19; 487–493.

317. Walters AS, Mandelbaum DE, Lewin DS, et al. Dopaminergic therapy in children with restless legs/periodic limb movements in sleep and ADHD. Dopaminergic Therapy Study Group. Pediatr Neurol 2000; 22(3); 182–186.

318. Simakojornboon N, Gozal D, Vlasic V, et al. Perodic limb movements in sleep and iron status in children. Sleep 2003; 26; 735–738.

319. Lazer R, Rowland L. Cramps. N Engl J Med 1971; 285; 31–40.
320. Hall AJ. Cramp and salt balance in ordinary life. Lancet 1947; ii; 231–233.
321. Leung AKC, Wong BE, Cho HYH, et al. Leg cramps in children. Clin Pediatr 1997; 36; 69–73.
322. Leung AKC, Wong BE, Chan PYH, et al. Nocturnal leg cramps in children: Incidence and clinical characteristics. J Natl Med Assoc 1999; 91; 329–332.
323. Norris FH Jr, Gasteiger EL, Chatfield PO. An electromyoraphic study of induced and spontaneous muscle cramps. Electroencephalogr Clin Neurophysiol 1957; 9; 139–147.
324. Jansen PH, Lecluse RG, Verbeek AL. Past and present understanding of the pathophysiology of muscle cramps: why treatment of varicose veins does not relieve leg cramps. J Eur Acad Derm Venereol 1999; 12(3); 222–229.
325. Man-Song-Hing M, Wells G, Lau A. Quinine for nocturnal leg cramps: a metaanalysis including unpublished data. J Gen Int Med 1998; 13(9); 600–606. Date of most recent update 2006; Database of Abstracts of Reviews of Effects 2007; 3. DARE-981581.
326. Vetrugno R, Provini F, Plazzi G, et al. Familial nocturnal facio-mandibular myoclonus mimicking sleep bruxism. Neurol 2002; 58; 644–647.
327. Herrera M, Valencia I, Grant M, et al. Bruxism in children: effect on sleep architecture and daytime cognitive performance and behavior. Sleep 2006; 29(9); 1143–1148.
328. Cheifetz AT, Osaganian SK, Allred EN, et al. Prevalence of bruxism and associated correlates in children as reported by parents. J Dent Child 2005; 72(2); 67–73.
329. Monaco A, Ciammella NM, Marci MC, et al. The anxiety bruxer child. A case-control study. Min Stomotol 2002; 51(6); 247–250.
330. Dooland KV, Townsend GC, Kaidonis JA. Prevalence and side preference for tooth grinding in twins. Aust Dent J 2006; 51(3); 219–224.
331. Malki GA, Zawawi KH, Melis M, et al. Prevalence of bruxism in children receiving treatment for attention deficit hyperactivity disorder: a pilot study. J Clin Pediatr Dent 2004; 29(1); 63–67.
332. Weideman CL, Bush DL, Yan-Go FL, et al. The incidence of parasomnias in child bruxers versus nonbruxers. Pediatr Dent 1996; 18(7); 456–460.
333. Ng DK, Kwok KL, Poon G, et al. Habitual snoring and sleep bruxism in a paediatric outpatient population in Hong Kong. Singapore Med J 2002; 43(11); 554–556.
334. Klackenberg G. Rhythmic movements in infancy and early childhood. Acta Pediatr Scand 1971; 224(Suppl 1); 74–82.
335. Hoban TF. Rhythmic movement disorder in children. CNS Spectrums 2003; 8(2); 135–138.
336. Laberge L, Tremblay R, Vitaro F, et al. Development of parasomnias from childhood to early adolescence. Pediatrics 2000; 106; 67–74.
337. Dyken ME, Lin-Dyken DC, Yamada T. Diagnosing rhythmic movement disorder with video-polysomnography. Pediatr Neurol 1997; 16; 37–41.
338. Kohyama J, Matsukura F, Kimura K, et al. Rhythmic movement disorder: polysomnographic study and summary of reported cases. Brain Devel 2002; 24; 33–38.
339. Manni R, Terzaghi M. Rhythmic movements during sleep: a physiological and pathological profile. Neurol Sci 2005; 26(Suppl 3); S181–S185.

340. Thorpy MJ, Glovinsky PB, Parasomnias. Psychiatr Clin North Am 1987; 10; 623–639.
341. Bombard JR, Sours JA, Spalter HF. Cataracts following chronic headbanging. Am J Psychiatr 1968; 125; 245–249.
342. Sorman GW. The headbanger tumor. Br J Plast Surg 1982; 35; 72–74.
343. Stuck KJ, Hernandez RJ. Large skull defects in a headbanger. Pediatr Radiol 1979; 8; 257–258.
344. Jackson MA, Hughes RC, Ward SP. "Headbanging" and carotid dissection. BMJ (Clin Res Ed) 1983; 287; 1262.
345. Mackenzie JM. "Headbanging" and fatal subdural hemorrhage. Lancet 1991; 338; 1457–1458.
346. Carlock KS, Williams JP, Graves GC. MRI findings in headbangers. Clin Imaging 1997; 21; 411–413.
347. Abe K, Amatomi M, Oda N. Sleepwalking and recurrent sleep-talking in children of childhood sleepwalkers. Am J Psychiatr 1984; 141(6); 800–801.
348. Hublin C, Kaprio J, Partinen M, et al. Sleep-talking in twins: epidemiology and psychiatric comorbidity. Behav Genet 1998; 28(4); 289–298.
349. Oswald I. Sudden bodily jerks on falling asleep. Brain 1959; 82; 92–103.
350. Fusco L, Pachatz C, Cusmai R, et al. Repetative sleep starts in neurologically impaired children: An unusual non-epileptic manifestation in otherwise epileptic subjects. Epilep Dis 1999; 1; 63–67.
351. Sander HW, Geisse H, Quinto C, et al. Sensory sleep starts. J Neurol Neurosurg Psychiatr 1998; 64; 690.
352. Montagna P, Provini F, Vetrugno R. Propriospinal myoclonus at sleep onset. Neurophysiol Clin 2006; 36(5-6); 351–355.
353. Coulter DL, Allen RJ. Benign neonatal myoclonus. Arch Neurol 1982; 32; 191–192.
354. Blennow G. Benign neonatal myoclonus. Acta Paediatr Scand 1985; 74; 505–507.
355. Shuper A, Mimouni M. Problems of differentiation between epilepsy and non-epileptic paroxysmal events in the first year of life. Arch Dis Child 1995; 73(4); 342–344.
356. Ramelli GP, Sozzo AB, Vella S, et al. Benign neonatal sleep myoclonus: An under-recognized, non-epileptic condition. Acta Paediatrica 2005; 94(7); 962–963.
357. Resnik TJ, Moshe SL, Perotta L, et al. Benign neonatal sleep myoclonus. Relationship to sleep states. Arch Neurol 1986; 43; 266–268.
358. DiCapua M, Fusco L, Ricci S, et al. Benign neonatal sleep myoclonus: clinical features and video-polygraphic recordings. Mov Disord 1993; 8; 191–194.
359. Alfonso I, Papazian O, Aicardi J, et al. A simple maneuver to provoke benign neonatal sleep myoclonus. Pediatrics 1995; 96(6); 1161–1163.
360. Gall J. "Binkie-Flutter", an apparently voluntary behavior of infants, possibly related to ibratory jaw movements in dogs: Report of 4 cases. Pediatrics 2005; 115(3); e367–e369. http://www.pediatrics.org/cgi/content/full/115/1/e367.
361. Goraya JS, Virdi V, Parmar V. Recurrent nocturnal tongue biting in a child with hereditary chin trembling. J Child Neurol 2006; 21; 985–987.
362. Johnson LF, KInsbourne M, Renuart AW. Hereditary chin-trembling with nocturnal myoclonus and tongue biting in dizygotic twins. Dev Med Child Neurol 1971; 13; 726–729.
363. Tuxhorn I, Hoppe M. Parasomnia with rhythmic movements manifesting as nocturnal tongue biting. Neuropediatrics 1993; 24(3); 167–168.

364. Blaw ME, Leroy RF, Steinberg JB, et al. Hereditary chin quivering and REM behavior disorder. Ann Neurol 1989; 26; 471.
365. Jarman PR, Wood NW, Davis MT, et al. Hereditary geniospasm: linkage to chromosome 9q13-q21 and evidence for genetic heterogeneity. Am J Hum Genet 1997; 61(4); 928–933.
366. Soland VL, Bhatia KP, Sheean GL, et al. Hereditary geniospasm: two new families. Mov Disord 1996; 11(6); 744–746.
367. Della Marca G, Rubino M, Vollono C, et al. Rhythmic tongue movements during sleep: A peculiar parasomnias in Costello syndrome. Mov Disord 2006; 21(4); 473–478.
368. Costello JM. A new syndrome. NZ Med J 1971; 74; 397.
369. Walters AS. Clinical identification of the simple sleep-related movement disorders. Chest 2007; 131(4); 1260–1266.
370. Sheik S, Stephen TC, Sisson B. Prevalence of Gastroesophageal reflux in infants with brief apneic episodes. Can Resp J 1999; 6; 401–404.
371. Lugaresi E, Cirignotta F. Hypnogogic paroxysmal dystonia: epileptic seizure or new syndrome? Sleep 1981; 4; 129.
372. Tinuper P, Cerullo A, Cirignotta F, et al. Nocturnal paroxysmal dystonia with short-lasting attacks: three cases with evidence for an epileptic frontal lobe origin of seizures. Epilepsia 1990; 31(5); 549–556.
373. Cohen HA, Ashkenazi A, Barzilai A, et al. Nocturnal acute laryngospasm in children: a possible epileptic phenomenon. J Child Neurol 2000; 15; 202–204.
374. Lombroso C. Pavor nocturnus of proven epileptic origin. Epilepsia 2000; 41(9); 1221–1226.
375. Huppertz HJ, Schulze-Bonhage A. Epileptic pavor nocturnus. Epilepsia 2001; 42(5); 704–705.
376. Malow BA. Paroxysmal events in sleep. J Clin Neurophysiol 2002; 19(6); 522–534.
377. Commission on Classification and Terminology of the International League Against Epilepsy. Proposal for revised classification of epilepsies and epileptic syndromes. Epilepsia 1989; 30; 389–399.
378. Andermann E, Andermann F, Silver K, et al. Benign familial nocturnal alternating hemiplegia of childhood. Neurology 1994; 44; 1812–1814.
379. Chaves-Vischer V, Picard F, Andermann E, et al. Benign nocturnal alternating hemiplegia of childhood: Six patients and long term follow-up. Neurology 2001; 57; 1491–1493.

5

Somatoform Disorder

INTRODUCTION TO SOMATOFORM DISORDERS

Somatization and conversion disorders comprise two identifiable entities for which, among other things, functional neurological deficits occur in the absence of an identifiable neurological disease or medical explanation. Common presentations of these pseudoneurological disorders are psychogenic non-epileptic seizures, psychogenic alterations in consciousness, and various forms of pseudoparalysis. Individual subjects will exhibit a panoply of seizure and post-ictal manifestations, many of which may be difficult to casually differentiate from true epileptic events. In that circumstance, EEG telemetry may be needed to secure the observed behavior as non-epileptic. Specific diagnosis will depend upon the identification of environmental and psychological factors at play that promote the development of these symptoms. The contextual presentation and the clarity with which the clinician explains and enlightens the subject will best determine the overall outcomes, not least of which will be the avoidance of inappropriate and potentially life-threatening medical intervention. Particularly challenging will be the not infrequent comorbidity of concurrent epilepsy and somatization and/or conversion disorder in the same individual.

THE CLINICAL PROBLEM AND EPIDEMIOLOGY

Somatoform disorder (Briquet's syndrome) is included in a group of clinical entities identified in common by the presence of physical symptoms suggesting a medical condition but are not fully explained by an underlying medical condition, substance, or other mental disorder.[1] The symptoms produce significant enough distress to impair function. If an underlying medical condition is identified, it is one that does not fully account for the degree of functional impairment encountered. These disorders occur frequently in children and are often transient in duration. In childhood, the developmental aspects of the child's maturational age impacts directly upon the subsequently manifest symptom complex. There is an additional impact upon this symptom complex, provoked by the child's reaction to the parental or guardian's response to these initial symptoms and the circumstances within which those symptoms developed. The most common somatoform physical symptoms (e.g., headache, stomach pain, limb pains, etc.) are provoked within the context of what is

referred to as an adjustment disorder. This is where combinations of psychological symptoms (anxiety, anger, etc.) and regressive behaviors develop in
response to common everyday life stresses. These reactions tend to be brief in
duration, equally represented between the genders, and with relatively simple
symptomatology. Conversion disorders (dissociative disorders) provoke more
significant physical symptoms (loss of function, pseudoneurological signs, etc.)
in the context of a more complex emotional stressor. This has a greater frequency among girls overall and more significantly so in preteen and teenage
age groups. Not uncommonly these too may be transient, particularly when
identified early and precipitating stressors are revealed and addressed. The
more chronic and severe aspects of the spectrum make up the diagnosable
somatoform disorders as defined by the DSM-IV-TR (Table 5-1).

Table 5-1 Somatoform Disorder

Diagnostic Criteria for Somatization Disorder (300.81)
1. History of many physical complaints beginning before age 30 years, occur over a period of
   years, result in treatment being sought or significant impairment in social, occupational,
   or other important areas of functioning
2. Each of the following at any time during the illness:
   (a) Four pain symptoms related to at least four different sites or functions
   (b) Two gastrointestinal symptoms other than pain
   (c) One sexual or reproductive symptom other than pain
   (d) One pseudoneurological symptom or deficit not limited to pain
3. Either (a) or (b)
   (a) After appropriate investigation, each symptom in criterion 2 cannot be fully
       explained by a known general medical condition or the direct effects of a substance
   (b) When there is a related general medical condition, the physical complaints or
       resulting impairments (social or occupational) are in excess of what would be
       expected from history, physical examination , or laboratory findings
4. The symptoms are not intentionally produced or feigned.

Diagnostic Criteria for Undifferentiated Somatoform Disorder (300.82)
1. One or more physical complaints
2. Either (a) or (b)
   (a) After appropriate investigation, the symptoms cannot be fully explained by a known
       general medical condition or the direct effects of a substance
   (b) When there is a related general medical condition, the physical complaints or result-
       ing impairments (social or occupational) are in excess of what would be expected
       from history, physical examination , or laboratory findings
3. The symptoms cause clinically significant distress or impairment in social, occupational,
   or other important areas of functioning
4. The duration of the disturbance is at least 6 months
5. The disturbance is not better accounted for by another mental disorder
6. The symptoms are not intentionally produced or feigned

Source: Modified from Reference.[1]

An important aspect of somatization disorders is that these are unintentional in nature (nonvolitional). The more severe end of the somatization
spectrum includes conversion disorder, pain disorder, hypochondriasis, and
body dysmorphic disorder.[1] Where there is insufficient criteria to satisfy a specific diagnosis, a "not otherwise specified" designation may be appropriate.
Illness falsification (Munchausen syndrome), malingering and by extension,
illness falsification disorder by proxy abuse (Munchausen by proxy, Meadow's
syndrome), all share the commonality of being an intentional production or
feigning of illness signs and symptoms.[1] In the case of illness falsification, the
intentional fabrication of symptoms and signs of illness is not due to external incentives prompting the individual to develop the symptom complex, but
rather there is an internal and subconscious psychological need to assume the
sick role.[1] In the circumstance of illness falsification by proxy, the perpetrator
presents a child for repeated medical evaluation of fabricated illness symptoms
and signs solely for the psychological benefit of the perpetrator. Malingering,
on the other hand, is a conscious and deliberate action to deceive in order to
gain some external incentive. These are all generally confirmed and revealed
by direct observation, objective evidence, and/or excluding other causes of
the symptoms. Other mental conditions that often include unexplained physical complaints are notable with major depressive disorders and anxiety
disorders.[1]

The appropriateness of the DSM-IV-TR criteria to diagnose childhood
somatization disorders can be questioned, although the diagnostic criteria
for conversion disorder may be more easily applicable (Tables 5-1 and 5-2).
The recognition of culturally sanctioned behaviors and experiences may also
help the clinician to understand the co-occurrence of particular presentations
(syncope, vertigo, seizures, blindness, paralysis, etc.) at specific times within
specific populations. The development of "mass hysteria" and other epidemics
of complex symptom presentations within communities, school settings, and
at cultural and religious gatherings should be taken into consideration.[2,3]
Although the majority of subjects suffering within the context of mass hysteria experience non-epileptic convulsive seizure events, sudden collapse with
little motor movement is not uncommon.[2,3] Long-term social and psychological consequences are often later expressed by those subjects. Mass hysteria has
been described in two main categories: mass motor hysteria, and mass anxiety
hysteria. Involuntary motor movements and dissociation, persisting for several
weeks and precipitated by social circumstances or stress, each characterize mass
motor hysteria. Mass anxiety hysteria arises from a falsely perceived sense of
danger. It is usually short-lived (hours to days), with a prominence of somatic
complaints expressed or exhibited.[3]

In the context of non-epileptic nonorganic phenomena with an "apparent" alteration of consciousness, somatoform disorders presenting as nonphysiologic non-epileptic seizures (NES), also referred to as psychogenic
non-epileptic seizures (PNES), is an important entity.[4,5] This type of somatoform disorder has even been reported as adult-onset breath-holding spells.[6]

Table 5-2 Conversion Disorder

Diagnostic Criteria for Conversion Disorder (300.11)

1. One or more symptoms or deficits affecting voluntary motor or sensory function that suggest a neurological or other general medical condition.
2. Psychological factors are judged to be associated with the symptom or deficit because the initiation or exacerbation of the symptom or deficit is preceded by conflicts or other stressors.
3. The symptom or deficit is not intentionally produced or feigned.
4. The symptom or deficit cannot, after appropriate investigation, be fully explained by a general medical condition, or by the direct effects of a substance, or as a culturally sanctioned behavior or experience.
5. The symptom or deficit is not limited to pain or sexual dysfunction, does not occur exclusively during the course of somatization disorder, and is not better accounted for by another mental disorder.

Specific type of symptom or deficit:

    With motor symptom or deficit
    With sensory symptom or deficit
    With seizures or convulsions
    With mixed presentation

Source: Modified from Reference.[1]

When PNES develop in a rather sophisticated individual, the clinical observations can be difficult to discriminate from true epileptic seizures.[5] Their resemblance to true epileptic seizures can sometimes only be distinguished by the absence of concomitant EEG epileptiform discharges during the event. These are reported to be as prevalent as 12%–21% of admissions to pediatric epilepsy monitoring units.[6–8] However, cumulative data from several large studies suggest a prevalence of recognized somatoform disorders presenting to epilepsy monitoring units to be about 4.7% (2.7%–8.1%, see Table 1-6). This lower incidence figure may be due to the nature of the referral population in that there are clearly a number of other "organic" and physiological entities, which may mimic epileptic seizures. The incidence of non-epileptic seizures in populations identified with somatoform disorders as a primary reason for referral may be quite different and helps to explain the divergence of quoted incidence figures. Although the term pseudoseizures may be accurate, care providers often misinterpret this to imply "feigned or put on." In response, patients and families often interpret this term as disparaging, or to mean "not real."[6,7] In reality, these are events that express a reaction to chronic or acute stress, which exceeds the capacity of the individual to adapt to it. Thus, these events are neither feigned nor intentional and are in fact very real. These stressors are often overlooked or denied by the patient and their family. Therefore, the terms psychogenic non-epileptic seizures (PNES), non-epileptic seizure (NES), or stress-related seizure are preferable.

Population studies of childhood somatoform disorders are few. A longitudinal study of the development of psychiatric disorders and need for mental health services in youth from 11 counties of western North Carolina was initiated in 1992 and conducted through 1996.[9] A representative sample of 4500 young people aged 9, 11, and 13 years was randomly selected, and parents were interviewed using validated screening tools such as the Child Behavior Checklist. All children scoring above a cutoff score (20, designed to include 25% of the population), and a 1 in 10 random sample of those scoring below the cutoff, were recruited for the longitudinal survey through age 16 years. Between 80% and 94% (3733) of the initial sample participated. The subsequent interviews utilized the Child and Adolescent Psychiatric Assessment (CAPA) to generate DSM-III diagnoses. Of the somatic complaints reported, the overall prevalence of musculoskeletal pains was 2.2%, stomach aches 2.8%, and headaches 10%.[9] The association between somatic complaints with depression and anxiety disorders was significantly higher in girls than boys, and the association of somatic complaints and disruptive behavior disorders, significantly higher in boys. More importantly, there were specific gender effects, with depressed girls having a four times greater prevalence of headaches and a thirteen times greater prevalence of musculoskeletal pains than nondepressed girls. Girls with anxiety disorder had a one hundred times greater prevalence of stomachaches and headaches combined. In boys, musculoskeletal pains were the only complaint associated with an emotional disorder.

In another large population study involving the Pediatric Research in Office Settings (PROS) network and the Ambulatory Sentinel Practice Network (ASPN), data from 21,065 patient visits concerning somatization in pediatric primary care settings reported by 395 clinicians representing 204 medical practices from 44 states, 4 Canadian provinces, and Puerto Rico, were analyzed.[10] Data collected included demographic characteristics, family functioning, child functioning, health care utilization, and psychiatric symptomatology utilizing The Pediatric Symptom Checklist (PSC). The risk of being a somatizer increased with age, from 0.99% of 4–5-year-olds to 2.5% of 11–15-year-olds ($p < 0.001$), and in girls of older age groups ($p < 0.001$).[8] From the entire group, 14.6% of all children and 50% of the somatizers screened positive for psychopathology. Families of somatizers were more likely to be classified as dysfunctional on the basis of these parental reports ($p < 0.001$).[10] The data again support the notion that unexplained somatic complaints might be within the context of a child with unrecognized but significant mental health needs, functional impairments, and familial dysfunction.

The exposure to an ill parent in childhood has been suggested to be a factor leading to the development of adult somatization disorder. The intergenerational transmission of somatization behavior has been studied by one group of investigators by means of a cross-sectional comparative design.[11] Three groups of mothers and their children 4–8 years of age—48 mothers suffering from chronic somatization, 51 mothers with chronic organic illness, and 52 healthy mothers—were observed and compared.[11] Somatizing mothers were more likely to report exposure to childhood neglect and to physical illness in a parent. The children of these somatizing mothers were more likely to have health problems and doctor visits than those children from the organically ill or healthy mothers.[11] This observation was further explored in the same groups by observing joint attention between mother-child pairs during play activities.[12] Structured play with and without a medical theme and snack time were observed and scored from videotaped play sessions. Results showed that somatizing mothers had less joint attention to their child at play than did the organically ill and healthy mothers. Somatizing mothers were more responsive to their child's bid for attention during medical theme play than at other times. The two studies taken together suggest that there may be a risk of somatization to be a learned response through modeling and reinforcement and not merely through innate psychopathology.[12] These observations have particular relevance with respect to non-epileptic seizures in that familial epilepsy or concurrent epilepsy within the same individual is not an uncommon association. This suggests the potential for a learned response by exposure within the appropriate environmental context.

Genetic contributions may also be a factor in the development of somatization disorders. Earlier research showed that somatization disorders tended to cluster in families as did several other disorders (i.e., alcoholism, antisocial personality disorder, ADHD).[13] Studies of monozygotic and dizygotic twins, however, have failed to demonstrate genetic links.[14–16] Prior experience of physical/sexual abuse in childhood have been strongly associated with somatization disorders in adulthood.[17] More recent studies of childhood somatization identify these factors as well but have not found this association to be as important or as constant.[18] A more complex interplay between remote trauma and more recent commonplace stressors of school, peer relationships, and family issues appear to have an equal or greater role in the acute precipitation of symptom presentation.

Conversion disorder is the psychiatric diagnosis most commonly associated with non-epileptic seizure phenomena. This is rare in children under age 8 years and most common in children 10 years of age through adolescence. As defined in Table 5-2, the symptom complex mimics a general medical condition and commonly takes on the character of a neurological disorder or neurological deficit.[1] Therefore, diagnostic accuracy is paramount and will inevitably involve some laboratory, neuroimaging, or neurophysiologic investigation in addition to psychiatric assessment. In a recent systematic literature review that included studies published since 1965 on the diagnostic outcome of adults with motor and sensory symptoms unexplained by disease, Stone and colleagues critically appraised this literature and carried out a multivariate, random effect, meta-analysis of the data.[19] They reported on 27 studies totaling 1466 patients with a median duration of follow-up of 5 years. There was a significant ($p < 0.02$) decline in the mean rate of misdiagnosis from the 1950s to the present day, declining from 29% in the 1950s to 4% (2%–6%) in the 1990s.[19] This decline was independent of age, sex, and duration of symptom and was probably due to improvements in study quality rather than improved diagnostic accuracy, arising from the introduction of brain imaging.[19]

The need to fully investigate children who present with conversion disorder symptoms should be tempered by the greater need to establish appropriate interventions. In a retrospective study of fifty-two pediatric patients with conversion disorders admitted to an Australian tertiary care teaching hospital over a 10-year interval, the typical child had multiple complaints, with pain (75%) and gait disturbances (69%) the most common combination.[20] Although 32/52 (62%) recovered by the time of discharge, those who underwent extensive investigation with difficulty in securing diagnosis were unaffected by treatment and experienced extremely lengthy hospitalizations (25%, average stay 31 days).[20] The polysymptomatic presentation of conversion disorder in children has been suggested to represent a unique entity of somatoform disorder with poorer prognosis and more past psychiatric and family problems.[21,22] Similar conclusions have been reached with a cohort of children who presented with PNES.[23] From among fifty-six children identified with PNES utilizing video-telemetry, 77% of subjects suffered from moderate to severe pain, most commonly headache (61%). Neck pain and backache were also common. Twenty-six of twenty-seven patients (96%) with persistent PNES, compared to seventeen (58%) whose PNES was resolved, experienced moderate to severe pain ($p < 0.001$).[23] Pain may be considered an under-recognized problem that occurs frequently and with significant severity among PNES patients. This feature suggests a commonality with somatoform disorders, not previously emphasized. Poorer outcomes have also been noted in adults who were originally diagnosed with conversion disorder and later reassessed as somatisizers upon long-term follow-up.[24]

Childhood conversion disorder generally carries a good outcome but has the potential to produce or uncover significant long-term comorbidities.[25–27] Upwards of 15% may continue to experience symptoms and fail to recover from their conversion disorder presentation over the long term. As many as 35% of children with conversion disorders will be diagnosed with mood or anxiety disorders 4 to 5 years later.[28] Population data are limited, however. The coexistence of medical causes, other mental health disorders, and culturally sanctioned behaviors makes epidemiological studies of conversion disorder in children difficult.[29] There are, however, several large-scale population surveys available. A population interview survey of 3021 randomly selected adolescents in Germany, followed over 3 years with longitudinal interviews using the Munich-Composite International Diagnostic Interview (MCIDI), supplemented by questions to cover DSM-IV and ICD-10 criteria for somatoform disorders, found that somatoform symptoms were quite prevalent among 14- to 24-year olds.[30] Fifty per cent of respondents reported a lifetime history of at least one somatoform symptom, and 10% experienced more than three.[30] Remarkably, similar findings have been reported from surveys of parents of preschool children in Spain and Sweden, with up to 15% reporting four symptoms within the prior 2 weeks.[31,32] The most commonly reported symptom was headache, followed by a lump in the throat and abdominal pain. Lifetime prevalence of any specific somatoform disorder was estimated to be 2.7%. The most prevalent somatoform disorders were pain disorder, with a lifetime risk of 1.7%, and conversion disorder, with an estimated lifetime risk of 0.4%.[30] In a retrospective chart review of an Iowan medical population, 11 subjects ages 9–20 years old were identified with conversion disorders from a total of 220,306 patients evaluated over a 2-year interval, equating to an approximate incidence rate of 2.4/100,000 per year.[33] A national surveillance study of childhood (<16 years old) conversion disorders in Australia has also recently been reported.[18] The survey compiled ascertainment reports through a voluntary reporting system of general practitioners and hospital emergency departments to the Australian Pediatric Surveillance Units (APSU).[18] Participation among Australia's 1050 pediatricians was 96% during the period of study (2002–2003). Diagnostic criteria conformed to that defined in the current DSM-IV-TR (see Table 5-2). Monthly e-mail prompts were sent to clinicians, and qualifying case questionnaires were subsequently reviewed and compiled. From an initial 310 reports, 194 confirmed conversion disorder cases were identified, resulting in a population (<16 years old) annual incidence of 2.3/100,000 (95% confidence interval[CI], 2.0–2.6/100,000). The reported incidence for children younger than 10 years was lower at 0.8/100,000 (95% CI 0.6–1.1/100,000). Most children (55%) presented with more than one symptom and 33% had three or more.[18] Importantly, there was an age-related difference in the rates of NES as a presentation of conversion symptom. NES was the presentation in only 11% of children less than 10 years old and 26% of those 10–16 years of age.[18] The presenting symptoms were often thought of as an acute response to a specific stressor; however, symptoms ranged in duration for up to 2 years before a diagnosis was established. The antecedent stressors most often identified in the Australian cohort were family separations or loss (34%), family conflicts or violence (20%), school and learning difficulties (14%), recent subject illness (8%), recent family member illness (7%), bullying (6%), sexual assault (4%), and others (7%).[18] These findings emphasize that more commonplace stressors may be significant triggers of conversion reactions as opposed to the prevailing and primary sexual abuse and trauma precipitants as previously held.[20,27]

The symptoms of conversion disorder must be associated with an identifiable stressor. When appropriate factors exist, the conversion symptoms evolve most often as neurological disturbances of voluntary motor function, sensory impairments, PNES, and respiratory and swallowing difficulties (see Table 5-3). Girls are affected in a ratio of 3:1 to boys in most series across all age groups. The timing of the stressor may bear some impact upon the severity of the conversion symptomatology. This is supported by the results of a recent comparative study of a group of fifty-four subjects with conversion disorder to a group of fifty control subjects with an affective disorder.[34] Each group was screened for life events experienced in the year before the symptom onset. Conversion subjects did not differ from control subjects in the number or severity of life events.[34] Conversion

Table 5-3 Primary Presentation of Conversion Disorder

Gender/ Symptom	Kozlowska[18] N = 194	Turgay[25] N = 137	Grattan- Smith[20] N = 52(54)*	Ho[36] N = 46	Pehlivanturk[28] N = 40
Boys	56 (29%)	38 (28%)	12 (25%)	9 (20%)	10 (25%)
Girls	138 (71%)	99 (72%)	39 (75%)	37 (80%)	30 (75%)
Disturbed Motor Function	124 (64%)	62 (45%)	36 (69%)	14 (22%)	4 (8.5%)
Motor Weakness	75 (39%)	2 (1.5%)	2 (4%)	0	0
Limb Paralysis	28 (14%)	2 (1.5%)	12 (23%)	7 (10%)	0
Abnormal Gait/Ataxia	73 (38%)	27 (20%)	36 (69%)	7 (10%)	0
Abnormal Movements	32 (16%)	13 (9%)	2 (4%)	1 (2%)	0
Abnormal Speech/Swallow	8 (4%)	18 (13%)	2 (4%)	0	0
Sensory Disturbances	46 (24%)	9 (6.5%)	40 (77%)	15 (32%)	4 (8.5%)
Paresthesia/ Anesthesia	23 (11%)	7 (5%)	40 (77%)	0	0
Visual Impairments	24 (12%)	2 (1.5%)	3 (6%)	1 (2%)	0
Hearing Impairments	5 (2%)	0	0	0	0
Non-Epileptic Seizures (PNES)	44 (23%)	63 (46.5%)	8 (15%)	15 (32%)	33 (83%)
Respiratory Difficulties	27 (14%)	3 (2%)	1 (2%)	0	0
Other	0	0	2 (4%)	0	0
Mixed/Combined Symptoms	106 (55% ≤ 3) 64 (33% >3)	0	40 (77%)	2 (4%)	1 (2.5%)

Source: Modified from References.[18,20,25,28,36]
Other = sneezing, PNES = psychogenic non-epileptic seizures.
* Two subjects had two separate conversion episodes.

subjects, however, showed a significant relationship between more recent life events and a greater severity of conversion symptoms. Especially contributing to this effect were life events with respect to work and relationships (family and interpersonal), particularly when these events occurred in the context of prior childhood or remote physical/sexual abuse.[34] These effects remained even after controlling for the previously found effects of childhood traumatization on the severity of conversion symptoms.[34] The findings implied that conversion symptoms may be precipitated by a composite of early and late life stressors that are best understood through mutifactorial stress models and not simply by the presence or absence of physical/sexual abuse.

The symptoms of conversion disorders are particularly distressing for the parents and care providers of the children so affected. There is a frequent observation that, distinct from the reaction of the parent, the affected children often exhibit an apparent lack of concern toward their own symptoms (la belle indifférence). This clinical recognition of apparent indifference to one's symptoms is often thought of as clinically meaningful. A systematic literature review evaluating the utility of this finding to discriminate between 356 reported patients with symptoms from conversion and symptoms from organic illness found that 21% of subjects with conversion disorder and 29% of subjects with organic disease displayed la belle indifférence, making it unhelpful as a clinical sign.[35] Whether the same would hold in pure childhood populations would be speculative at this point, but probable, given our current limited data.[36–38]

OVERVIEW: PATHOPHYSIOLOGY AND MECHANISMS

The underlying causes and mechanisms of somatoform and conversion disorders are neither well studied nor well understood. Brain activation studies using functional MRI techniques (fMRI) in several small cohort studies of subjects displaying different conversion disorder symptomatology when compared to normal control subjects have described similar patterns of results.[36–40] These studies have demonstrated a paradoxical inhibition of the expected normally activated cortical regions and involved neural networks with concurrent increased activation within the frontal lobes, particularly the left inferior region.[36–40] This region of the frontal lobe may be needed to specifically inhibit those cortical and subcortical regional circuits involved in the deficient function expressed by the conversion symptomatology. This overall pattern of inferior frontal lobe activation has been demonstrated in subjects, with visual loss and concomitant paradoxical inhibition of the corresponding visual cortex, cognitive processing impairments with concomitant paradoxical inhibition of the corresponding association areas, and motor weakness and paralysis with concomitant paradoxical inhibition of the corresponding motor cortexes and pathways.[39–42]

The roles of genetics, coupled with environmental factors, appear to have a significant impact upon the expression of somatic symptoms and potentially upon conversion disorder in particular. Genetic polymorphisms have been identified within the promoter region of the serotonin transporter gene, and the catechol-O-methyltransferase (COMT) and tryptophan hydroxylase-2 (the rate-limiting enzyme for serotonin biosynthesis) genes.[43–45] Individuals with each of these genetic variations have been associated with the behavioral traits for greater anxiety and liability to react to hardship with greater degrees of emotional distress. Individuals with both the serotonin transporter gene polymorphism and each of the other gene variants (COMT and tryptophan hydroxylase-2) experience greater reductions in concomitant serotonin neurotransmitter uptake as a physiological consequence, and an even greater anxiety response to provoked behavioral responses. The combination of the low-expressing alleles of the serotonin transporter gene coupled with lower COMT activity yielded greater sensitivity to pain stress and diminished up regulation of opiod release.[46] These sensitivities are evident not only on clinical examination but also, now, by metabolic brain imaging and neurophysiologic testing.[44–46] Neuroimaging has identified greater amygdala activation using C^{11} carfentanil imaging during anxiety, and increased neurophysiological event-related potentials (ERPs) of neural activity at 240 ms during a passive emotional picture perception task. Combinations of these anxiety-enhancing genetic variations in the serotonin transporter and tryptophan hydroxylase-2 genes appear to be additive in modulating the sensory encoding of affective stimuli, physiologically identified using these techniques.[44–46]

Family coping styles and the effects of modeling are likely another potent influence on individuals who develop somatoform disorders. As commented upon earlier, the effects of learned behaviors transmitted as a function of exposure to somatization behavior cannot be overlooked.[11,12] Within the context of the family, there is the structure of an expected response to specific exposures such as illness and stress. There has been identified the familial clustering of somatization disorders, with higher rates of somatic complaints reported by the children of parents with somatization disorders.[47,48] The parents of children with somatic complaints have been noted to exhibit overprotectiveness, and thus may foster greater dependency from the child due to a perceived child vulnerability.[20] Whether this perception and adaptation serves some other function within the context of family dynamics (e.g., parental conflict avoidance) is unknown, but has been postulated.[49,50] There may be an underlying inability or poorer qualitative ability to effectively cope with a presented stress, where coping is a voluntary effort to regulate emotion, physiology, thought, or behavior. The stressful exposure induces physiologic responses; an individual may actively attempt to modify these responses, make efforts to accommodate to these physiologic changes by means of acceptance or distraction, or passively cope by means of avoidance. When the presented stress exceeds the ability of the child to cope, maladaptive strategies may be invoked—this may be unknowingly or knowingly sanctioned by the family.[38,50–52] Longitudinal studies of adults with somatic disorders note increased symptoms with greater emotional upheaval.[53] These studies have also suggested that more prior childhood illness and a parental "lack of care" contribute to the chronicity of somatization and continued failure to adopt neutralizing coping strategies.[53,54] In a recent study of young adults who were previously evaluated for recurrent abdominal pain in earlier childhood, when compared to control adults who were participants in a previous childhood study of tonsillectomy and adenoidectomy, investigators found a strong specific association between recurrent abdominal pain and adulthood anxiety.[55] The development of later anxiety and mood disorders in prior childhood somatisizers has been strongly emphasized in longitudinal population follow-up studies and literature reviews.[27,55–61] For a summary of the factors discussed in the foregoing sections, see Table 5-4.

Table 5-4 Factors Involved with Somatoform Disorder

Family Predispositions and Precipitants

- Parental history of somatization
- Parental history of mood disorder
- Parental/family discord
- Parental perception of vulnerable child
- Limited parental-child communication

Child Predispositions and Precipitants

- Social difficulties
- Academic problems
- Life stressors
- Physical illness
- Prior physical/sexual abuse
- Self perception of vulnerability
- Inadequate coping skills
- Genetic predisposition to mood disorders
- Learned somatization behavior

Maintaining Factors

- Reinforcement of sick role
- Avoidance of family tensions
- Avoidance of life stressors
- Evolution of mood disorder
- Enhancement of maladaptive coping mechanisms

Source: Modified from References.[59,60]

THE CLINICAL CONDITIONS AND TREATMENTS: NON-EPILEPTIC SEIZURES

Somatoform disorders of childhood may evolve several neurological presentations, especially within the framework of a conversion disorder. As described in the preceding sections, the most common presentations include a loss of voluntary motor function, or gait disturbance, frequently with a concurrent complaint of pain. A number of rather unusual neurological presentations have been reported, with only a few potentially misinterpreted as epileptic (Table 5-5). It is important to keep perspective in that although the foregoing discussion has been targeted toward nonphysiologic events, there are clearly many more physiologic phenomena that also bear potential confusion with epileptic seizures, and hence this book. There are a number of terms used interchangeably throughout the literature, which in some circumstances have been imprecise, misinterpreted, and at times considered pejorative. The terms stress seizures and psychogenic non-epileptic seizures (PNES), meaning that these are nonphysiologic non-epileptic events, are preferred rather than the terms pseudoseizures, psychogenic seizures, and hysterical attacks.

Table 5-5 Conversion Disorder Nonphysiologic Neurological Presentations

Disturbed Voluntary Motor Function

- Gait abnormality (ataxia)
- Limb paralysis
- Paraplegia
- Abnormal movements (tremor, twitches, posturing, "tics")
- Abnormal speech
- Abnormal swallow ("Globus hystericus")

Disturbed Sensory Function

- Visual abnormality (blindness, visual field deficits, obscurations, diplopia, triplopia, pallinopsia)
- Ocular abnormality (convergence spasm, strabismus, ptosis, abnormal ocular movements, pupillary disturbances)
- Anesthesia
- Paresthesia
- Vertigo
- Altered taste, hearing, smell, balance

Non-Epileptic Seizures

- Motor convulsions
- Staring spells
- Stuttering
- Altered mental states
- Syncope
- Narcoleptic events

Respiratory Abnormalities

- Dyspnea
- Hyperventilation
- Breath-holding spells
- Cough
- Hiccoughs

Others

- Urinary retention
- Hypergraphia

Source: Modified from References.[6, 18, 20, 25, 28, 36, 62–81]

The true frequency of PNES in childhood is not definitively known. A compilation of diagnoses encountered in reports from large pediatric epilepsy-monitoring units identify PNES in 12%–21% of cognitively normal referred subjects who are definitively diagnosed after EEG recording the events in 8% (Table 1-3).[82–87] This prevalence figure is somewhat lower when subjects are cognitively impaired, approximating 4.7% (range 2.7%–8.1%, see Table 1-7).[6–8, 87–93] These prevalence rates are in contrast to the calculated 39.9% (range 15%–83%) reported in representative reports of series of pediatric subjects evaluated for a conversion disorder specifically (Table 5-3).[18,20,25,28,36,94] These overall estimates are even higher in adult populations, with an estimated prevalence of PNES identified at epilepsy centers of 15%–30%.[95,96] This equates with a population prevalence of about 2–33/100,000 persons.[95,96] The concurrent diagnosis of true epilepsy complicated by superimposed PNES is more difficult to clearly articulate for pediatric subjects, but has been reported to be about 10%–18%.[82,97,98] Epilepsy, PNES, and developmental delays have been clearly identified in one study, which reported the prevalence to be 4.8%.[82] Estimates for adults with concurrent epilepsy and PNES have been similar to those of the pediatric series, about 9%–15%.[98,99] Previously reported higher estimates have been based upon dubious interpretation of interictal EEG findings.[100]

The diagnosis of PNES on clinical grounds and history alone in most instances is difficult. Often the initial intervention for a suspected seizure begins at the subject's home by virtue of emergency medical personnel or within the confines of the emergency department. Initial descriptions may be provided by distraught family members or available only through second-hand written descriptions of limited detail. Even with direct observation, occasionally the event can be sophisticated enough to be persuasive for true epileptic seizures in the absence of concurrent video-EEG monitoring. More importantly, however, there is always a need to be diagnostically certain so as to be able to present the problem cogently with the subject and family. Mere clinical pronouncements, as in the days of Charcot, will likely not suffice.[101]

The clinical manifestations of PNES can resemble the semiology of virtually any epileptic-type seizure. Published pediatric series offer clinical descriptions that divide more frequently into varying types of motor manifestations than nonmotor behaviors (Table 5-6).[79,80,82,92,94,102–106] However, the frequencies are approximations because both the descriptions and extracted frequencies reflect the type of behavior being studied in specific ages and circumstances and not consecutive subjects. The duration of the PNES events were quite variable from mere seconds, particularly in regard to head drops, staring, and eye-rolling behaviors, to as long as 35 minutes for "generalized" convulsive-type motor movements. Overall, motor events tend to be long (i.e., greater than 3–5 minutes). The frequency was also variable, ranging from multiple daily events to as infrequent as every 3–4 months. Children under 10 years of age most often display staring behavior or some rhythmic rocking with unresponsiveness. Older children more often engage in greater motor involvement.

Subjects commonly will announce the beginning of an event as they begin to perceive aura symptoms of tingling, numbness, or lightheadedness. Observations have been emphasized concerning a slow crescendo quality to the events, where one particular activity will be evident for several minutes, gradually intensify, then often evolve to dominate another body part, or change movement pattern. Alternatively, sudden starts and stops may predominate. Forced eye closure with active opposition to opening has been noted in an

Table 5-6 Pediatric PNES Manifestations

Clinical Descriptions	Range of Observed Frequencies (%)
Altered Mental Status	8–60
Staring Spells	8–60
Unresponsiveness	0–18
Vocalizations	0–23
Groaning/Shrieking	0–36
Hyperventilation	6–18
Limb Movements	0–32
In-Phase and Out-of-Phase	41–60
Jerking	32–48
Kicking	0–2
Stiffening	0–2
Thrashing	41–60
Generalized Body Movements	41–60
Collapsing	0–48
Limpness	10–45
Stiffening	0–2
Jerking	0–14
Thrashing	0–15
Tremulousness	0–15
Rolling Side-to-Side	0–14
Pelvic Thrusting	0–14
Eye/Eyelid Movements	0–5
Upward	
Fluttering	
Head/Neck Movements	
Side-to-Side	
Flexion Extension	
Pseudo-Status Epilepticus	

Source: Modified from References.[79,80,82,92,94,102–108]

adult series of subjects with PNES, whereas no epileptic seizures, either partial or generalized, were associated with forceful eye closure in 408 studied events by DeToledo and colleagues.[107] Recorded epileptic attacks were also associated with a stereotypic involvement of facial muscles: (1) eyes are usually wide open, (2) the eyebrows are elevated during the tonic stage in a frowning appearance, and (3) there is rhythmic blinking occurring synchronously with clonic movements.[107] Deviations from these patterns of facial muscle activation should raise suspicion of PNES. The observation of forceful eye closure as a reliable indicator of PNES was affirmed in another study with fifty of fifty-two subjects who had their PNES recorded on video-telemetry.[108] When compared to true epileptic events, forceful eye closure was noted in only 4 of 156 other subjects whose epileptic events were recorded by Chung et al.[108]

Even when epileptic seizures occurred during sleep, the subjects open their eyes.[108] A recent pediatric study has also suggested eye closure to be a reliable sign of non-epileptic but physiologic events in infants.[109] In a retrospective video-telemetry review of eye-opening behavior during seizures recorded in infants, the authors found that of 91 seizures in 69 infants, the eyes were open in 85 (93.4%) cases. They concluded that infants whose eyes are closed throughout the paroxysmal event are most likely not having seizures.[109] Although this type of analysis has not been reproduced in older children, similar conclusions have been implied based on observed clinical experiences. Postictal behavior has also not been reported to be homogeneous across series but most frequently has been described as being heralded by some period of weakness, dull responsiveness, or unresponsiveness. Not infrequently, older subjects engage in frank combativeness.

Prolonged PNES events, or "psychogenic status epilepticus," have been infrequently reported in the pediatric age group. However, some series of PNES cohorts note that the maximum duration of the events exceeds 10 minutes.[94, 102] There are two teenagers (18 and 19 years old) described within an adult series, and two additional series of six and ten children, respectively, treated within an emergency department setting, who have been described with psychogenic status epilepticus.[81, 81, 110, 111] The majority of those children were repeatedly treated with intravenous drugs, and several were exposed to invasive diagnostic procedures as part of their acute evaluations.[81, 110, 111] The occurrence of prolonged staring spells may be identified as PNES if there is preserved responsiveness to touch, concurrent body rocking, and/or absence of body twitches, upward eye movements, play interruption, or urinary incontinence.[112, 113]

Unfortunately, an accurate history of the actual observed events may contain any attribute of true epileptic seizures. There are no specific prodrome, ictal or postictal characterizations that are diagnostic. A combination of clinical characteristics will be sufficiently suggestive to allow a presumptive identification of PNES; however, the use of ancillary diagnostic procedures will be additionally helpful.[114] The post-ictal measurement of an increased prolactin level has been utilized to distinguish epileptic seizures from PNES.[114–116] Prolactin is normally produced and released by the anterior pituitary under the modulating influence of the prolactin-releasing factor and prolactin-inhibiting factor, each of which in turn are activated by serotonergic and dopaminergic inputs, respectively.[115] As a result, drugs that act by increasing serotonin or as a dopamine antagonist will increase prolactin, and those compounds with the opposite actions will inhibit prolactin release. A rise in serum prolactin of at least twofold and typically five- to tenfold amount ($\geq$130–260 ng/mL) maximizes at 20–30 minutes after an epileptic-generalized convulsive seizure when compared to baseline (24 hours or more prior), and falls back to baseline 1–2 hours afterwards.[115, 117–121] Convulsive epileptic seizures must extend over a period of at least 10 seconds and be accompanied by a change of consciousness in order to precipitate a measurable change in prolactin levels. This increase in prolactin is nearly constant in 90%–100% of generalized tonic-clonic convulsive seizure subjects studied. An increase in serum prolactin may be sensitive for epileptic seizures; however, the absence of a rise in serum levels is not necessarily an indicator of PNES.[122] Alterations in serum prolactin are not appreciated after myoclonic or absence seizures, including absence status epilepticus, and only minimally (≤ 13 ng/mL) after febrile convulsions, syncope, and febrile illnesses in children.[122] Prolactin measurements in relation to partial epileptic seizures are more variable in response and degree of change.[123–126] A rise in prolactin, at least twofold, from baseline has been reported in 40%–80% of complex partial seizures and 10% of simple partial seizure subjects studied.[123–126] Electrographic seizure discharges from the mesial temporal lobe in particular are likely to produce elevations in prolactin levels.[126] Measurements of other serum biomarkers (e.g., cortisol, growth hormone, endogenous opiods, beta-lipoprotein, vasopressin, adrenocorticotropic hormone, and thyrotropin) also rise in response to stress states, including syncope, cluster headaches, myocardial ischemia, and after epileptic seizures, but not after PNES.[119–121, 123, 124] Serum creatine kinase is also elevated after generalized tonic-clonic convulsions, but not after partial, absence, or PNES.[127] The use of suggestion techniques to provoke PNES has been utilized in the past but has been called into question on ethical grounds.[128] Saline infusions and the topical application of an alcohol patch have each had prior widespread use, with resulting provocation of typical PNES in 77%–82% of so tested subjects, including children.[104, 129, 130] Despite the specificity of these procedures nearing 100%, this act of subject deception and the avoidance of informed consent calls into question any benefit to the subject with underlying mental health issues by exposing them to a greater potential mental health harm.[128] An alternative suggestion technique, which involves full informed consent of the subject, is the use of hypnosis. With regard to children, a child assent process with parental consent can be obtained. Hypnosis is performed after a determination of whether and how suggestible the subject will be to hypnosis.[131] Obtaining a hypnotic induction score in older children, followed by the process of hypnosis with concurrent video-telemetry, is preferred.[131] If during the procedure a typical event is induced, then review with family members will allow definitive confirmation of the event as PNES. This technique can then be utilized to further teach the subject to discriminate between non-epileptic and epileptic events as well as terminate those that are PNES.

Many patients with non-epileptic seizures have concurrent epilepsy, which makes their treatment a challenge. These children will often suffer the comorbidities of depression, anxiety, dependency, and behavior problems. Differentiating epileptic from PNES in this circumstance may be difficult. Patients may initially respond to antiepileptic drug therapy only to require ever-escalating doses and additional drugs because of continued "breakthrough" seizures. PNES should be considered in clinical instances where unexpected poor seizure control develops in the face of adequate antiepileptic drug levels, inconsistent

or ever-evolving seizure patterns, or a marked change in their seizure semiology, especially in the face of consistently normal EEG recordings. In this
circumstance, video-telemetry recording of an event may be the best and only
way to definitively determine the correct diagnosis. The coexistence of epilepsy
and PNES in children is not well defined. Of fifty-three subjects less than 20
years of age whose seizures were recorded with video-telemetry by Holmes
and colleagues, 8/11 (73%) had ictal recordings of both epileptic seizures and
PNES.[103] In another study of children under 10 years of age, 60 subjects underwent video-telemetry recording; 9/60 (15%) had epileptic seizures recorded
and 24/60 (40%) had PNES recorded. However, no subject had both.[106] More
recent and larger series in children identify both epileptic and PNES in about
10%–18%.[82,97,98]

Although the gold standard of PNES diagnosis is the recording of a typical event with concurrent video-telemetry, the specificity of the EEG findings
is not always definitive.[132–134] The initial suspicion of PNES is a clinical one,
and the subsequent video-telemetry is most often obtained in order to confirm
this clinical suspicion. Pitfalls in diagnosis can fall under three main reasons:
(1) the ictal EEG recording is over-read as abnormal when it is in fact a normal variant or nonspecific, sharply contoured background rhythm, or alpha
rhythm fragment; (2) the ictal recording is not recognized as a rhythmic movement artifact; (3) the ictal recording of certain true epileptic seizures do not
reflect up to the routine surface EEG. The former two circumstances will incorrectly "diagnose" epilepsy when in fact theses are PNES events, whereas this
later circumstance results in a misdiagnosis of PNES when in fact there is
true epilepsy.[133,134] The epileptic seizures most often apt to be underidentified
are simple and complex partial epileptic seizures. A wide array of stereotyped
clinical behaviors may be associated with simple partial seizures but without
any alteration in consciousness, thus arousing suspicion that these are PNES.
Complex partial seizures, on the other hand, are not infrequently associated
with bizarre behavior; emotional outbursts and vocalizations when initiated
from the frontal lobe may not be reflected well and identified by surface EEG
recording techniques.[134]

Psychotherapeutic evaluation and interventions can have success in resolving the problems contributing to PNES.[7] If no concurrent epilepsy exists,
withdrawal of antiepileptic drugs should be undertaken. Consultation with
the child's school nurse and administrators will be needed to assure "normalized" activity. A recent follow-up survey of 50 children with "pseudoseizures"
put on appropriate drug treatment and/or psychotherapy for 3 months found
that thirty-six (72.0%) remitted, ten (20.0%) showed a decrease in frequency,
and four (8.0%) did not improve.[94] Poorer outcomes were correlated to longer
duration of the condition before diagnosis.[94] In an earlier study of eighteen
children compared to twenty adults diagnosed with PNES followed at the same
epilepsy monitoring unit, long-term follow-up disclosed significant differences
in outcomes.[26] At 1, 2, and 3 years after diagnosis, 73%, 75%, and 81% of
the children and adolescents had resolution of their PNES attacks at these

follow-up times compared to only 25%, 25%, and 40%, respectively, in the adult cohort at the same time intervals postdiagnosis.[26]

Similar good outcomes have been noted by other authors, citing resolution rates of 45%–95% (average 77%) within 6 weeks to 4 years.[8, 25–28, 130] Important factors in contributing to poorer outcomes have been identified as delay in diagnosis, younger age at onset, and high PNES frequency. Outcomes appear to better when psychiatric care and counseling are instituted early.

Psychiatric interventions are paramount to effective intervention and good outcome. The PNES may serve the patient as a defense mechanism against personal insecurities and anxiety. This is a maladaptive defense mechanism that must be supplanted with a substitution that the patient can rely on (i.e., continued care and support by the physician). The child and family must be supported through the transition into more appropriate behavioral strategies. An explanation of the diagnosis, emphasizing that the symptoms are a stress-induced involuntary physical manifestation, and a reassurance that a life-threatening or serious neurological disorder is not present will be necessary but not likely to completely satisfy the parents and child. The parent must be aided in understanding that there has been no neurological disease. Testing may be needed to objectify this for them. That is why video-telemetry can be useful as both a diagnostic and therapeutic tool. The parents can view the PNES events with assurance that a non-epileptic event excludes the diagnosis of epilepsy. Identification of possible stressors is important. These may be proximate to the presentation of symptoms or potentially in the remote past. Often there is a combination of factors contributing to the presentation at hand. Psychiatric examination for possible underlying diagnoses such as depression, anxiety disorder, or other mood disorder is necessary. The identification of other possible triggers (family discord, parental stress, physical/sexual abuse, etc.) and addressing their impact and management will also need to be accomplished. Emphasizing wellness and focusing the family's energies on developing better coping strategies rather than a cure in some instances may be a good approach. For the child with comorbid epilepsy, they should be encouraged to try and identify whether each event is an epileptic or a non-epileptic seizure. With nonjudgmental encouragement, many children will be readily able to make that distinction and exert some control over their illness. Cognitive behavioral therapy and appropriate psychopharmacologic medication for anxiety, depression, and other coexistent psychopathology needs to be managed by appropriate mental health professionals.[114, 135]

REFERENCES

1. *Diagnostic and Statistical Manual of Mental Disorders (DSM-IV-TR)*, 4th edition, text revision, Arlington, VA: American Psychological Association, 2000; 485–517.
2. Roach ES, Langley RL. Episodic neurological dysfunction due to mass hysteria. Arch Neurol 2004; 61; 1269–1272.
3. Wessley S. Mass hysteria: two syndromes? Psychol Med 1987; 17; 109–120.

4. Holmes GL, Sackellares JC, McKiernan J, et al. Evaluation of childhood pseudoseizures using EEG telemetry and videotape monitoring. J Pediatr 1980; 97; 554–558.

5. Metrick ME, Ritter FJ, Gates JR, et al. Nonepileptic events in childhood. Epilepsia 1991; 32; 322–328.

6. Inagaki T, Mizuno S, Miyaoki T, et al. Breath-holding spells in somatoform disorder. Int J Psychiatry 2004; 34(2): 201–205.

7. Wood BL, Haque S, Weinstock A, et al. Pediatric stress-related seizures: conceptualization, evaluation, and treatment of nonepileptic seizures in children and adolescents. Curr Opin Pediatr 2004; 16(5); 523–531.

8. Bhatia MS, Sapra SMA. Pseudoseizures in children: a profile of 50 cases. Clin Pediatr 2005; 44(7); 617–621.

9. Egger HL, Costello EJ, Erkanli A, et al. Somatic complaints and psychopathology in children and adolescents: Stomach aches, musculoskeletal pains, and headaches. Am Acad Child Adolesc Psychiatr 1999; 38(7); 852–860.

10. Campo JV, Jansen-McWilliams L, Comer DM, et al. Somatization in pediatric primary care: Association with psychopathology, functional impairment, and use of services. J Am Acad Child Adolesc Psychiatry 1999; 38(9); 1093–1101.

11. Craig TKJ, Cox AD, Klein K. Intergenerational transmission of somatization behavior: a study of chronic somatizers and their children. Psychol Med 2002; 32(5); 805–816.

12. Craig TKJ, Bialas I, Hodson S, et al. Intergenerational transmission of somatization behavior: 2. Observations of joint attention and bids for attention. Psychol Med 2004; 34; 199–209.

13. Wender PH, Klein DF. *Mind, Mood, and Medicine.* New York: Meridian Publishing, 1981.

14. Torgersen S. Genetics of somatoform disorders. Arch Gen Psych 1986; 43; 502–505.

15. Fritz GK, Fritsch S, Hagino O. Somatoform disorders in children and adolescents: a review of the past 10 years. J Am Acad Child Adolesc Psychiatry 1997; 36(10); 1329–1338.

16. Reilly J, Baker GA, Rhodes J, et al. The association of sexual and physical abuse with somatization: characteristics of patients presenting with irritable bowel syndrome and non-epileptic attack disorder. Psychol Med 1999; 29(2); 399–406.

17. Roelofs K, Keijsers GP, Hoogduin KA, et al. Childhood abuse in patients with conversion disorder. Am J Psychiatr 2002; 159(11); 1908–1913.

18. Kozlowska K, Nunn KP, Rose D, et al. Conversion disorder in Australian pediatric practice. J Am Acad Child Adolesc Psychiatry 2007; 46(1); 68–75.

19. Stone J, Smyth R, Carson A, et al. Systematic review of misdiagnosis of conversion symptoms and "hysteria". BMJ 2005; 331(7523); 989–996.

20. Grattan-Smith P, Fairley M, Procopis P. Clinical features of conversion disorder. Arch Dis Child 1988; 63(4); 408–414.

21. Murase S, Sugiyama T, Ishii T, et al. Polysymptomatic conversion disorder in childhood and adolescence in Japan. Early manifestation or incomplete form of somatization disorder? Psychother Psychosom 2000; 69(3); 132–136.

22. Leary PM. Conversion disorder in childhood-diagnosed too late, investigated too much. J R Soc Med 2003; 96; 436–438.

23. Ettinger AB, Devinsky O, Weibrot DM, et al. Headaches and other pain symptoms among patients with psychogenic non-epileptic seizures. Seizures 1999; 8(7); 424–426.

24. Kent DA, Tomasson K, Coryell W. Course and outcome of conversion and somatization disorders. A four-year follow-up. Psychosom 1995; 36(2); 138–144.
25. Turgay A. Treatment outcome for children and adolescents with conversion disorder. Can J Psychiatry 1990; 35; 585–588.
26. Wyllie E, Friedman D, Luders H, et al. Outcome of psychogenic seizures in children and adolescents compared with adults. Neurology 1991; 41; 742–744.
27. Wyllie E, Glazer JP, Benbadis S, et al. Psychiatric features of children and adolescents with pseudoseizures. Arch Pediatr Adolesc Med 1999; 153(3); 244–248.
28. Pehlivanturk B, Unal F. Conversion disorder in children and adolescents: clinical features and comorbidity with depressive and anxiety disorders. Turk J Pediatr 2000; 42; 132–137.
29. Cassady JD, Kirschke DL, Jones TF, et al. Case series: Outbreak of conversion disorder among Amish adolescent girls. J Am Acad Child Adolesc Psychiatr 2005; 44(3); 291–297.
30. Lieb R, Pfister H, Mastaler M, et al. Somatoform syndromes and disorders in a representative population sample of adolescents and young adults: prevalence, comorbidity and impairments. Acta Psychiatr Scand 2000; 101; 194–208.
31. Domenech-Llaberia E, Jane C, Canals J, et al. Parental reports of somatic symptoms in preschool children: Prevalence and associations in a Spanish sample. J Am Acad Child Adolesc Psychiatry 2004; 43; 598–604.
32. Fichtel A, Larson B. Psychosocial impact of headache and comorbidity with other pains among Swedish school adolescents. Headache 2002; 42; 766–775.
33. Thomasson K, Kent D, Coryell W. Somatization and conversion disorders: comorbidity and demographics at presentation. Acta Psychiatr Scand 1991; 84; 288–293.
34. Roelofs K, Spinhoven P, Sandijck P, et al. The impact of early trauma and recent life-events on symptom severity in patients with conversion disorder. J Nerv Ment Dis 2005; 193; 508–514.
35. Stone J, Smyth R, Carson A, et al. La belle indifférence in conversion symptoms and hysteria: systematic review of misdiagnosis of conversion symptoms and "hysteria." Br J Psychiatry 2006; 188; 204–209.
36. Ho AMW, Ransby MJ, Farrell K, et al. Psychological assessment and treatment of non-epileptic seizures and related symptoms in children and adolescents. In *Non-Epileptic Seizures*. Eds: JR Gates, AJ Rowan. Boston MA, Butterworth-Heinemann, 2000; 207–226.
37. Lach LM, Peltz L. Adolescents' and parents perception of non-epileptic seizures: A retrospective and qualitative glance. In *Non-Epileptic Seizures*. Eds: JR Gates, AJ Rowan. Boston MA, Butterworth-Heinemann, 2000; 227–236.
38. Wood BL, Haque S, Weinstock A, et al. Pediatric stress-related seizures: conceptualization, evaluation, and treatment of non-epileptic seizures in children and adolescents. Curr Opin Pediatr 2004; 16(5): 523–531.
39. Werring DJ, Weston L, Bullmore ET, et al. Functional magnetic resonance imaging of the cerebral response to visual stimulation in medically unexplained visual loss. Psychol Med 2004; 34; 583–589.
40. Ron MA. Explaining the unexplained: understanding hysteria. Brain 2001; 124, 1065–1066.
41. Spence SA, Crimlisk HL, Cope H, et al. Discrete neurophysiological correlates in prefrontal cortex during hysterical and feigned disorder of movement. Lancet 2000; 355, 1243–1244.

42. Tardif HP, Barry RJ, Fox AM, et al. Detection of feigned recognition memory impairment using the old/new effect of the event-related potential. Int J Psychophysiol 2000; 36, 1–9.

43. Lesch, KP, Bengel D, Heils A, et al. Association of anxiety-related traits with a polymorphism in the serotonin transporter gene regulatory region. Science 1996; 274(5292); 1527–1531.

44. Diatchenko L, Nackley AG, Slade GD, et al. Maixner W. Catechol-O-methyltransferase gene polymorphisms are associated with multiple pain-evoking stimuli. Pain 2006; 125(3); 216–224.

45. Herrmann MJ, Huter T, Muller F, et al. Additive effects of serotonin transporter and tryptophan hydroxylase-2 gene variation on emotional processing. Cerebral Cortex 2007; 17(5); 1160–1163.

46. Xu K, Ernst M, Goldman D. Imaging genomics applied to anxiety, stress response, and resiliency. Neuroinformatics 2006; 4(1); 51–64.

47. Cloninger C, Reich T, Guze S. The multifactorial model of disease transmission: III. Familial relationship between sociopathy and hysteria (Briquet's syndrome). Br J Psychiatry 1975; 127; 23–32.

48. Livingston R. Children of people with somatization disorder. J Am Acad Child Adolesc Psychiatry 1993; 32; 536–544.

49. Mullins LL, Olson R. Familial factors in the etiology, maintenance, and treatment of somatoform disorders in children. Fam Syst Med 1990; 8; 159–175.

50. Wood B. Physically manifested illness in children and adolescents: a biobehavioral family approach. Child Adolesc Psychiatr Clin North Am 2001; 10; 543–562.

51. Compas BE, Thomsen AH. Coping and responses to stress among children with recurrent abdominal pain. J Devel Behav Peds 1999; 20(5); 323–324.

52. Thomsen AH, Compas BE, Colletti RB, et al. Parent reports of coping and stress responses in children with recurrent abdominal pain. J Ped Psychol 2002; 27(3); 216–226.

53. Craig TK, Boardman AP, Mills K, et al. The South London Somatisation Study. I: Longitudinal course and the influence of early life experiences. Br J Psychiatry 1993; 163; 579–588.

54. Craig TK, Drake H, Mills K, et al. The South London somatisation study. II. influence of stressful events, and secondary gain. Br J Psychiatry 1994; 165(2); 248–258.

55. Campo JV, DiLorenzo C, Chiappetta L, et al. Adult outcomes of pediatric recurrent abdominal pain: do they just grow out of it? Pediatrics 2001; 108(1); e1–6. http://www.pediatrics.org/cgi/content/full/108/1/e1.

56. Santalahti P, Aromaa M, Sourander A, et al. Have there been changes in children's psychosomatic symptoms? A 10-year comparison from Finland. Pediatrics 2005; 115; e434–e442. http://www.pediatrics.org/cgi/content/full/115/4/e434.

57. Egger HL, Angold A, Costello J. Headaches and psychopathology in children and adolescents. J Am Acad Child Adolesc Psychiatr 1998; 37; 951–958.

58. Egger HL, Costello EJ, Erkanli A, et al. Somatic complaints and psychopathology in children and adolescents: stomach aches, musculoskeletal pains and headaches. J Am Acad Child Adolesc Psychiatr 1999; 38; 852–860.

59. Eminson DM. Somatising in children and adolescents. 1. Clinical presentations and aetiological factors. Adv Psychiatr Treat 2001; 7; 266–274.

60. Eminson DM. Somatising in children and adolescents. 2. Management and outcomes. Adv Psychiatr Treat 2001; 7; 388–398.

61. Spierings C, Poels PJ, Sijben N, et al. Conversion disorders in childhood: a retrospective follow-up study of 84 inpatients. Dev Med Child Neurol 1990; 32(10); 865–871.

62. Keane JR. Triplopia: thirteen patients from a neurology inpatient service. Arch Neurol 2006; 63(3); 388–389.

63. Keane JR. Neuro-ophthalmic signs of hysteria. Neurology 1984; 34; 127.

64. Luzza F, Pugliatti P, DiRosa S, et al. Tilt-induced pseudosyncope. Int J Clin Pract 2003; 57(5); 373–375.

65. Grubb BP, Gerard G, Wolf DA, et al. Syncope and seizures of psychogenic origin: identification with head-upright tilt table testing. Clin Cardiol 1992; 15; 839–842.

66. Petersen MEV, Williams T, Sutton R. Psychogenic syncope diagnosed by prolonged head-up tilt testing. Q J Med 1995; 88; 209–213.

67. Mathias CJ, Deguchi K, Bleasdale-Barr K, et al. Familial vasovagal syncope and pseudosyncope: observations in a case with both natural and adopted siblings. Clin Auton Res 2000; 10; 43–45.

68. Mathias CJ, Deguchi K, Schatz I. Observations on recurrent syncope and presyncope in 641 patients. Lancet 2001; 357; 348–353.

69. Roach ES, Langley RL. Episodic neurological dysfunction due to mass hysteria. Arch Neurol 2004; 61; 1269–1272.

70. Hicks JA, Shapiro CM. Psuedo-narcolepsy: case report. J Psychiatr Neurosci 1999; 24(4); 348–350.

71. Krahn LE. Reevaluating spells initially identified as cataplexy. Sleep Med 2005; 6(6); 537–542.

72. Stein MT, Harper G, Chen J. Persistent cough in an adolescent. J Dev Behav Pediatr 1999; 20(6); 434–436.

73. Boeble M. Interactional treatment of intractable hiccups. Fam Process 1989; 28(2); 191–206.

74. Mari F, DiBonaventura M, Vanacore N, et al. Video-EEG study of psychogenic nonepileptic seizures: differential characteristics in patients with and without epilepsy. Epilepsia 2006; 47(Suppl 5); 64–67.

75. Holmes GL, Sackellares JC, McKiernan J, et al. Evaluation of childhood pseudoseizures using EEG telemetry and videotape monitoring. J Pediatr 1980; 97; 554–558.

76. Metrick ME, Ritter FJ, Gates JR, et al. Nonepileptic events in childhood. Epilepsia 1991; 32; 322–328.

77. Inagaki T, Mizuno S, Miyaoki T, et al. Breath-holding spells in somatoform disorder. Int J Psychiatry 2004; 34(2); 201–205.

78. Vossler DG, Haltiner AM, Schepp SK, et al. Ictal stuttering: A sign suggestive of psychogenic nonepileptic seizures. Neurology 2004; 63; 516–519.

79. Benbadis SR. Hypergraphia and the diagnosis of psychogenic attacks. Neurology 2006; 67(1); 904.

80. Burnum JF. La maladie du petit papier. Is writing a list of symptoms a sign of an emotional disorder? N Engl J Med 1985; 313; 690–691.

81. Holtkamp M, Othman J, Buchheim K, et al. Diagnosis of psychogenic Nonepileptic staus epilepticus in the emergency setting. Neurology 2006; 66; 1727–1729.

82. Kotagal P, Costa M, Wyllie E, et al. Paroxysmal nonepileptic events in children and adolescents. Pediatr 2002, 110(4); e46–e51. http://www.pediatrics.org/cgi/content/full/110/4/e46.

83. Gibbs J, Appleton RE. False diagnosis of epilepsy in children. Seizure 1992; 1; 15–18.

84. Stroink H, van Donselaar CA, Geerts AT, et al. The accuracy of the diagnosis of paroxysmal events in children. Neurology 2003; 60; 979–982.

85. Uldall P, Alving J, Hansen LK, et al. The misdiagnosis of epilepsy in children admitted to a tertiary epilepsy centre with paroxysmal events. Arch Dis Child 2006; 91; 219–221.

86. Beach R, Reading R. The importance of acknowledging clinical uncertainty in the diagnosis of epilepsy and non-epileptic events. Arch Dis Child 2005; 90; 1219–1222.

87. Bye AM, Kok DJ, Ferenschild FT, et al. Paroxysmal non-epileptic events in children: a retrospective study over a period of 10 years. J Paediatr Child Health 2000; 36(3); 244–248.

88. Hindley D, Ali A, Robson C. Diagnoses made in a secondary care "fits, faints, funny turns" clinic. Arch Dis Child 2006; 91; 214–218.

89. Ferrie CD. Preventing misdiagnosis of epilepsy. Arch Dis Child 2006; 91; 206–209.

90. Desai P, Talwar D. Non-epileptic events in normal and neurologically handicapped children: A video-EEG study. Pediatr Neurol 1992; 8; 127–129.

91. Holmes G, McKeever M, Russman B. Abnormal behavior or epilepsy? Use of long-term EEG and video monitoring with severely to profoundly mentally retarded patients with seizures. Am J Ment Ret 1983; 87(4); 456–458.

92. Neill JC, Alvarez N. Differential diagnosis of epileptic versus pseudoepileptic seizures in developmentally disabled persons. Appl Res Ment Ret 1986; 7(3); 285–298.

93. Donat JF, Wright FS. Episodic symptoms mistaken for seizures in the neurologically impaired child. Neurology 1990; 40(1); 156–157.

94. Bhatia MS, Sapra SMA. Pseudoseizures in children: a profile of 50 cases. Clin Pediatr 2005; 44(7):617–621.

95. Benbadis SR, Hauser WA. An estimate of the prevalence of psychogenic non-epileptic seizures. Seizure 2000; 9; 280–281.

96. Benbadis SR, O'Neill E, Tatum WO, et al. Outcome of prolonged EEG-video monitoring ata typical referral center. Epilepsia 2004; 45; 1150–1153.

97. Devinsky O, Sanchez-Villsenor F, Vazquez B, et al. Clinical profile of patients with epileptic and Nonepileptic seizures. Neurology 1996; 46; 1530–1533.

98. Benbadis SR, Agrawal V, Tatum WO. How many patients with psychogenic Nonepileptic seizures also have epilepsy? Neurology 2001; 57; 915–917.

99. Lesser RP, Lueders H, Dinner DS. Evidence for epilepsy is rare in patients with psychogenic seizures. Neurology 1983; 33; 502–504.

100. Benbadis SR, Tatum WO. Overinterpretation of EEGs and misdiagnosis of epilepsy. J Clin Neurophys 2003; 20(1); 42–44.

101. Havens LL. Charcot and hysteria. J Nerv Ment Dis 1966; 141; 505–516.

102. Kramer U, Carmant L, Riviello JJ, et al. Psychogenic seizures: video telemetry observations in 27 patients. Pediatr Neurol 1995; 12; 39–41.

103. Holmes G, Sckellares JC, McKiernan J, et al. Evaluation of childhood pseudoseizures using EEG telemetry and videotape monitoring. J Pediatr 1980; 97; 554–558.

104. Wyllie E, Friedman D, Rothner D, et al. Psychogenic seizures in children and adolescents: outcome after diagnosis by ictal video and electroencephalographic recording. Pediatrics 1990; 85; 480–484.

105. Brunquell P, Mc Keever M, Russman BS. Differentiation of epileptic from nonepileptic head drops in children. Epilepsia 1990; 31(4); 401–405.
106. Duchowny MS, Resnick TJ, Deray MJ, et al. Video EEG diagnosis of repetitive behavior in early childhood and its relationship to seizures. Pediatr Neurol 1988; 4(3); 162–164.
107. DeToledo JC, Ramsay RE. Patterns of involvement of facial muscles during epileptic and Non-epileptic events: review of 654 events. Neurology 1996; 47; 621–625.
108. Chung SS, Gerber P, Kirlin KA. Ictal eye closure is a reliable indicator for psychogenic seizures. Neurology 2006; 66; 1730–1731.
109. Korff CM. Nordli DR Jr. Paroxysmal events in infants: persistent eye closure makes seizures unlikely. Pediatrics 2005; 116(4); e485–e486. http://www.pediatrics.org/cgi/content/full/116/4/e485.
110. Selbst SM, Clancy R. Pseudoseizures in the pediatric emergency department. Pediatr Emerg Care 1996; 12(3); 185–188.
111. Pakalnis A, Paolicchi J, Gilles E. Psychogenic status epilepticus in children: psychiatric and other risk factors. Neurology 2000; 54; 969–970.
112. Rosenow F, Wyllie E, Kotagal P, et al. Staring spells in children: Descriptive features distinguishing epileptic and Non-epileptic events. J Pediatr 1998; 133; 660–663.
113. Leis AA, Ross MA, Summers AK. Psychogenic seizures: ictal characteristics and pitfalls. Neurology 1992; 42; 95–99.
114. Barry JJ, Sanborn K. Etiology, diagnosis, and treatment of non-epileptic seizures. Curr Neurol Neurosci Reports 2001; 1; 381–389.
115. Pritchard PB. The role of prolactin in the diagnosis of non-epileptic seizures. In *Non-Epileptic Seizures*. Eds: JR Gates, AJ Rowan. Boston MA, Butterworth-Heinemann, 2000; 93–100.
116. Zelnick N, Kahan L, Rafael A, Besner I, Iancu TC. Prolactin and cortisol levels in various paroxysmal disorders in childhood. Pediatr 1991; 88(3); 486–489.
117. Trimble M. Serum prolactin in epilepsy and hysteria. BMJ 1978; 2; 1682.
118. Abbott RJ, Browning McK, Davidson DLW. Serum prolactin and cortisol concentrations after grand mal seizures. J Neurol Neurosurg Psychiatry 1980; 43; 163–167.
119. Pritchard PB, Wannamaker BB, Sagel J, et al. Serum prolactin and cortisol levels in evaluation of pseudoepileptic seizures. Ann Neurol 1985; 18; 87–89.
120. Aminoff MJ, Simon RP, Wiedemann E. The hormonal responses to generalized tonic-clonic seizures. Brain 1984; 107; 569–578.
121. Berkovic S. Clinical and experimental aspects of complex partial seizures. Doctor of Medicine thesis, University of Melbourne. In *A Textbook of Epilepsy*. 3rd edition. Eds: J Laidlaw, A Richens, and J Oxley. New York, Chuchill Livingstone, 1988.
122. Yerby MS, vanBelle G, Fiel PN, et al. Serum prolactin in the diagnosis of epilepsy: sensitivity, specificity, and predictive value. Neurology 1987; 37; 1224–1226.
123. Culebras A, Miller M, Bertram L, et al. Differential response of growth hormone, cortisol, and prolactin to seizures and to stress. Epilepsia 1987; 28; 564–570.
124. Rao ML, Stefan H, Bauer J. Epileptic but not psychogenic seizures are accompanied by simultaneous elevation of serum pituitary hormones and cortisol levels. Neuroendocrinology 1989; 49; 33–39.
125. Wyllie E, Lueders B, MacMillan JP, et al. Serum prolactin levels after epileptic seizures. Neurology 1984; 34; 1601–1604.
126. Sperling MR, Pritchard PB, Engel J, et al. Prolactin in partial epilepsy: an indicator of limbic seizures. Ann Neurol 1986; 20; 716–722.

127. Wyllie E, Lueders H, Pippenger C, et al. Postictal creatine kinase in the diagnosis of seizure disorders. Arch Neurol 1985; 42(2); 123–126.

128. Stagno SJ, Smith ML. The use of placebo in diagnosing psychogenic seizures: who is being deceived? Sem Neurol 1997; 17; 213–218.

129. Walczak TS, Williams DT, Berten W. Utility and reliability of placebo infusion in the evaluation of patients with seizures. Neurology 1994; 44; 394–399.

130. Lancman ME, Asconape JJ, Graves S, et al. Psychogenic seizures in children: long term analysis of 43 cases. J Child Neurol 1994; 9; 404–407.

131. Barry JJ, Atzmon O, Morrell MP. Discriminating between epileptic and non-epileptic events: the utility of hypnotic seizure induction. Epilepsia 2000; 41; 81–84.

132. Sirven JI, Glosser DS. Psychogenic Non-epileptic seizures. Theoretic and clinical considerations. Neuropsychiatr, Neuropsychol, Behav Neurol 1998; 11(4); 225–235.

133. Benbadis SR. The EEG in Non-epileptic seizures. J Clin Neurophysiol 2006; 23(4); 340–352.

134. Finlayson RE, Lucas AR. Pseudoepileptic seizures in children and adolescents. Mayo Clin Proc 1979; 54; 83–87.

135. James A, Soler A, Weatherall R. Cognitive behavioral therapy for anxiety disorders in children and adolescents. The Cochrane Database of Systematic Reviews 2005; 4; CD004690.

6

Factitious Disorders

INTRODUCTION TO FACTITIOUS DISORDERS

Factitious epilepsy is one of the most difficult, potentially sinister, and often difficult to conclusively prove conditions mimicking epileptic seizures. By the very nature of the disorder, the individual perpetrator engages in a medical pretense of volitional deception. Non-epileptic seizures are but one of a myriad of other medical conditions, symptoms, and signs frequently intentionally feigned. In the context of children, parents and guardians may perpetuate a feigned illness in their child by the commission of pediatric condition falsification. In this instance, the parent or caretaker may be diagnosed with factitious disorder by proxy and is engaged in Munchausen syndrome by proxy abuse (MBPA). These parents may employ a simple fabrication of symptoms and signs and as such may report "epileptic" seizures rather easily. Typically, these events are not witnessed by any other observer and defy objective assessments. In a more extreme form of cruelty, the parent may engage in behaviors to inflict actual illness or signs of illness (e.g., suffocate a child to induce seizures or apnea) in order to objectify the complaint. The following chapter discusses the spectrum of this entity, and enumerates important clues to its identification and appropriate responses for intervention.

THE CLINICAL PROBLEM AND EPIDEMIOLOGY

When evaluating a pediatric neurological condition, factitious disorders are not initially thought of. Many of the symptoms and signs we consult upon and manage are never witnessed firsthand. Rather, patients and parents report descriptions of these, or if fortuitous, a home video recording may be provided for examination. Physical or psychological symptoms and signs that are intentionally produced or feigned in order to assume a sick role characterize factitious disorders (FD). This fabrication and falsification is done in the absence of external gain or incentive (Table 6-1).[1] This later point distinguishes the actions of those with FD from malingering, where there is some external gain sought after or an intention to avoid something unwanted. There are other factors more complex than mere secondary gain, which motivate individuals with FD. It is not simply a disorder of adults either, as there is ample evidence to acknowledge its existence in both children and adolescents.[2–4] The evolution of the clinical terminology will be briefly reviewed below.

Table 6-1 Factitious Disorder

Diagnostic Criteria for Factitious Disorder (300.16, 300.19)

1. The intentional production or feigning of physical or psychological signs or symptoms.
2. The motivation for the behavior is to assume the sick role.
3. External incentives for the behavior (such as economic gain, avoiding legal responsibility, or improving physical well-being, as in malingering) are absent.

Code based on type:

    With predominantly psychological signs and symptoms
    With predominantly physical signs and symptoms
    With combined psychological and physical signs and symptoms

Source: Modified from Reference.[1]

It was in 1951 that Dr. Richard Asher identified and named the medical condition "Munchausen syndrome," which we now refer to as factitious disorder.[5] It was some 25 years later that Dr. Roy Meadow identified the "Munchausen syndrome by proxy."[6] Munchausen syndrome was a reference to patients who Asher described as having imposed self-inflicted injuries and their attempts to "trick" the doctors into believing that they were suffering from an organic illness by their lavish stories, pretense, and lies. The appellation was rooted in the book of embellished tales written anonymously by a geologist, Rudolf Erich Raspe, in 1785.[7] In his book, Raspe attributed the adventurous exploits of his protagonist to the unknowing, unsuspecting, and nonfictional person of Baron H. Carl Freiedrich Munchausen, who was born in Hanover, Germany, in 1720. Over his lifetime, Munchausen developed a reputation as having a penchant to tell grandiose stories about his military exploits in Russia. This reputation attracted the elite and aristocrats of the time to dine with him in order to experience firsthand a master storyteller. Raspe apparently had been at several of these dinners, and when he fell upon financial difficulty, he published a book of his favorite stories for money, *Baron Munchausen's Narrative of his Marvelous Travels and Campaign in Russia*.[7] Thus, the syndrome bearing Munchausen's name was a reference to the analogous fabrications made by both Asher's patients and those attributed to Munchausen himself. There is a long debate within the literature about the inappropriateness of the reference and the ultimate abandonment of the name as a medical term.

Meadow, in his report of two children who were repeatedly made ill at the hands of their mothers, coined the phrase "Munchausen syndrome by proxy" in 1977.[6] The parental-induced illnesses prompted numerous potentially harmful treatments and investigations. One child endured twelve hospitalizations and six procedures under anesthesia that recurred over a period of several years during which the signs and symptoms were fabricated. The second child's reported misery culminated in death as a result of chronic salt poisoning and hypernatremic dehydration. This has been referred to as

Meadow's syndrome, or Polle syndrome, but is now called pediatric condition falsification.[7,8] The condition is defined as the fabrication of symptoms and falsification of records and samples to feign illness in the child (or person under the care of the perpetrator).[8] Illness can also be fabricated through simulation and the production of symptoms in the child (e.g., suffocation in order to produce an "epileptic" seizure), depression of consciousness or apnea being the most common neurologic presentation.[9–16] In international nonindustrialized nations, descriptions of induced apnea are notably absent, however.[16] The utilization of these terms were further refined by a multidisciplinary group of the American Professional Society on the Abuse of Children (APSAC).[17,18] The resultant definitions were designed to elucidate two discrete concepts: the maltreatment of the child, and the motivations of the perpetrator. Factitious disorder by proxy is the diagnostic label for the psychiatric disorder of a perpetrator who deliberately feigns or induces illness in a child for the purpose of fulfilling a psychological need (Table 6-2).[19] The actual abuse of the child is the pediatric condition falsification. Therefore, the commission of pediatric condition falsification by an adult or caretaker diagnosed with FD by proxy is engaged in MBPA. When the abuse of the child is done for external reasons or secondary gain, it is more appropriately considered as "malingering by proxy." Parents may have other psychiatric conditions that result in their engagement in pediatric condition falsification but not in order to satisfy a psychological need (e.g., psychosis, anxiety disorder, etc.) and thus would not clearly meet the definition of factitious disorder by proxy.[19] Therefore, for diagnostic accuracy, it is important to understand the nature and intent of the abuse.[20] Specific inclusion and exclusion criteria have been implored in order to more systematically identify the adults who engage in this type of child abuse.[21]

The epidemiology of FD in children and adolescents is limited. A literature review encompassing 30 years was reported by Libow, in which a compilation of children less than 18 years of age who intentionally falsified symptoms of illness was analyzed.[2] From forty-two cases (mean age 13.9 years) of whom 71% were female, the most commonly reported false or induced illnesses were fever, ketoacidosis, purpura, and infections. These were induced by injection,

Table 6-2 Factitious Disorder by Proxy

Diagnostic Criteria for Factitious Disorder (300.16, 300.19)

1. The intentional production or feigning of physical or psychological signs or symptoms in another person who is under the individual's care.
2. The motivation for the perpetrator's behavior is to assume the sick role by proxy.
3. External incentives for the behavior (such as economic gain, avoiding legal responsibility, or improving physical well-being, as in malingering) are absent.
4. The behavior is not accounted for by another mental disorder.

Source: Modified from Reference.[7]

ingestion, and self-inflicted bruising. The mean duration of the deception was 16 months (maximum of 5 years) before being detected.[2] Many of the children were fascinated with health care and had parental coaching or support in perpetrating the factitious illness. This and other reports have identified a willingness of the children to submit to procedures and endure interventions while maintaining the deception.[2–4] There is clearly a similarity to the symptom elaboration seen in somatisizers as well as that of malingering. In fact, there may well be an overlap of the presentation. It is the actual intent of the subject that is the determining feature that allows specific categorization. This intent may not be straightforward to discern. Certainly, for children, the need to assume a sick role may have intended and unintended secondary gains, such as the reception of focused attention, school absences, a sense of empowerment, perhaps desired treatments (pain medication), and special care arrangements (private hospital room, play therapist, etc.). All of these are desirable and pleasant. Importantly, the identification of children who engage in illness falsification may allow for an intervention before chronic FD results in unnecessary invasive interventions and the creation of symptoms that can have potentially life-threatening consequences and death. Such was the fate of an individual who repeatedly self-induced syncopal convulsions with combined forced valsalva and carotid massage.[22] This is an important corollary (Table 6-3). There is data to support the contention that some adults who engage in illness falsification have had experience as illness falsifiers when they were children themselves. More compelling is the fact that several cases have been reported where these individual children were the earlier victims of MBPA or experienced encouragement to falsify illness through caregiver collusion.[23]

The epidemiology of MBPA has been better evaluated than FD. Several large-scale literature reviews have been published within the industrialized and nonindustrialized countries. There is some variability to the types of symptom

Table 6-3 Factitious Disorder in Children

Difficulties in Identification of Childhood and Adolescent Illness Falsification

- Overlap among malingering, illness falsification disorder, Munchausen by proxy
- Limited psychological study of the childhood perpetrators
- Children's motivations and intentions are difficult to assess
- Apparent secondary gain for the child is almost unavoidable
- Physician denial about the child's intent and gravity of the symptoms

Potential Origins of Childhood and Adolescent Illness Falsification

- Learned behavior
- Symptom coaching or collusion from caregiver
- Prior victimization
- Developmental vulnerability

Source: Modified from Reference.[23]

falsification presented, although the caregiver profiles remain similar. Under an active reporting system in the United Kingdom and Republic of Ireland, the established annual incidence of Munchausen syndrome by proxy is 0.5/100,000 for children under 16 years of age, with a peak incidence of 2.8/100,000 children in the first year of life.[13] This reporting system had a high capture rate (94%) and did include three forms of abuse: Munchausen by proxy, nonaccidental poisoning, and nonaccidental suffocation.[13] The perpetrator and case profiles are summarized in Table 6-4.[13, 16, 24, 25] Data extrapolated from the United

Table 6-4 Summary Profiles of cases of Munchausen by Proxy

Characteristic*	Feldman[16] N = 122	Rosenberg[24] N = 117	Sheridan[25] N = 451	McClure[13] N = 128
Years Encompassed	1987–2001	1966–1987	1972–1999	1992–1994
Survey Type	Literature review	Literature review	Literature review	Prospective Reports
Population	Non- (UK, US, C, NZ, A)	English speaking	English speaking	UK & Ireland
Perpetrator				
Mother	86%	98%	76.5%	85%
Father	4%	1.5%	6.7%	4.6%
Other Relative	2%	–	–	1%
Parental Significant other	4%	–	–	2%
Health Care Field	–	30%	14.2%	–
Admitted Guilt	–	22%	11.1%	–
Court Conviction	–	8%	5.1%	–
Abused Themselves	–	–	21.7%	–
Munchausen Syndrome or Features	–	24%	29.3%	–
Victims				
Gender	54% male	46% male	52%	47% males
Mean Age at Diagnosis	<3yo (26%)	39.8 months	48.6 months	20 months
	3–12yo (52%)			
	>12yo (12%)			<5yo (77%)
Mortality	–	9%	6%	6.2%
Prior Sibling(s) Abuse/Death	3.2%/–	"several"/8.6%	61.3%/25%	41%/18%

Source: Modified from References.[13, 16, 24, 25]

Notes: UK—United Kingdom, US—United States, C—Canada, NZ—New Zealand, A—Australia.

* Where data is known.

Kingdom survey by Schreier and applied to the United States population has estimated about 200 cases per year.[26] Whether these figures are generated from countries other than western industrialized, or English-speaking or not, they are, at best, underestimates of the problem. Discussants agree overall that, although these figures are estimations, this is still a relatively rare form of child abuse.

Some additional points bear emphasis. As has been pointed out in previous literature, mothers are the primary perpetrators of this form of child abuse. Mothers dispense abuse equally between their children's genders, whereas fathers are three times more likely to abuse their sons.[25] It is common for mothers to have had training or have worked within the healthcare establishment and to develop some degree of medical sophistication. These mothers appear to be very attentive and caring but are capable of not only ignoring their children but also subjecting them to the cruelest of abuses (e.g., suffocation, intravenous injection of feces, etc.). Moreover, up to 25% of siblings within the family of a child who has been diagnosed with MBPA have succumbed to prior illnesses without identification of cause, and a further 61% may be victims of other types of abuse. Although the mortality of victims of MBPA is estimated at about 6%–9%, it may be considerably higher (33%) if the additional deaths caused by suffocation and poisoning are included.[13,24,25] Virtually all children suffer severe long-term psychological morbidity, and many suffer injury from the abuse itself or from the coincident medical procedures undertaken. There have been often noted unusual deaths and illnesses in family pets and a high frequency of reported house fires in their households.[15] These features are also characteristic in cases where the father has been the perpetrator.[14,15] Overall, the profile in men appears not unlike those for the women who perpetrate factitious illness abuse in their children.

The symptom presentations in children who are victims of MBPA can be quite broad and often multiple. Rosenberg and Sheridan listed 68 and 101 different symptom presentations, respectively.[25,26] The ten most common symptoms are presented in Table 6-5. A compilation of the the most common

---

Table 6-5 Most Frequent Symptoms of Factitious Disorder by Proxy

- Bleeding (18%–44%)
- Seizures (17.5%–42%)
- Apnea (15%–26.8%)
- Diarrhea (11%–20%)
- Anorexia/feeding problems (2%–24.6%)
- Unconsciousness/CNS depression (3.3%–19%)
- Vomiting (4.9%–10%)
- Fever (8.6%–10%)
- Cyanosis (4%–11%)
- Rash (3.3%–9%)

Source: Modified from References.[24,25]

Table 6-6 Neurological Symptoms of Factitious Disorder and Factitious Disorder by Proxy

Factitious Disorder (induced by drugs, self-inflicted injury, and fabrication)

- Seizures
- Paralysis
- Pain disorders
- Head trauma
- Pupillary abnormalities
- Klein-Levin syndrome
- Myopathy
- Myelopathy
- Dystonia and involuntary movement disorders
- Baroreflex failure
- Syncope

Factitious Disorder by Proxy (descending frequency) (induced by non-accidental suffocation, poisoning, neglect, and fabrication)

- Apnea
- Seizures
- Behavioral changes/hyperactivity
- Pain disorders/headache
- Developmental delays
- Lethargy
- Unconsciousness/CNS depression
- Speech & hearing problems
- Ataxia
- Dizziness/vertigo
- Fatigue
- Involuntary movements/tremors
- Hallucinations
- Nystagmus
- Learning disability

Source: Modified from References.[3,11–13,22,24,25,28–34]

neurological symptoms of both FD and MBPA from the literature is listed in Table 6-6.[27]

OVERVIEW: PATHOPHYSIOLOGY AND MECHANISMS

Most MBPA perpetrators are women, usually the child's mother. These women are often engaging and overly willing to submit their children to investigation. They are a constant presence with the child, participating in every aspect of care and hospital evaluation. Their spouses, on the other hand, are often very passive and generally not at home very much. More striking is their desire and attempts to develop relationships with the medical staff on all levels. They may insist on helping the nurses perform their duties, invite themselves to share conversation and meals, engage in social contacts with the staff outside of the healthcare facility, and traverse the typical separations of parent and providers.[35, 36] This insistence on the part of these mothers to be part of the care team often triggers uneasiness in the healthcare personnel. This behavior is in distinction to those patients with FD, who are often perceived as difficult.[36] These parents care for their children within the hospital with characteristic excessive doting. Despite this apparent front of excessive attention to their child, covert video has documented clear neglectfulness and overt cruelty.[35] These mothers are very accepting of rather dire medical diagnoses and rarely upset at the possibility of serious medical consequence.[36] The maternal perpetrators of abuse commonly (24%–29%) have factitious disorder or somatization disorders themselves.[24, 25]

Fathers who engage in MBPA are a small minority, estimated to be 1.5%–7% of all identified perpetrators.[13, 16, 24, 25] Their personality is in distinct contrast to that of the typical mother. The fathers have been described as more demanding, and ready to complain to authorities about care provision while in hospital. They too remain with the child constantly, but are not interested in becoming an assistant in the care provided by hospital staff. They also have a high frequency of FD.[14, 15] The mortality for children associated with abuse incurred at the hands of the father would appear to be greater than for mothers, but the case numbers are too few to clarify this with certainty. Meadow reported that eleven of fifteen children who suffered MBPA by their fathers died after tolerating repeated smothering and poisonings.[15]

These parents, mother or father, appear to commit the acts of abuse without specific provocation. The child's behavior or state of health has not been shown to be a determinant as to whether an act will be incited. However, each parent will typically react with great anger and indignation when nondiagnostic test results are presented. This emotional response may be amplified and convert to rage and or suicidal behavior when the parent is confronted with the conclusion that they have been the perpetrator of an abusive relationship with their child.[8]

The underlying pathogenesis of MBPA is evolving within the psychiatric field. Several mechanistic factors appear central to the development of the disorder and include (1) the mother's own prior experience of abuse, (2) a pathological relationship with her child, and (3) the positive effect of the medical care system upon them.[37]

A prior history of Munchausen syndrome or personal abuse has been identified commonly in the perpetrators. Bools and colleagues interviewed nineteen of forty-seven mothers studied after the diagnosis had been made. These women commonly divulged (79%) their own prior childhood experiences of physical and sexual abuse.[38] This frequency of prior abuse in the perpetrators has been previously reported to be lower (21%–30%) when the data is not specifically sought after by directed interview.[24, 25] This background of prior abuse may continue to predispose these women to feelings of isolation and diminished self-worth. This in turn may be one driving factor in the psychological causes of their actions.

The pathological relationship of the perpetrator mother and her child has been suggested to be one of manipulating the child in order to gain access to the medical complex for her own personal gratification.[35] This idea is somewhat contrary to the prior concept of an overly protective parent and her perception of the child as vulnerable. Contrary to the overprotection afforded the vulnerable child, these women engage in brutal cruelty proven without doubt via covert video surveillance.[11, 12]

How the medical establishment confers a positive reinforcement for the perpetrator's behaviors is likely from a complex interplay of multiple factors. There is clearly a general ambience of caring and support within the hospital and from hospital personnel. These mothers may thrive on the enhanced feeling of self-worth and importance given to them and the data they provide during often-prolonged medical investigation without clear solution.[39] This sense of worth and importance may be enhanced as the severity of the abusive events escalate and the more urgent need for further evaluation is realized. These mothers derive a sense of worth and importance when told that they are strong to be able to endure such dire problems without medical explanation in their child. Additionally, there is an element of gratification for the mother to know that she has been successfully concealing the truth from more learned opponents.[39] These mothers seem to engage in a one-upsmanship at deceiving the medical investigators.

Many of these mothers carry significant psychopathological diagnoses. In the large review by Sheridan, nearly 30% (132/451) of mothers had characteristics suggestive of Munchausen syndrome.[25] A further 22.8% (103/451) had another psychiatric diagnosis, most often depression or personality disorder.[25] In Bools and colleagues' study of interviews from 47 mothers diagnosed with MBPA, there were 72% (32/47) who had a history of somatoform or FD, 26/47 (55%) had a history of self-injury, and 10/47 (21%) were substance and alcohol abusers.[38] Notably, 17/19 (36% of all mothers studied) who were interviewed 1–15 years after original identification as MBPA also had concurrent personality disorders, defined as predominantly borderline and histrionic types.[38] As previously emphasized, these mothers are profoundly needy. Psychotherapy has determined that both rage and extremely low self-esteem couple to induce the degree of abuse these mothers engage in.[35, 39] These character traits, with the added distortions of their thoughts and coping with their actions by way of denial, perpetuate a near delusional state. Authors have suggested that they go on pathologically lying about their actions to a degree that allows them to believe that their child actually has an organic illness.[37]

THE CLINICAL CONDITION AND TREATMENTS: MUNCHAUSEN SYNDROME BY PROXY ABUSE

The evaluation of any child who has a difficulty in reconciling neurological disorder with paroxysmal features will at some point suggest MBPA. A number of warning signs have been suggested, which should alert the physician to this possibility (Table 6-7). An important clinical concept is that this is a pediatric diagnosis and not solely a psychiatric one. This is to say that it is incumbent upon pediatricians and pediatric specialists alike to be vigilant for the warning signs of this abuse disorder in their pediatric patients.

Suspicion for the possibility of MBPA is the first step in identification (Table 6-7). A thorough and careful scrutiny of all original medical records and test results, with an independent analysis of their validity and interpretation must be undertaken. This is necessary in order to identify false and fabricated statements of fact given by the perpetrator. Even when MBPA is suspected, the diagnosis can be difficult. Careful identification of those complaints that are real and those that are fabricated, as well as those which occur only in the mother's presence and those that have been witnessed by others, will provide support for additional covert investigation. Details about the family, its social, medical, and psychiatric history, should be verified from independent sources. Clarification about the exact neurological occurrences and their relationship to the mother's behavior and whereabouts need to be determined. The confirmation of laboratory and other testing data as being fabricated and not authentic may be possible if specifically sought after and all pertinent specimens are obtained and thoroughly examined. The identification of poisons, whether they are in small quantities of rare toxins or massive quantities of common remedies and household items (e.g., antihistamines, salt, bleach, etc.) will need to be specifically tested for.[13,31,40] A case of MBPA in brothers has been reported, where the elder of the two died at the hands of a maternally

Table 6-7 Warning Signs of Munchausen by Proxy Abuse

- Recurrent symptoms without identifiable cause
- Symptoms that are rare, unusual, or do not make sense
- Symptoms that baffle experienced clinicians
- Seizures (symptoms) with no response to treatment
- Seizures (symptoms) that occur only in the presence of the parent
- Inevitable intolerance to every prescribed treatment or intervention
- Discrepancies between presented history and documented facts
- Inconsistencies between presented history and clinical findings
- Overly attentive parent never away from the child while hospitalized
- Parent who is uncharacteristically accepting of the child's illness without worry
- Parent with prior medical training or experience
- Prior history of SIDS or other unexplained death in a sibling

Source: Modified from Reference.[10]
Note: Multiplicity of warning signs is most concerning.

administered poison, but unrecognized at the time of illness investigation. It was identified 14 years later in the younger brother who was being cared for in the terminal stages of what was thought to be mitochondrial encephalopathy lactic acidosis and stroke-like episodes (MELAS).[40] This poisoning was unequivocally shown to be secondary to chronic salicylates, opioids, and benzodiazepine toxicity before the second child succumbed. The second step in proving the abuse is to separate the caretaker from the child and observe for symptom relief (Table 6-8). Even this intervention does not always preclude the continuation of symptoms, particularly if chronic poisoning is the mode of abuse. Thus, continued suspicion and scrutiny is required.[40] When evaluating for an episodic phenomenon such as seizures, long observation periods and/or prolonged video monitoring may be needed. Covert video surveillance can be diagnostically enlightening, but must be done with careful attention to the safety of the child.[11,12] A retrospective review of forty-one hospitalized cases of suspected MBPA evaluated in hospital under covert video surveillance confirmed twenty-three diagnoses. The video recording was critical to obtain an unequivocal diagnosis of MBPA in more than 56% of the cases.[41] Importantly though, in four other cases, the parents were proven innocent.[41]

It has been debated as to whether the involvement of a child psychiatrist early in the evaluation process may be beneficial in the process of diagnosing MBPA. Their expertise will allow the managing physician to help understand the relationship of the mother with the child. This may also allow for the potential of psychiatric intervention at the point where the mother is confronted with evidence of the fraud and abuse if this is ultimately determined. Psychiatric evaluation of the mother–child dyad, however, should not be the way to exclude MBPA.[37,41] This type of evaluation does help to possibly discern a maternal motivation (i.e., a self-centered unmet psychological need).[18] Furthermore, there is the potential for an experienced consultant unfamiliar with the family and circumstances to be less readily manipulated by the perpetrator and thus better able to offer an unbiased opinion.

Once irrefutable evidence is obtained that the perpetrator is fabricating, falsifying, or inducing the symptoms of the child, confrontation of the

Table 6-8 Course of Action in Suspected Munchausen by Proxy Abuse

- Separate child from parent in hospital setting
- Collect and safeguard all specimens and records
- Crosscheck accuracy and veracity of all elements of the health history
- Verify temporal relationship of symptoms, signs, and parental presence
- Confirm recorded observations
- Enlist child psychiatrist
- Employ covert video monitoring
- Involve appropriate child protection services/authorities

Source: Modified from Reference.[10]
Note: Multiplicity of warning signs is most concerning.

perpetrator with this knowledge is advocated.[26, 37] This should be done by the managing physician with the support of the child psychiatrist. It would be rare for the mother (perpetrator) to admit their actions upon being confronted; more usual would be a firm but calm denial. Clearly, some mothers will become extremely agitated, depressed, or suicidal and will be in need of immediate psychiatric support or hospitalization.[26, 37] The ultimate goal of confrontation is to protect the child from further abuse, and thus appropriate protective services will need to be immediately involved. Psychiatric intervention for the mother acutely may also be needed. Long-term psychotherapeutic interventions for these mothers has had limited study, but has been advocated in a minority of cases where the perpetrator is highly motivated to confront their difficulties.[39]

The outcomes of those children who are thankfully identified as having suffered as victims of fabricated illness have been mixed. As many as 6%–9% of children will die as a result of the abuse, with as many as 8% of survivors suffering permanent disfigurement or physical impairment in function.[24, 25] In a large cohort of 54 children studied in follow-up 1–14 years (mean 5.6 years) after illness fabrication had been identified, Bools and colleagues found that 30/54 (55%) were living with their biological mothers and the remaining 24/54 (45%) were with other family members or in foster care.[42] Significant emotional and conduct disorders were identified in the children within each group, thirteen living with their biological mothers and fourteen not living with their biological mothers. Of these 27 children, 17/27 (63%) were not improving despite interventions, and 10/27 (37%) were improving.[42] Those children who improved with intervention tended to be younger than those who were not improving. Some positives that encouraged improvement were (1) continued positive input from the father of three children, (2) successful short-term foster care before return to the biologic mothers of five children, (3) mothers involved in a long-term therapeutic intervention from a social worker for three children, (4) successful remarriage of two mothers, (5) early adoption of three children, and (6) long-term foster care placement for one child.[42] It is important to note that some of these children who remained with their biologic mothers continued to be the subject of their mothers' fabrications even years after the initial identification.[43] Remarkably, 41/56 (73%) had been subsequently identified with failure to thrive, nonaccidental injury, inappropriate medication ingestion, neglect, or subject to more than one fabrication. Of equal importance was the fact that of the 103 siblings from these index cases, there were data available from 82 that supported similar abuse exposure in these siblings.[43] There were 39% (32/82) who had been the subject of fabricated illnesses, and 17% (14/82) who had suffered from failure to thrive, nonaccidental injury, inappropriate medication ingestion, or neglect.[43]

Berg and Jones have reported better outcomes after an intensive, multidisciplinary, in-hospital family intervention program.[44] They reported on the outcomes of sixteen treated families hospitalized for up to 4 months (mean 7½ weeks), at an average of 27 months postdischarge. There were no ongoing concerns for 9/16 families, mild concerns for 5/16 families, and serious concerns about the mental health of the mother in 2/16 families, although no overt abuse was suspected or identified.[44]

REFERENCES

1. *Diagnostic and Statistical Manual of Mental Disorders (DSM-IV-TR)*, 4th edition, text revision, Arlington, VA: American Psychological Association 2000; 485–517.
2. Libow JA. Child and adolescent illness falsification. Pediatrics 2000; 105; 336–342.
3. Ballas S. Factitious sickle cell acute painful episodes: a secondary type of Munchausen syndrome. Am J Hematol 1996; 53; 254–258.
4. Christopher KL, Wood RP, Ekert RC, et al. Vocal cord dysfunction presenting as asthma. N Engl J Med 1983; 308; 1566–1570.
5. Asher R. Munchausen's syndrome. Lancet 1951; I; 339–341.
6. Meadow R. Munchausen by proxy: the hinterland of child abuse. Lancet 1977; ii; 343–345.
7. *Diagnostic and Statistical Manual of Mental Disorders (DSM-IV-TR)*, 4th edition, text revision, Am Psych Assoc, Arlington, VA. 2000; 781.
8. Galvin HK, Newton AW, Vandeven AM. Update on Munchausen syndrome by proxy. Curr Opin in Pediatr 2005; 17(2); 252–257.
9. Meadow R. Fictitious epilepsy. Lancet 1984; ii; 25–28.
10. Meadow R. Munchausen syndrome by proxy. Arch Dis Child 1982; 57; 92–98.
11. Southall DP, Stebbens VA, Rees SV et al. Apnoeic episodes induced by smothering: two cases identified by covert video surveillance. BMJ 1987; 294; 1637–1641.
12. Rosen CL, Frost JD, Bricker T, et al. Two siblings with cardiorespiratory arrest: Munchausen syndrome by proxy or child abuse? Pediatrics 1983; 71; 715–720.
13. McClure RJ, Davis PM, Meadow SR, et al. Epidemiology of Munchausen syndrome by proxy, non-accidental poisoning, and non-accidental suffocation. Arch Dis Child 1996; 75; 57–61.
14. Makar AF. Munchausen syndrome by proxy: father as perpetrator. Pediatrics 1990; 85; 370–373.
15. Meadow R. Munchausen syndrome by proxy abuse perpetrated by men. Arch Dis Child 1998; 78(3); 210–216.
16. Feldman MD, Brown RM. Munchausen by proxy in an international context. Child Abuse Negl 2002; 26(5); 509–524.
17. Ayoub CC, Alexander R. Definitional issues in Munchhausen syndrome by proxy. Am Prof Soc Abuse of Child 1998; 11; 7–10.
18. Ayoub CC, Alexander R, Beck D, et al. APSAC Taskforce on Munchausen by Proxy, Definitions Working Group. Position paper: Definitional issues in Munchhausen syndrome by proxy. Child Maltreat 2002; 7(2); 105–111.
19. Fisher JA. Investigating the Barons: narrative and nomenclature in Munchausen syndrome. Perspectives Biol Med 2006; 49(2); 250–262.
20. Schreier H. Munchausen by proxy defined. Pediatrics 2002; 110(5); 985–988.
21. Rogers, R. Diagnostic, explanatory, and detection models of Munchausen by proxy: extrapolations from malingering and deception. Child Abuse Negl 2004; 28(2); 225–238.
22. Lai CW, Ziegler DK. Repeated self-induced syncope and subsequent seizures. Arch Neurol 1983; 40; 820–823.
23. Libow JA. Beyond collusion: active illness falsification. Child Abuse Negl 2002; 26; 525–536.

24. Rosenberg DA. Web of deceit: a literature review of Munchausen syndrome by proxy. Child Abuse Negl 1987; 11; 547–563.
25. Sheridan MS. The deceit continues: an updated literature review of Munchausen syndrome by proxy. Child Abuse Negl 2003; 27; 431–451.
26. Schreier H. Munchausen by proxy. Curr Probl Pediatr Adolesc Health Care 2004; 34; 126–143.
27. Tellioglu T, Oates JA, Biaggioni I. Munchausen's syndrome presenting as baroreflex failure. New Engl J Med 2000; 343(8); 581.
28. Meadow R. Neurological and developmental variants of Munchausen syndrome by proxy. Devel Med Child Neurol 1991; 33; 267–272.
29. Heubrock, D. Munchhausen by proxy syndrome in clinical child neuropsychology: a case presenting with neuropsychological symptoms. Child Neuropsychol 2001; 7(4); 273–285.
30. Jungheim K. Badenhoop K. Ottmann OG. Usadel KH. Kleine-Levin and Munchausen syndromes in a patient with recurrent acromegaly. Eur J Endo 1999; 140(2); 140–142.
31. Bauer M. Boegner F. Neurological syndromes in factitious disorder. J Nerv Ment Dis 1996; 184(5); 281–288.
32. Rashid N. Medically unexplained myopathy due to ipecac abuse. Psychosomatics 2006; 47(2); 167–169.
33. Papadopoulos MC, Bell BA. Factitious neurosurgical emergencies: report of five cases. Br J Neurosurg 1999; 13(6); 591–593.
34. Fehnel CR, Brewer EJ. Munchausen's syndrome with 20-year follow-up. Am J Psychiatry 2006; 163(3); 547.
35. Schreier H. On the importance of motivation in Munchhausen syndrome by proxy: the case of Kathy Bush. Child Abuse Negl 2002; 26; 537–549.
36. Zitelli BJ, Seltman MF, Shannon RM. Munchausen's syndrome by proxy and its professional participants. Am J Dis Child 1987; 141; 1099–1102.
37. Forsyth BWC, Asnes AG. Munchausen syndrome by proxy. In *Lewis's Child and Adolescent Psychiatry*. Eds: FR Volkmar, M Lewis, 4th edition. Philadelphia, PA, Lippincott Williams & Wilkins, 2007; 719–727.
38. Bools CN, Neale B, Meadow R. Munchausen syndrome by proxy: A study of psychopathology. Child Abuse Negl 1994; 18; 773–788.
39. Nicol AR, Eccles M. Psychotherapy for Munchausen by proxy. Arch Dis Child 1985; 60; 344–348.
40. Schreier H, Ricci L. Follow-up of a case of Munchausen by proxy syndrome. J Am Acad Child Adolesc Psychiatry 2002; 41(12); 1395–1396.
41. Hall DE, Eubanks L, Meyyazhagan S, et al. Evaluation of covert video surveillance in the diagnosis of Munchausen syndrome by proxy: lessons from 41 cases. Pediatrics 2000; 105(6); 1305–1312.
42. Bools CN, Neale BA, Meadow SR. Follow up of victims of fabricated illness (Munchausen syndrome by proxy). Arch Dis Child 1993; 69; 625–630.
43. Bools CN, Neale BA, Meadow SR. Co-morbidity associated with fabricated illness (Munchausen syndrome by proxy). Arch Dis Child 1992; 67; 77–79.
44. Berg B, Jones D. Outcome of psychiatric intervention in factitious illness by proxy (Munchausen's syndrome by proxy). Arch Dis Child 1999; 81; 465–572.

7

Movement Disorders

INTRODUCTION TO MOVEMENT DISORDERS

Not surprisingly, the misidentification of all types of involuntary movements as possibly epileptic in origin is common. This extends directly from the fact that many epileptic seizure types have associated rhythmic and stereotyped motor movements and behaviors. Partial seizures in particular present with a varied array of involuntary motor activity without alterations in consciousness. Thus, the mere presence or absence of an altered state of consciousness will not be sufficient to differentiate epileptic from non-epileptic motor movements. In addition, there exists a unique grouping of involuntary movement disorders that have a paroxysmal character similar to the nature of epileptic seizure events. Even more similar is the fact that both epilepsy and non-epileptic involuntary movement disorders often coexist with both underlying static and progressive neurological diseases. However, specific clinical features, characteristic presentations, and associated symptoms will better enable the clinician to discriminate from epilepsy the various movement disorders.

THE CLINICAL PROBLEM AND EPIDEMIOLOGY

Unusual and involuntary movements are a common and an often perplexing problem in childhood. There are a number of physiologic and developmental types of movements recognized at various ages. These are camouflaged within a landscape of both static and progressive neurological disorders that are produced by a myriad of genetic, metabolic, and acquired etiologies. The clarity of any movement's evolution, the descriptive precision of the movement's character during observation, and the completeness of the subject's clinical and family history will often determine whether the movement in question is ultimately pathologic or not.

Abnormal movements are generally nonvoluntary and unintentional; however, not all nonvoluntary unintentional movements are abnormal.[1,2] Consider, for example, reflexive or automatic movements such as sneezing, blinking, and breathing. None of these are abnormal, but are clearly nonvoluntary and unintentional. Although an individual may exert variable degrees of influence over the frequency, intensity, and excursion of these movements, they inevitably occur. The clinician must extract a careful history to clarify the exact description and setting in which the movement occurs. This will allow

217

Table 7-1 Clinical Approach to History

Key Clinical Components of History

- What are the characteristics of tone, posture and movement exhibited?
- Is the movement "fast" or "slow"?
- Is the movement large or small in amplitude, arrhythmic or rhythmic, stereotyped or not?
- What is the quality of the movement: intermittent (repetitive), continuous (without stopping), episodic (paroxysmal) or sustained?
- Does it occur with wakefulness, at sleep or both, at rest or with action?
- Is the movement suppressible by the child or stop with distraction?
- Are there vocalizations?
- Is there a sensory component?
- Is the movement complex or involve self-mutilation?
- Are there or have there been any associated neurological and or systemic abnormalities?
- Is there a familial pattern to the abnormality?
- Is there familial consanguinity?
- Were there any significant perinatal, natal or postnatal complications or findings?
- Have there been periods of encephalopathy, convulsions, ocular abnormalities or rashes?
- What was the age of onset?
- Does the character of the movement evolve over a period of time (minutes, hours, day-night)?
- Has the character of the movement evolved over time?
- What has been the chronological evolution of the abnormality?
- Are there any specific precipitants (drugs, exercise, infection etc.) or palliatives (rest/sleep, food)?

Key Clinical Components of Examination

- Careful general examination
- Carefully directed observation of all limb, face, ocular and trunk movements
- Observance of body posture at rest, with action, and when suspended
- Direct the child to move limbs toward a target, write/draw, run, climb, and ambulate on toes/heels/and in tandem
- Distract the child and startle the child
- Standard neurological examination

the correct identification (Table 7-1). Abnormal movements may be apparent only under certain circumstances and visible at variable frequencies, "intermittent" being multiple times per hour or day with periods of time when it is not observable, "continuous" being present nearly always, and "paroxysmal" being evident infrequently, usually episodically once a day or less. Similarly, the rhythm of the movement offers an important identifying characteristic. The regularity and predictability of a movement or lack thereof serves to further classify the quality of the movement (Table 7-2).

These clinical descriptors allow an organization of movements into discrete symptom entities, which can then be further etiologically examined.

Automatic movements are those that are performed or occur without conscious effort. These may be learned behaviors or reflex in nature. These

Table 7-2 Movement Hallmark Characterizations

Rhythmic	Arrhythmic	Intermittent	Continuous	Paroxysmal
Tremor	Myoclonus	Chorea	Athetosis	Dystonia
Stereotypy	Tic	Ballismus	Myokymia	Dyskinesias
Segmental	Athetosis	Dystonia	Dystonic	Tic
myoclonus	Dystonia	Akathasia	reactions	Stereotypy
	Periodic sleep		Torticollis	Hyperekplexia
	movements			
	Hyperekplexia			
	Akathasia			

Source: Modified from References.[2–4,5]

can often accompany an abnormal movement in an effort to mask or cover it up. An extension of this automatic movement is the notion that a sensory stimulus may at times induce an automatic movement. Therefore, an unpleasant unwanted sensation or inner tension such as can occur with restless legs syndrome, akathasia, or motor/vocal tics will result in the abnormal movement and an accompanying automatic masking movement. There can be some degree of supressibility if the individual so chooses, but often it is only temporary or incomplete. Similarly, habit movements and stereotypies can be suppressed unconsciously when the child is distracted while engaging in them. This character helps to distinguish them from other types of abnormal involuntary movements that are typically neither suppressible nor distractible.

The types of individual involuntary movements observed in children are equivalent to those identified in adulthood with additional neurodevelopmental and transient entities (Table 7-3).[1,2]

Although the majority of these are not usually confused as epileptic, many are evaluated initially as potentially epileptic or occur in the context of an underlying childhood neurodevelopmental disorder and or epilepsy. A number of different types of paroxysmal movements are additionally exhibited predominantly in childhood and not seen in adulthood. The primary type of movement should be first determined; then the possible specific etiologic disorder can be more readily defined later. A flow diagram of the commonly encountered types of movements (Figure 7-1) is offered with some helpful decision points to allow better characterization of the observed movement.[1] These decision points are inserted at the most unique and often defining feature that allows diagnosis. It must be said that not all movements will fit cleanly into this schema but this should serve as a basic foundation from which to evaluate the movement. The classic separation of abnormal movements into hyperkinetic and hypokinetic forms can be helpful as a starting point. The term dyskinesia is used as a synonym for hyperkinetic movements in general. Hypokinetic movements are characterized by a scarcity of movement accompanied by bradykinesia, the slowed and diminished amplitude of a voluntary movement. This can be manifest by a masked facies (hypomimia), diminished blinking,

Table 7-3 Major Types of Movements

Movement	Description and Characterization	Distribution	Common Etiologies	Examples
Akathasia	An inner feeling of general restlessness or sensation of discomfort relieved by movement. Complex, stereotyped, suppressible, occasionally rhythmic	• Focal • Generalized • Vocalized	Iatrogenic: drug withdrawal (antidopaminergics, dopamine depleting)	• Pacing, squirming, fidgeting • Crossing–uncrossing legs • Humming
Athetosis	An abnormal slow writhing continuous movement from co-contractions of agonist and antagonist muscles with dispersion into muscles not required for the provoked assumption of posture or voluntary movement	• Focal (distal limbs) • Generalized	Acquired basal ganglia injury (cerebral palsy)	Overflow writhing and stiffening when attempting to speak
Ballismus	A severe form of chorea with excessive, involuntary, stereotyped, nonrhythmic, large-amplitude flailing movements of the proximal limbs	• Segmental (hemibody, bilateral limbs) • Generalized	Contralateral subthalamic nucleus injury	Violent limb and body thrashing

Term	Description	Classification	Etiology	Features
Chorea	Excessive, involuntary, stereotyped, nonrhythmic, small-amplitude dancing movements of the distal limbs and face, with motor impersistence. (Inability to maintain a muscular contraction continually and smoothly)	• Focal (distal limbs, face) • Generalized	• Lesions of the ventral thalamus and striatum, with overactive dopaminergic activity; e.g., post-streptococcal • Genetic	• Unsustainable tongue protrusion • "Milkmaid" hand grasp • Fidgety-type seated position
Dyskinesia	The broad category of hyperkinetic movements and specific paroxysmal disorders (PKC, PDC, PED, PHD, CSE, ICCA, RE-PED-WC)	• Focal • Generalized	• All within this column • Genetic	See first column
Dystonia	An abnormal sustained co-contraction of agonist and antagonist muscles not required for the assumption of a normal posture or voluntary movement. Often results in twisting and an abnormal posture. Spontaneous and action induced	• Focal • Segmental • Generalized • Vocalized	• Iatrogenic: drug administration (antidopaminergics, dopamine depleting) • Acquired basal ganglia injury (cerebral palsy) • Genetic	• Hand and foot postures • Blepharospasm • Dysphonia • Trunkal twisting

continued

Table 7-3 continued

Movement	Description and Characterization	Distribution	Common Etiologies	Examples
Myoclonus	A sudden, brief, synchronized, shock-like contraction of a muscle or group of muscles resulting in a nonrhythmic repetitive jerky movement. Massive myoclonus involves the entire body at once	• Focal • Segmental • Generalized	• Acquired injury (hypoxic-ischemic, hypoglycemia, etc.) to the cortex and subcortical motor pathways • Iatrogenic: drug administration (antiepileptics-diphenylhydantoin) • Metabolic (renal and hepatic failure) • Neuromuscular (SMA) • Genetic (Angelman syndrome)	• Asterixsis • Polyminimyoclonus of outstretched hands and fingers in SMA • Limb and facial jerks after profound hypoxicischemic encephalopathy • Ocular myoclonus (slow, conjugate vertical oscillations) • Ocular myorhythmia (slow, conjugate horizontal oscillations)
Myokymia	A fine rippling or quivering contraction of a muscle. Distuishable from a benign fasciculation only by EMG examination	Focal (facial region)	Pontine lesions (tumor, demyelination, stroke)	Twitching of the orbicularis oculi

Opsoclonus	Chaotic, irregular, continuous, brief ocular movements, often accompanied by body myoclonus and ataxia	Focal	• Metabolic (neuroblastoma, opsoclonus-myoclonus-ataxia syndrome) • Immune-mediated	Quick, chaotic dysconjugate eye movements
Stereotypy	A repetitive, stereotyped, rhythmic movement that stops with distraction or engagement	• Focal • Segmental • Generalized	Idiopathic (autistic, cognitively impaired, and normal children)	• Head banging • Hand flapping • Body rocking • Thumb sucking • Trichotillomania
Tics	An involuntary, stereotyped, nonpurposeful, often rhythmic, repetitive movement or sound that can be voluntarily suppressed. These can be transient or chronic, simple or complex, single or multiple, with or without combinations of movements and or sounds indistinguishable from normal voluntary movements and sounds	• Focal • Segmental • Generalized	• Genetic • Metabolic disease and CO poisoning • Acquired or precipitated by encephalitis, trauma, medications (neuroleptics, psychostimulants, anticholinergics, tricyclics, and sympathomimetics)	• Head shaking • Neck craning • Arm and finger flicking or stretching • Grimacing • Blinking or eye rolling • Body tensing and slamming • Vocalizations and expletives

continued

Table 7-3 continued

Movement	Description and Characterization	Distribution	Common Etiologies	Examples
Tremor	A stereotyped, rhythmic, and oscillatory involuntary movement. Can be seen at rest, with action, or sustention against gravity. It is produced by abnormal alternating contractions of agonist and antagonist muscles	• Focal • Segmental	• Genetic • CNS disease and neurodegeneration (cerebellar, SN, dentato-rubro-olivary complexes, etc.) • Neuropathy • Acquired or precipitated by encephalitis, trauma, stroke, medications (neuroleptic, psychostimulants, and sympathomimetics)	• Hand oscillations upon extension or at rest • Vocal quivering when speaking • Head titubations while seated upright, standing, or walking • Head and body shuddering while seated

Source: Modified from References.[1–4,5,6]
Notes: Focal = small segments of the body at one time (voice, palate, tongue, mouth, fingers, toes, hands, feet, face, shoulder, etc.); Segmental = larger two contiguous regional portions of the body or a whole extremity (head and shoulders, whole limb, trunk and legs, etc.); Generalized = focal and both axial and appendicular segments simultaneously; PKC = paroxysmal kinesiogenic and nonkinesiogenic choreo-athetosis/dystonia; PDC = paroxysmal dystonic choreo-athetosis; PED = paroxysmal exercise-induced dystonia; PHD = paroxysmal hypnogogic nocturnal dyskinesia; CSE = paroxysmal choreo-athetosis and spasticity; ICCA = infantile convulsions and paroxysmal choreo-athetosis; RE-PED-WC = Rolandic epilepsy-paroxysmal exercise-induced dystonia and writer's cramp; SMA = spinal muscular atrophy with polyminimyoclonus; EMG = electromyography; SN = substantia nigra.

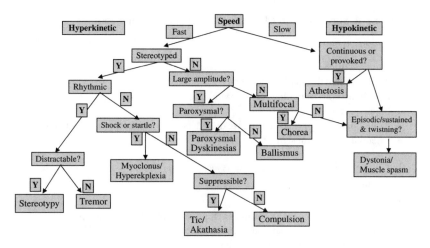

Figure 7-1. Childhood Movements Decision Algorithm Y—"yes", N—"no". (Source: Modified from Reference.[1])

drooling, soft speech (hypophonia), and loss of speech inflection (aprosody). Hypokinetic movement disorders are also often accompanied by rigid hypertonia, the "lead-pipe" quality with a regularly interrupted resistance to passive movement, "cogwheeling." However, the vast majority of movements seen in children are distinctly hyperkinetic as Parkinson's disease and Parkinsonism are less frequently encountered in youth. Tics and movements associated with cerebral palsy (dyskinesia, athetosis, muscle spasms, dystonia, etc.) would clearly predominate childhood referrals. Furthermore, involuntary movements may have overlapping qualities with each other that are not necessarily mutually exclusive, and specific etiologic causes often produce a multiplicity of abnormal movements. The observance of movements only in sleep but not during wakefulness suggests the presence of a sleep-related movement disorder such as hypnogogic dyskinesias, sleep starts, or periodic limb movements of sleep (see Chapter 4). This distinction of being evident only in sleep should be carefully differentiated from movements that persist intermittently during wakefulness and into sleep. There are only a select few abnormal movements that conform to this later pattern myoclonus (including ocular and palatal) and myokymia (fine muscle rippling). Less frequently muscle spasms, chorea, and tics may also be able to be noted to do this but not characteristically in most patients.[2,3]

Abnormal movements are not necessarily disorders themselves but rather are symptoms of possible underlying disease or a developmental process. Therefore, not only the predominant movement but also other associated movements, examination findings, age, and past and family histories need to be integrated in order to determine the appropriate investigative focus. Many clinical features will allow identification of those disorders that are unique to childhood and potentially among those that are benign and transient (Tables 7-4 and 7-5).

Table 7-4 Some Benign Movement Disorders of Childhood

Neonates – Infants

- Neonatal jitteriness
- Benign neonatal (sleep) myoclonus
- Hereditary chin trembling (geniospasm)
- Binkie flutter
- Benign paroxysmal extraocular gaze disorders (tonic upgaze, tonic downgaze)
- Essential setting-sun sign

Infants – Children

- Shuddering spells
- Spasmus nutans
- Benign myoclonus of early infancy (benign non-epileptic infantile spasms)
- Tonic reflex seizures in early infancy
- Benign paroxysmal torticollis of infancy
- Transient and paroxysmal dystonia of infancy
- Sandifer's syndrome
- Laryngeal dyskinesia
- Stool-holding stiffening spells
- Gratification disorder
- Stereotypies
- Benign nocturnal alternating hemiplegia of childhood
- Diaphragmatic flutter
- Fever-precipitated myoclonus, ballismus, and tremor with effects on stereotypies
- Otitis media spells

Children – Adolescents

- Transient tics
- Non-epileptic head drops
- Childhood head tremor
- Essential palatal tremor

Source: Modified from References.[2,4,5,7–15]

Once a movement is characterized and a benign entity cannot confidently be identified, then an alternative etiology must be considered with appropriate evaluation undertaken if needed. It is useful to organize these etiologies into primary, idiopathic, or hereditary disorders and secondary, acquired, or iatrogenic ones for the predominant types of movement present (Table 7-6).[2,4,5,7–12]

Although there are many movement disorders in children considered primary or genetic in origin, the majority are secondary to another acquired cause: infectious, postinfectious, metabolic, iatrogenic, toxic, and/or destructive. A multitude of additional genetic and neurometabolic diseases induce various types of movements (Table 7-7).[2,4,5,7–12,16]

The following tables are extensive but should not be considered complete. These are provided so as to expose the scope and breadth of the potential causes of both acute and chronic progressive entities. A full discussion of all these

Table 7-5 Some Movement Disorders with Onset and Predominance in Childhood

Neonates – Infants

- Hyperekplexia
- Infantile chorea with severe bronchopulmonary dysplasia
- Paroxysmal dyskinesias

Infants – Children

- Cardiac surgery-induced choreoathetosis
- Bobble-head doll syndrome
- Myoclonus-dystonia syndrome
- Opsoclonus-myoclonus-ataxia syndrome
- Paroxysmal dyskinesias

Children – Adolescents

- Paroxysmal dyskinesias
- Tourette's syndrome
- Diaphragmatic flutter
- Hereditary chin trembling (geniospasm)

Source: Modified from References.[2,4,5,7–13]

Table 7-6 Some Etiologic Examples of Childhood Involuntary Movements

Primary Movement	Idiopathic/Genetic Etiologies	Secondary Etiologies
Athetosis/Dystonia	Idiopathic torsion dystonia	*Post Infectious/Immune-Mediated*
	Transient dystonia of infancy	HIV/toxoplasmosis
	Paroxysmal torticollis of infants	*Metabolic*
	Dopa-responsive dystonia	Glutaric aciduria
	Childhood-onset Parkinson disease	Hartnup disease
		Creatine deficiency
	Juvenile parkinsonism	Biotinidase deficiency
	Krabbe leukodystrophy	Homocystinuria
	Pelizaeus-Merzbacher disease	Kernicterus
	Neuronal ceroid lipofuscinosis	*Iatrogenic/Intoxication*
	Wilson's disease	Levodopa/carbidopa
	Lesch-Nyhan disease	Metaclopromide
	Leigh's disease (striatal necrosis)	Gabapentin
		Cetirizine (H-1 receptor antagonist)
		SSRIs
		Anticholinergic withdrawal
		Neuroleptics/antidopaminergics

continued

Table 7-6 continued

Primary Movement	Idiopathic/Genetic Etiologies	Secondary Etiologies
	Alternating hemiplegia	Calcium channel blockers
		Lithium
		Contraceptives
		Ischemic/Vascular
		Cerebral palsy
		Thalamic/striatal infarction
Ballismus/Chorea	Benign hereditary chorea	*Post Infectious/ Immune-mediated*
	Pregnancy	Syndenham's chorea
	Wilson's disease	Infectious mononucleosis
	Huntington's disease	Mycoplasma encephalitis
	Canavan spongy degeneration	Herpes simplex encephalitis
		HIV/toxoplasmosis
	Neuronal ceroid lipofuscinosis	Fever induced (ballismus/tremor/myoclonus)
	Lesch-Nyhan disease	*Metabolic (genetic)*
	Ataxia-telangiectasia	Biopterin deficiency
	Friedreich ataxia	Creatine deficiency
	Neuroacanthocytosis	Glutaric aciduria
	Leigh's disease (striatal necrosis)	Diabetes mellitus (hyperglycemia)
		Ischemic/Vascular
		Moya moya disease
		Post-cardiac surgery-induced chorea
		BPD-associated chorea-myoclonus
		Anticardiolipin syndrome
		SLE
		Subthalamic/striatal infarction
		Iatrogenic/Intoxication
		CO poisoning
		Phenytoin
		Ethosuximide
		Gabapentin
		Isoniazid
		SSRIs
		Lithium
		Oral contraceptives
		Levodopa, dopaminergics, dopamine-blocking agents
		Pemoline, methylphenidate, amphetamines
		Antihistamines
		Anticholinergics

Mercury
Tricyclic antidepressants

Dyskinesia (paroxysmal)	Paroxysmal torticollis of infants	*Post Infectious/Immune-mediated*
	Benign paroxysmal tonic upgaze	Mycoplasma encephalitis
		HIV/toxoplasmosis
	PKC	*Metabolic (genetic)*
	PKD	Thyrotoxicosis
	PED	Cystinuria
	PHD	Hartnups disease
	CSE	Hypoglycemia
	ICCA	Non-ketotic hyperglycinemia
		Pyruvate decarboxylase deficiency
	RE-PED-RE	*Ischemic/Vascular*
	PKAN	Cerebral hypoxic-ischemic injury
		Thalamic infarction
		Iatrogenic/Intoxication
		Gabapentin
		Hydantoin
		Metaclopromide
		Neuroleptics/antidopaminergics
		Methylphenidate
		Pemoline
		Carbamazepine
		Clonazepam
Myoclonus	Physiologic	*CNS Tumor*
	Hiccups	Opsoclonus-myoclonus-ataxia syndrome
	Anxiety induced	*Post Infectious/Immune-Mediated*
	Exercise induced	Opsoclonus-myoclonus-ataxia syndrome
	Essential	Herpes simplex encephalitis
	Benign myoclonus of infancy	Subacute sclerosing panencephalitis
	Benign neonatal sleep myoclonus	HIV/toxoplasmosis
	Hereditary chin trembling	Fever induced (ballismus/tremor/myoclonus)
	Hyperekplexia	*Metabolic (genetic)*
	Neuronal ceroid lipofuscinosis	Non-ketotic hyperglycinemia
	Gaucher disease	Multiple carboxylase deficiency
	Wilson's disease	Biotin deficiency
	Sialidosis	Vitamin B-12 deficiency
	Friedreich ataxia	

continued

Table 7-6 continued

Primary Movement	Idiopathic/Genetic Etiologies	Secondary Etiologies
		Hepatic & renal failure
		Dialysis syndrome
	Huntington's disease	Post-hypoglycemic encephalopathy
	PKAN	*Ischemic/Vascular*
	MERRF	Cerebral hypoxic-ischemic
	Leigh's disease (striatal	injury
	necrosis)	*Iatrogenic/Intoxication*
		Heavy metals (manganese, lead, etc.)
		Bismuth
		Morphine
		SSRIs
		Tricyclic antidepressants
		Levodopa, dopaminergics
		Carbamazepine
		Lithium
		Valproate
		Phenytoin
Tremor	Physiologic	*CNS Tumor*
	Essential	Bobble-head doll syndrome
	Shuddering spells	*Post Infectious/Immune-Mediated*
	Essential palatal tremor	Guillain-Barre syndrome
	Spasmus nutans	HIV/toxoplasmosis
	Neonatal jitteriness	Influenza
	Benign familial chorea	Fever induced
	Juvenile Parkinsonism	(ballismus/tremor/myoclonus)
	Juvenile Huntington disease	*Metabolic (genetic)*
	Wilson's disease	Phenylketonuria
	Hereditary motor & sensory	Hyperthyroidism
	neuropathies	Hypoglycemia
	PKAN	Vitamin B-12 deficiency
	Diaphragmatic flutter	*Ischemic/Vascular*
		Cerebral hypoxic-ischemic
		injury
		Iatrogenic/Intoxication
		Valproate
		Carbamazepine
		Ethosuximide
		Lamotrigine
		Bronchodilators (B-adrenergics)
		Levodopa, dopaminergics
		Iron overdose
		Mercury

Lithium

Pemoline, methylphenidate, caffeine,
amphetamine, theophylline

Antihistamines

Corticosteroids

Tricyclic antidepressants

Source: Modified from References.[2, 4, 5, 7–13, 16–19]
Notes: SSRI = serotonin reuptake inhibitors; BPD = brochopulmonary dysplasia; SLE = systemic
lupus erythematosis; PKC = paroxysmal kinesiogenic and non-kinesiogenic choreo-athetosis/dystonia;
PDC = paroxysmal dystonic choreo-athetosis; PED = paroxysmal exercise-induced dystonia;
PHD = paroxysmal hypnogogic nocturnal dyskinesia; CSE = paroxysmal choreo-athetosis and
spasticity; ICCA = infantile convulsions and paroxysmal choreo-athetosis; RE-PED-WC = Rolandic
epilepsy-paroxysmal exercise-induced dystonia and writer's cramp; PKAN = Pantothenate
kinase-associated neurodegeneration, previously known as Hallervorden-Spatz disease;
MERRF = mitochondrial epilepsy with ragged red fibers.

Table 7-7 Some Neurometabolic Movement Disorders Primarily of Childhood

Primary Disorders

1. Tourette's syndrome
2. Wilson's disease
3. Hyperekplexia
4. Lesch-Nyhan disease
5. Spinal muscular atrophy (SMA) associated polyminimyoclonus

Hypokinetic-rigid syndromes and dystonias associated with metabolic diseases

1. Biotinidase deficiency
2. Pediatric neurotransmitter diseases
3. Spinocerebellar degenerations
4. Lysosomal storage diseases
   - Niemann-Pick type C disease
   - Neuronal Ceroid Lipofucinoses
   - Juvenile GM1 and GM2 gangliosidosis
   - Metachromatic leukodystrophy
   - Krabbe's disease
   - Pelizaeus-Merzbacher disease
5. Organic aminoacidopathies
   - Phenylketonuria
   - Glutaric aciduria
   - Homocysteinuria
   - Methylmalonic acidemia
   - Tryptophan deficiency (Hartnup's disease)
   - Others

continued

Table 7-7 continued

6. Mitochondrial disorders
   - Leigh's disease
   - MELAS
7. Neuraxonal dystrophy
8. Ataxia-telangiectasia
9. Dopa-responsive dystonia (with marked diurnal fluctuation)
10. Machado-Joseph disease
11. Subacute sclerosing panencephalitis
12. Neuroacanthocytosis
13. Juvenile idiopathic parkinsonism
14. Dentatorubro-pallidoluysian atrophy
15. Pantothenate kinase-associated neurodegeneration (PKAN)
16. Huntington disease
17. Others

Secondary to other neuroanatomic disturbances

1. Kernicterus
2. Cerebral palsy
3. Hydrocephalus
4. CNS tumors
5. Post-encephalitis
6. Drugs and intoxications
7. Others

Unknown pathophysiology for associated movement disorders

1. Alternating hemiplegia of childhood
2. Rett's syndrome

Source: Modified from References.[2,4,5,7–10,16]
Notes: MELAS = mitochondrial encephalomyopathy lactic acidosis and stroke-like episodes;
PKAN = Pantothenate kinase-associated neurodegeneration, previously known as Hallervorden-Spatz disease.

entities is beyond the focus of this text; however, those entities, both benign and unique to childhood, with the potential to be confused as epileptic will be described further in the subsequent text.

Involuntary movements of all types are often identified and considered as possibly epileptic in origin. Series of children referred for EEG telemetry have stratified a number of involuntary movement types that can be specified in a majority of these cases. By the nature of the examination the population being evaluated is biased toward those children with a primary concern of epilepsy. Nonetheless, these surveys suggest an approximate prevalence of involuntary movements that approaches 10.6%–19.5% in telemetry referral centers.[20–30] The higher percentage figure is observed in those children who have additional underlying neurocognitive impairments. These figures contrast with an approximate prevalence of involuntary movements noted in only

4.5% of children referred for a clinical evaluation of non-epileptic events and not epilepsy specifically.[27] The actual incidence and prevalence within the general population are not available. The referral population studies are dependent upon the underlying etiology and specific disorders attracting evaluation. Population studies of cerebral palsy (CP) subjects, for example, have demonstrated a rather stable incidence rate of 1.7–2.0 per 1000 surviving live births.[31–37] Among these surviving children with CP, the dyskinetic form of the disorder occurs in a full 8%–15% of all cases.[32, 38] Dyskinetic CP comprises involuntary movements and postures, abnormal fluctuations of tone, and a persistence of primitive motor responses.[32, 38] Important points can be drawn from the data presented in Table 7-8.

In comparison to adult movement disorder clinic populations, the overall prevalence of childhood tic disorders and stereotypies are more commonly referred and diagnosed. There is a preponderance of hypokinetic-rigid syndromes and Parkinson's disease noted in the adult series and by contrast the majority of movement disorders seen in children are hyperkinetic. Perhaps a more intriguing group of children are those who manifest benign and often-transient involuntary movements.[9, 10] These children are otherwise normal but present with a rather broad array of observable focal, segmental, and generalized events (Table 7-4). Their overall prevalence is unknown but likely underidentified given the transient (duration <1 year) and benign nature of their appearance. In a pediatric movement disorder clinic series from Spain, of 356 patients evaluated (excluding CP, tics/Tourette's syndrome, and iatrogenic movements), 67 (19%) were transient, unassociated with neurological disease, and thus benign by definition.[9] The majority (76%) had the onset of the disorder under 1 year of age and 50% began within the first 3 months of life.[9] The most common types of transient movement were various types of dystonia, tremor, and myoclonus. These readily recognizable disorders obviate the need for further investigation or intervention.

Population surveys have identified tics as the most predominant childhood movement disorder with up to 12%–24% of school-aged children exhibiting them.[13, 39, 40] Although many are transient, those that endure and become chronic or develop into Tourette's syndrome may have a prevalence closer to 0.5%–6%.[13, 40] An overall population prevalence of Tourette's syndrome has been recently estimated to be 1–10 per 1000.[40–43] These estimates have been derived from combined school-based samples of over 6000 children in Rochester, NY, and Sweden, utilizing parent and teacher questionnaires, applying DSM-IV criteria.[40–43] An important aspect of the prevalence data is the ascertainment of an even significantly higher frequency of tics found in 27% of 341 special education students compared with only 19.6% of 1255 regular education students in an unselected community school-based sample.[42] Children in addition to adults suffer movement disorders as a result of severe head trauma. The incidence of posttraumatic tremor has been noted in over 45% patients of whom up to 18% may exhibit forms of posttraumatic dystonia.[44–47]

Table 7-8 Incidences of Various Movement Disorders Identified in EEG Telemetry Series Compared to Movement Disorder Clinics

Non-Epileptic Events	EEG Telemetry Series of Neurologically Normal Children[20–26] N = 1211*	EEG Telemetry Series of Neurologically Abnormal Children[20, 22, 27–30] N = 532*	Movement Disorder Clinic for Children[2] N = 684†	Movement Disorder Clinic for Adults[5] N = 21,766‡
Encountered Abnormal Movements	129 (10.6%)	104 (19.5%)	684 (100%)	21,766 (100%)
Specific Movement Diagnoses:				
(Tics/Tourette Syndrome)	57 (44.1%)	42 (40.3%)	261 (39%)	1,022 (4.7%)
(Nonspecific and Mixed Movements)	NS	32 (30.7%)	53 (8%)	434 (2.0%) "psychogenic"
(Tremor/Shuddering)	26 (20.1%)	25 (24%)	129 (19%)	3,013 (13.9%)
(Myoclonus)	7 (5.4%)	19 (18.2%)	19 (2%)	547 (2.5%)
(Dystonia/Posturing)	14 (10.8%)	36 (34.6%)	162 (24%)	6,798 (31.3%)
(Paroxysmal dyskinesias/torticollis)	4 (3.1%)	3 (2.9%)	NS	169 (1.5%)
(Stereotypies/Habit and Self-Stimulatory Behaviors)	14 (10.8%)	16 (15.4%)	NS	163 (0.7%)
(Paroxysmal Gaze/Eye Movements)	2 (1.6%)	29 (27.9%)	NS	NS
(Chorea/Ballism)	NS	NS	34 (5%)	658 (3.1%)
(Tardive Syndromes/Dyskinesias)	NS	NS	NS	583 (2.7%)
(Parkinson's Disease)	NS	NS	NS	7,564 (32.9%)

Source: Modified from References.[2,5,20–30]

Notes: NS = not specified.

* From among all non-epileptic events assessed only, excludes diagnosed epilepsy patients.

† Excludes iatrogenic movement disorders and cerebral palsy patients.

‡ Data combined from two large clinic populations (Columbia University Medical Center, NY, and Baylor College of Medicine, Houston) that include multiple movements per patient.

OVERVIEW: PATHOPHYSIOLOGY AND MECHANISMS

The basal ganglia (BG) and their connections are the primary subcortical nuclei responsible for motor function (Figures 7-2 and 7-3). BG are comprised of the caudate, putamen, nucleus accumbens (these three make up "the striatum"), globus pallidus, and olfactory tubercle with the integrally and functionally related substancia nigra (SN) and subthalamic nucleus (SubTN).[48] There is a dense array of neuronal architecture whereby the striatum, composed mostly of medium spiny neurons, receives inputs from the cortex and dopamine-containing projections from the SN. These spiny neurons also receive inputs from excitatory glutaminergic inputs from the thalamus, γ-aminobutyric acid (GABA) inhibitory inputs from the GP and other adjacent spiny striatal

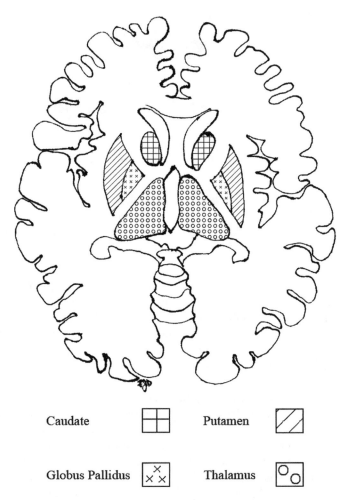

Caudate   Putamen

Globus Pallidus   Thalamus

Figure 7-2. Axial Brain Sketch Through the Level of Thalami and Basal Ganglia.

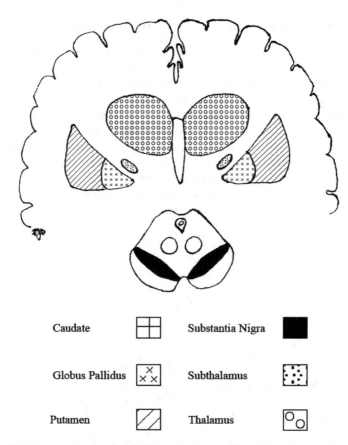

Figure 7-3. Coronal Brain Sketch Through Level of Basal Ganglia and Subthalamic Nuclei with Corresponding Region of Projections into Midbrain at Level of Red Nuclei.

neurons and local inhibitory interneurons, and cholinergic input from striatal interneurons. The medium spiny neurons contain GABA and thus their outputs are inhibitory. The SubTN receives excitatory glutaminergic projections from several areas of the cortex with prominent influence from the frontal and motor cortexes in addition to inhibitory GABA projections from the GP. The SubTN itself projects primarily glutaminergic excitatory outputs to other BG nuclei (Table 7-9).

The pathophysiology of movement disorders is a summation of a complex series of inputs and outputs that result from overactivation, underactivation, or derangement of this precisely integrated system of motor execution. These perturbations can be the result of destructive, infiltrative, irritative, metabolic, inflammatory, and other causes. A simplified schema (Figure 7-4) is presented based upon popular acceptance.[52–55] In this model, the direct pathway is composed of glutaminergic outputs from the cortex that are directly targeted to the putamen (P) of the striatum, thalamus (T), and the internal division of the

Table 7-9 Neurotransmitters of the Basal Ganglia

Neurotransmitter	Main Projections
Acetylcholine	*Excitatory* Striatal interneurons to other interior striatal medium spiny neurons
Dopamine	*Potentiates the inputs to D1 and inhibits those to D2 recepotors* Mesencephalostriate projections from SNpc to D1 & D2 receptors within the striatum
γ-aminobutyric acid (GABA)	*Inhibitory* Projections from each striatum, GPi, GPe to T and striatum and GPi
Glutamate	*Excitatory* Corticostriate projections from the cerebral cortex to the striatum and SubTN Thalamostriate projections from the T to the striatum Thalamocortical projections from the T to the frontal motor cortex
Serotonin	*Excitatory* Projections from the dorsal raphe nuclei to SubTN and striatum
Neuropeptides (enkephalin, dynorphin, substance P)	Contained within separate populations of medium spiny neurons along with GABA. Dynorphin and substance P are contained within neurons that express D1 receptor-type and enkephalin is contained within neurons that express D2 receptors. Both populations serve as inhibitory projections to the GPi and SNpr "direct pathway" and to the GPe "indirect pathway."

Source: Modified from References.[8,48,49–51]
Notes: GPe = globus pallidum externa GPi = globus pallidum interna, SNpc = substantia nigra pars compacta, SNpr = substantia nigra pars reticulata, SubTN = subthalamic nucleus, T = thalamus.

globus pallidus (GPi). An indirect pathway involves a loop from the P, external division of the globus pallidus (GPe), SubTN, GPi, and T. The substancia nigra pars compacta (SNpc) provides dopaminergic-modulating inputs.[52–55] Dopamine enhances the putaminal neurons of the direct pathway via activation of their D2 receptors and inhibits putaminal neurons of the indirect pathway via activation of their D1 receptors. The D1 receptor family (includes D1 and D5 receptors) potentiates the effects of cortical inputs to the striatum, whereas the D2 family (includes D2, D3, and D4 receptors) diminishes them.[52–55] As a result of these dual pathways working in tandem, voluntary movements can be facilitated through the direct pathway and unwanted movement inhibited by the indirect pathway.[49,50,55] This direct pathway has a net excitatory output

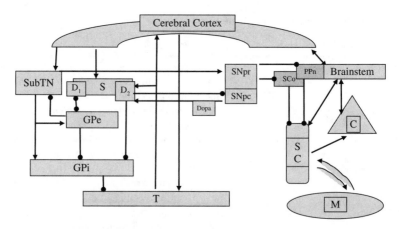

Figure 7-4. Functional Organization of the Corticobasal Ganglia Motor Network.
(Source: Modified from References.[6, 42, 47–49])
Notes: BS = brainstem
C = cerebellum
Dopa – (dopamine) = line
D_1, D_2=dopamine receptors types 1 and 2
GABA (g-aminobutyric acid) = lines with filled circle [(−) net inhibitory effect]
Glutamic acid = lines with arrowhead [(+) net excitatory effect]
GPe = globus pallidum externa
GPi = globus pallidum interna
M = muscle
PPn = pedunculopontine nucleus
S = striatum
SC = spinal cord
SCo = superior colliculus
SNpc = substantia nigra pars compacta
SNpr = substantia nigra pars reticulacta
SubTN = subthalamic nucleus
T = thalamus

with only a limited and primary inhibition targeted upon the globus pallidus, whereas the indirect pathway has a net inhibitory output. The balance of these two pathway outputs result in voluntary movement and an alteration in their net outputs or oscillation in them can result in abnormal movement.[49–51,55] In hyperkinetic movement disorders, there is decreased activity of the SubTN, which serves to disinhibit GPi output to thalamocortical projections, thus enhancing movement, whereas in hypokinetic movement disorders, a decrement in dopamine projected from the SN to the P augments inhibition of the GPe, which disinhibits the SubTN. This subsequent disinhibition then results in excessive excitation of the GPi and the SNpr, which in turn inhibits the thalamocortical and brainstem motor projections via the superior colliculus (SCo) and pedunculopontine nucleus (PPn) to diminish movement.[49–51,55] It is thus the failure to inhibit unwanted movements and/or the failure to facilitate wanted voluntary movements, which result from disorders affecting the basal ganglia.[49,50,55]

The genesis of movement disorders can be on the basis of many different mechanisms and locations within the motor-generating systems. These can occur from neuronal destruction within single populations of cells and locations or from multifocal and global injury. Genetically programmed cell death, toxin-induced injury, or excessive receptor activation (inhibitory and excitatory) could all potentially induce involuntary movement under the appropriate circumstance. Anatomic localization of the "lesion" has an imperfect correlation with the observed movement abnormality; however, there are some general conclusions, notwithstanding. Lesions of the caudate will often produce effects upon affect and behavior as well as induce both chorea and dystonia.[56] Putaminal lesions induce pareses and dystonia; subthalamic lesions will induce hemiballismus if unilateral and chorea or ballismus if bilateral.[55,56,57] Globus pallidus and SNpc lesions will typically induce dystonia.[56–58] Involuntary ocular movements can have lesion localization within the SNpr.[59] It should be recognized, however, that disturbances or lesions in several different nuclei could induce some or multiple abnormal movements. Thus, the specificity of the nuclei involved may not always be unique to those correlated above. For example, putaminal lesions can produce both chorea and ballismus in the context of hyperglycemia and diabetes mellitus, and chorea-dyskinesia can be induced by mitochondrial disorders such as Leigh's encephalopathy, affecting both globus pallidi and putamen.[6, 17–19]

THE CLINICAL CONDITIONS AND TREATMENTS

Most involuntary movements in children can be recognized as such and not confused as epileptic. Those movements with a stereotyped rhythmic quality (tremor) or a shock/startle-like quality (myoclonus) are most apt to mimic true epileptic movements. Sudden sustained postures and the observation of unusual eye movement and gaze positions may also mimic epilepsy in the appropriate contexts. The patient's age will have an important impact upon the likelihood of clinical misinterpretation, especially for parents. Parental descriptions given to clinicians will often, therefore, be shaded toward an epileptic quality because epilepsy as an entity may be more commonly appreciated in comparison to involuntary movement disorders per se. In the following sections emphasis will be placed first upon those benign entities recognized in children with the greatest potential to be confused as epileptic and then subsequently upon those that are fairly unique in childhood (see Tables 7-4 and 7-5).

Neonates and Infants

Jitteriness

Infants can display a bewildering array of unusual but normal movements and postures. From among these a number of specific and discrete clinical entities have been identified. Benign neonatal jitteriness, a form of high-frequency tremor, is identifiable in the majority of neonates (preterm and term), with maximal expression between the ages of 2–8 months of life, with a gradual decline in prevalence over the first year of life.[60,61] From sample 936 healthy full-term infants, 44% displayed varying degrees of the jitteriness.[61] These infants were typically the most active or sleepy and differentiated from the quiet resting group.[61] These infants were also noted to be somewhat more difficult to console and visually less attentive.[61] Preterm infants born to mothers with pre-eclampsia appear to be especially likely to demonstrate jitteriness. In a small comparative study of premature infants, the authors found that 75% of sixteen newborns born to pre-eclamptic mothers compared to none of those thirty-two born of normotensive mothers were jittery.[62]

In jittery infants, an initial termination of the movements may be followed by resumption a month or two later for several weeks before ultimate resolution, and only 10% exhibit persistence of the movement beyond the first year.[60,61,63] It can be recognized as quick, jerky, fragmentary movements that may migrate to different limbs with involvement of the face, particularly the chin, often in clusters of activity.[60,61,63,64] This can be precipitated by loud sounds, simple touch, with crying or manifest spontaneously. Similar jitteriness may be secondary to hypoxic-ischemic encephalopathy, hypoglycemia, hypocalcemia, and drug withdrawal (marijuana, cocaine, selective serotonin reuptake inhibitors, narcotics, etc.), but other clinical indicators and pertinent history will be evident.[61,64–66] The excursion of the movement is suppressible with limb restraint, but the proximal initiating jerk may still be felt. There are no associated eye movement abnormalities with benign jitteriness; however, eye movement abnormalities and behavior-state disturbances may be noted with the other etiologies.

The long-term outcomes of otherwise healthy preterm and term infants with jitteriness are excellent. The mean resolution of jitteriness is 7.2 months, with over 80% experiencing resolution by 9 months of age.[60,63]

Both benign neonatal sleep myoclonus and Binkie-flutter are described in Chapter 4, and the reader is referred to that discussion.

Hereditary Chin Trembling

This is a rare autosomal-dominant condition that has been reported in about twenty-seven families worldwide since the initial description in 1894 under the description of "geniospasm."[67,68] There may be a much higher prevalence secondary to under-recognition to date. This is best characterized as a form of chin myoclonus with brief, jerky, pseudorhythmic up and down chin movements superimposed upon a quivering lower lip. The quivering can be observed from birth and usually becomes more prominent with age.[69,70] There are families with affected children whose movements also diminished and terminated in adolescence.[70] The quivering can occur in discrete bouts and may be intense enough to impair speaking, such that children in reported families have described social embarrassment as a result.[70] The movement can neither be voluntarily initiated nor suppressed, may be intensified with anxiety and emotion, and usually remains persistent during sleep. No additional neurologic or involuntary movements are associated with the disorder. Individuals may have the myoclonus triggered by tapping the mentalis muscle.

Neurophysiologic studies using EMG of the mentalis muscle during bouts of quivering have recorded the myoclonus in arrhythmic frequencies of 5.7–10.3 Hz range.[69] Other neurophysiologic measures, SEP, EEG, EMG needle studies, transcranial magnetic stimulation, palmomental reflex, and others, have all been normal.[69] The disorder has been linked to chromosome 9q13-q21.[71] However, there are families who do not have this linkage, indicating evidence for genetic heterogeneity.[72]

Treatments with various benzodiazepines for this disorder have been largely unsuccessful or show only modest benefit. The application of periodic botulinum toxin injections into the mentalis muscle has proved effective for suppression of the movements.[69]

Paroxysmal Extraocular Gaze Deviations

There are several benign and transient paroxysmal extraocular gaze deviations observed with reasonable frequency in infancy. These deviations by their nature are often incorrectly considered as a partial manifestation of an epileptic event. Descriptions have included periods of tonic upward gaze, tonic downward gaze, skew deviations, ocular flutter, and opsoclonus.[73–83] The most commonly identified ocular movements are tonic upward deviations (TUD). These infants display eye movements that conform to the following clinical characteristics: (1) TUD typically last minutes to hours and rarely days, identified as intermittent discrete events; (2) there is downbeat nystagmus observable on downward gaze; (3) the infants have normal horizontal eye movements; (4) TUD disappear with sleep, worsen with fatigue; and (5) TUD begin in the first 6–12 months of life, with spontaneous remission in 3–4 years.[73–78] Children may have ataxia accompany the deviation but otherwise show no functional disturbances during the deviations. There may be an accompanying oscillating head tilt to compensate sustained visual attention on a target during the ocular deviation. Although many children are neurodevelopmentally normal, in one series 50% had language and psychomotor delays.[73,76] Individual patients have been described with neurodevelopmental abnormalities and concurrent periventricular leukomalacia on MRI.[79] An additional family with autosomal-dominant inheritance has been reported.[80] Levodopa responsiveness has been observed.[74,80]

Children who display tonic downward deviations (TDD) have clinical movements that conform to the following: (1) TDD typically last several seconds in duration but occur multiple times per day, (2) many children also have an accompanying horizontal strabismus, (3) TDD are often precipitated with sudden movement of the child, by stimulation, or with initiating feeding, (4) TDD can be identified in both neurodevelopmentally normal and abnormal term infants, and preterm infants by 36 weeks corrected age, and

(5) TDD spontaneously remits within 6 months in healthy term infants and by 3 years in preterm infants.[81–83] In neurologically impaired infants, neuroimaging has demonstrated gliosis and encephalomalacia of the optic pathways and occipital cortices.[83] There has been an additional report of two normally developed infants born without any complications at full term who showed benign "setting sun" phenomenon (TDD) immediately after birth. Each child developed brief episodes of downward gazing during sucking and crying, with complete resolution by 7 months old. One of the children had them remit transiently at 3 months only to reappear at 6 months, then disappear permanently by 7 months.[84]

An underlying mechanism for the appearance and then disappearance of these gaze deviations in otherwise normal infants, particularly premature infants, has been posited to be a delayed maturation and consequent dysfunctional persistence of the extrageniculocalcarine visual pathways.[81] This delay in maturation enhances the maladaptive persistence of the subcortical extrageniculocalcarine visual system, which subserves vertical gaze during the period of normal myelination of the optic nerves, tracts, and visual pathways. Therefore, its inappropriate activation accentuates the initiation of vertical eye movements.

Infants and Children

Shuddering Spells

Shuddering spells (attacks) are a common infantile form of essential tremor.[85] Tremor being a to-fro, oscillatory, stereotyped, rhythmic movement is readily identified, although the physical distribution of shuddering, even in families with essential tremor, makes recognition for parents difficult.[86] Shuddering spells typically appear at about 6 months of age, are usually abrupt in onset, and are reminiscent of a sudden shivering-type movement while the child is seated.[87] There is no associated loss of awareness. The child appears as if an "ice cube was dropped down their back," with a sudden upright stiffening, grimace, and eye-widening look, accompanied by head and trunk shivering. The head will oscillate vertically in a "yes-yes" direction, most often as the infant appears to simultaneously grimace and straighten upright. These movements are very quick, lasting only a few seconds, with an EMG-recorded frequency of 10 Hz.[88] Individual episodes may occur as frequently as ≥100 times during the day, with long intervening intervals where they are unobserved.[88] There is often associated tremor or similar phenomena in family members.[85,89] These attacks generally resolve over the later half of the first year of life but may extend into early childhood.[88] Children with shuddering may later develop more archetypal manifestations of essential tremor involving the upper extremities (95%) and/or the head with or without accompanying dystonia.[85,89] The cerebellum and cerebellar outflow pathways are thought to be the anatomical regions responsible.[90] Some medications can precipitate involuntary movement including tremor. Common among those precipitants include infants exposed in utero to cocaine or selective serotonin reuptake inhibitors, children consuming stimulant medications, caffeine, nicotine, bronchodilators, and valproic acid. Laboratory investigation is generally not necessary; however, inexperienced clinicians may commonly confuse these attacks with infantile spasms and pursue an EEG prompted by the description alone. The confusion should be minimal because these are both descriptively and phenomenologically distinct. Treatment is also not usually needed. The use of clonazepam, β-adrenergic blocking agents (propranolol, timolol), and primidone has been successful. Consideration for the use of gabapentin may also be expected to be beneficial if a physiological relationship to essential tremor, orthostatic tremor, and orthostatic myoclonus exits.[85,91–93]

Spasmus Nutans

This is a unique form of self-limited ocular nystagmus identified only in children. It is characterized by the concurrent combination of conjugate, asymmetric, bilateral, horizontal, rapid, fine ocular oscillations (11–15 Hz), accompanied by head tilt and a compensatory head tremor of 2–4 Hz.[94,95] The head tremor is in opposition to the direction of nystagmus and in negation to the movement of the eyes. Rarely, the nystagmus is in a vertical direction, and although bilateral and asymmetric, monocular nystagmus may occur in isolation or prior to involvement of both eyes. Onset is usual within the first year of life (4–12 months) but may develop up to 3 years of age. Gradual reduction and disappearance is observed over a few months but may be as long as 2–3 years.[94,96]

The underlying pathophysiology for the movement is unknown. Similar clinical findings have been recognized with monocular visual loss and intracranial visual pathway lesions (optic nerve glioma, chiasmatic glioma, leukoencephalopathy).[96] Data from a study of 277 children presenting with congenital nystagmus revealed that in 24/277 (8.6%) it was asymmetric and in only seven (29% of asymmetric nystagmus subjects and 2.5% of the total) was it a diagnosis of spasmus nutans, based upon normal neuroimaging, visual evoked potential (VEPs), and electroretinograms (ERGs).[97] Of the remaining 19/24 with asymmetric nystagmus, twelve had intracranial pathology and five had retinal diseases (albinism, cone-rod dystrophy, or cone dysfunction). In a retrospective review of twenty-two children identified with spasmus nutans, only three had no ocular or intracranial pathology. Visual acuity was reduced in 75% of eyes at presentation and 58% of eyes at follow-up. Strabismus and refractive error was ultimately identified in over 30%.[98]

Optic pathway tumors, leukoencephalopathy, oculomotor apraxia, cerebellar vermian hypoplasia, and retinal disease have all been identified as the cause of asymmetric nystagmus.[96–100] Those children without such pathology identified after specific investigation are correctly identified as having spasmus nutans. There are no diagnostic signs that can differentiate patients with spasmus nutans with or without underlying pathology.[96] Although the estimated frequency of these associated pathologies is not known, there is sufficient data to support the continued use of routine neuroimaging (MRI) and neuro-ophthalmologic evaluation of those infants clinically suspected to have spasmus nutans. Attention for refractive correction in idiopathic cases is also needed. An interesting treatment trial in children with congenital nystagmus has demonstrated improvement in visual acuity, reduction in nystagmus intensity, and improved foveation with the use of both gabapentin and memantine.[101] Their utility in spasmus nutans is postulated but not yet studied.

Benign Myoclonus of Early Infancy (Benign Non-epileptic Infantile Spasms)

This is an important clinical entity to recognize in that confusion with a more ominous pathogenesis can be avoided. These infants may manifest clusters of massive clonic movements.[102–104] These contractions are longer lasting, 2–4 seconds, than cortical myoclonic contractions of epileptic infantile spasms, which are 20–75 ms. The spasm involves the trunk and bilateral upper and lower limbs in extension or flexion. The usual onset age is within the first 3–15 months of life. A normal EEG during an ictal series of "spasms" as well as interictally defines the disorder. The most important feature, without which a clinical distinction can only be presumed, is the normal ictal EEG. Development is normal prior to, during, and after termination of their clinical expression assuring benign prognosis.

The initial description of sixteen infants in 1977 showed spasms occurring during wakefulness, with normal interictal EEGs and clinical resolution within several months.[102] However, eleven of the sixteen were treated with anticonvulsants including corticotrophin, although the authors believed that these represented a distinct entity, not merely a favorable West's syndrome.[103] The phenomenon was further characterized subsequently in five additional infants as a paroxysmal, shudder-type movement involving mainly the trunk, sometimes the head, associated with tonic limb contractions of variable intensity with concurrent normal EEG video-telemetry monitoring during clusters of spasms.[103] Polygraphic recording during the spasms identified the tonic component of the limb contraction. Resolution of spasms without treatment was spontaneous in all five within 2 weeks to 10 months.[103] A review of forty-six published cases and an additional six cases has been recently published.[104] All long-term clinical follow-up assessments of these infants have been normal.[104]

Tonic Reflex Seizures of Early Infancy

Tonic reflex seizures of early infancy are a unique and rarely described entity of young infants, beginning at 1–3 months of age.[105, 106] These are sudden episodes of tonic arched posture with concurrent four-limb extension and abduction, most obvious in the arms, with associated apnea and cyanosis, without loss of consciousness. The episodes have been recorded with concurrent video-telemetry and last 3–10 seconds with normal ictal and interictal EEG. The episodes appear only while being held upright and are triggered by sudden change in posture (forward, upward, downward).[105,106] Some events have been triggered while parents carried their infants down a set of stairs. The episodes are often followed by a brief period of crying but no loss of consciousness. There is complete resolution of the episodes over a period of 1–2 months after onset and normal long-term neuro-developmental outcome has been observed with follow-up over 2–13 years.[105,106]

There have been only a few cases (<20) reported in the literature; however, the phenomenon may be much more frequent than identified or recognized as a different syndrome. These posturing events bear resemblance to an exaggerated physiologic startle response (Moro reflex) and to reflex behavior observed in infants with brief epochs of gastroesophageal reflux. These are distinct from the sustained, unusual, and abnormal postures associated with Sandifer's syndrome. Similarly, reflex epileptic myoclonus and tonic infantile spasms are important entities to differentiate from these. The clinical hallmarks of brief duration, a stereotyped easily elicited trigger mechanism, and the transient nature in an otherwise normal infant should prompt consideration of benign tonic reflex seizures. An EEG during the event will be diagnostic.

Benign Paroxysmal Torticollis of Infancy

This entity is listed here because it is most often recognized as a movement disorder. It will also be considered under the heading of migraine equivalents.

Benign paroxysmal torticollis (BPT) is defined by self-limited, recurrent, stereotyped episodes of torticollis without lateral predilection, often associated with pallor, hypotonia, vomiting, and apathy.[107–112] There is no loss of awareness but an unsteady gait and trunkal instability with resistance to head straightening are notable. Concurrent awkward trunk and pelvic postures with frank ataxia have been described additionally as the main features.[108] The events last from minutes, to several hours, to days with recurrences one to three times per month.[107–111] Sleep can often help terminate the event. Most children who develop BPT do so within the first 3 months of life, but onset before age 3 years is expected.[107–110]

There is either ultimate resolution or evolution into paroxysmal vertigo or more typical migraine headaches after age 5 years.[107,108,113] In some children there is a family history of similar events, which implies a possible genetic link.[108,111,114] A surface EMG study of one child during an episode disclosed continuous electrical discharges within the contracted ipsilateral sternocleidomastoid and contralateral trapezius muscles, which suggests that the occurrence was dystonic in origin.[115] However, dystonia can be an atypical motor aura prior to migraine. The relationship to vestibular dysfunction remains a possibility as suggested by previous abnormalities in auditory and vestibular function testing.[107,108]

Reports of several children are now available with family histories of familial hemiplegic migraine with ataxia.[116] In these subjects the propensity for atypical auras is usual and important in that calcium channel dysfunction has been suggested to contribute to its development. CACN1A gene mutations on

chromosome 19 have been found in more than half of the families with hemiplegic migraine and episodic ataxia syndromes.[116] These syndromes have both
shared symptoms and calcium channel dysfunction, with the potential involvement of the cerebellum in common. This structure has been postulated to serve
as the genesis of the dystonia associated with BPT. Now, several children with
BPT and family members with familial hemiplegic-ataxia migraine have also
been found to harbor the *CACN1A* mutation.[117]Neuroimaging, CSF analysis,
and neurotransmitter measurement as well as EEG recordings are normal. No
specific treatment is of proven benefit; however, antimigraine therapies have
been more commonly utilized (see Chapter 8).

Paroxysmal and Transient Dystonia of Infancy

Paroxysmal and transient dystonia of infancy is a subtle postural abnormality
that is exhibited in otherwise healthy preterm infants and to a lesser degree full
term infants.[118–121] This is manifest as sudden and briefly assumed dystonic
postures especially when the infant is attempting a voluntary activity against
gravity. This can be best observed when the infant is suspended vertically or
seated and reaching motions are initiated. The excessive amount of postural activity can be seen as sudden and excessive arm extensions and assumed
arching or trunk and neck hyperextension postures.[118–121]

   These hyperextension postures have been studied in a small cohort of twelve
preterm infants by simultaneous video and surface EMG analyses compared to
ten full terms.[122] The postural dysfunction was not related to the presence of
hyperextension at earlier ages, to the neurological outcomes at a corrected age
of 18 months, or to lesions found on neonatal brain ultrasound scans. Seven
of the infants had normal examinations, and five demonstrated only minor
abnormalities such as mild leg hypertonia, mild diffuse hypotonia, or asymmetry in posture and motility.[122] These minor abnormalities were attributed to
deficiencies in the "fine-tuning" of postural activity when engaged in voluntary
tasks.[122] Findings such as these do not predict long-term motor deficits and
became less evident over time.[118, 121] Term infants may display similar dystonic
postures ("transient idiopathic dystonia of infancy") in a focal or segmental
distribution with eventual disappearance. The trunk as well as the limbs in
isolation or on one side may be affected.[123, 124] These postures are most often
notable in the first year of life, usually by 5–9 months of age, and rarely later.
Hyperpronation of the forearm, equinovarus of the foot, episodic opisthotonus, and mild tremor can all be manifest.[123, 124] Sleep brings relief from
the postures, as does voluntary activity with the affected extremity. Curiously,
quiet rest and distraction from affected limb use accentuates the abnormal posture. The remainder of the examination is normal and the posturing tends to
wane over the second year of life, although the earlier the onset the longer the
observed duration.[123, 124]

   A more paroxysmal character to infantile dystonia has been observed and
reported infrequently ("transient paroxysmal dystonia of infancy").[125] This
paroxysmal dystonia lasted from a few minutes to several hours of either

symmetrical or asymmetrical upper limb posturing, described in a report of nine cases.[125] Several attacks were noted each day. As the attacks lengthened, the frequency tended to diminish until resolution by 8–22 months in seven of the nine infants.[125] These infants all had normal neurodevelopmental examinations and outcome at the time of report.

Sandifer's Syndrome/Gastroesophageal Reflux Dystonia

Sandifer's Syndrome describes a phenomenon in infants and children whereby gastroesophageal acid reflux (GER) will induce or trigger dystonic postures (dyspeptic dystonia).[126–129] These postures include torticollis, retrocollis and, at times, opisthotonus. The unusual and paroxysmally assumed postures have been described in association with writhing limb movements, hypotonia, and gurgling sounds. The most dramatic presentation of GER may be an "apparent life-threatening event" (ALTE). In infants this is typically associated with feeding and vomiting, whereas in older children emesis may not always be apparent. Although this association is often cited, in realty it is rarely a proven etiology. However, in the context of preserved consciousness, the child with GER may much more frequently be observed to turn upside down or assume other bizarre body contortions in an effort to relieve what is interpreted to be chest or abdominal pain during the events of acid reflux.

The syndrome has been described in the context of hiatal hernia and is noted in a high proportion of neurologically abnormal infants.[126,128,129] The resultant posturing is thought to be a direct result of acid (pH<4) inducing an esophageal sensory reflex motor response to the head and neck musculature. Esophageal dilation and accentuation of peristalsis and esophageal spasm have also been observed as contributing to the triggering mechanisms of the observed posturing.[130,131] Neither the prevalence of the syndrome nor a homogeneous mechanism is known, however.

A recent study of twelve children referred for investigation of GER found that the presence of acid reflux was a necessary component to the induction of dystonic posturing.[132] The investigation used combined 24-hour esophageal impedance-pH measurements with a single catheter containing six impedance channels and one pH sensor, with the impedance channels spanning from the pharynx to the distal esophagus. Three of the twelve children had no demonstrable association between GER and posturing, and 5/12 had Sandifer's syndrome (i.e., acid (pH<4) GER-induced posturing) recorded. There was resolution of symptoms in these eight children with proton pump inhibitor treatment.[132] The remaining four children interestingly developed dystonic posturing events associated with nonacid reflux that also resolved with antireflux treatment. The authors speculated that this bolus-induced reflux dystonia (BIRDy) may represent a newly described subgroup of weak-acid/non-acid bolus-induced reflux disease in infants.[132] A similar effect upon peristalsis has been suggested previously.[130,131] The same syndrome has also been rarely reported to occur in breast-fed infants as well.[133]

GER may additionally present in infants as inspiratory stridor secondary to laryngeal dyskinesia.[14] The stridor is present during calm breathing at rest, crying, or in sleep. This may be suggestive of possible brainstem dysfunction but is actually due to paradoxical vocal cord adduction during inspiration in the absence of vocal cord paralysis. The laryngeal dyskinesia and, consequently, the stridor resolve over the latter half of the first year of life, unrelated to treatment of GER. When the same inspiratory stridor occurs due to paradoxical vocal cord adduction during inspiration in the absence of vocal cord paralysis in adolescents and adults, the mechanism is felt to be functional or factitious (Munchausen's stridor).[134]

Stool-holding Stiffening Spells

An unusual cause of non-epileptic movement or posturing has been recently described, the child engaging in stool holding. Four children (3–13 months) were variously described with "seizures" due to an individually stereotyped set of behaviors each child engaged in.

The tonic postures included flexing of the legs with "pushing forward" of the upper body, flushing, and a blank stare.[135] In some episodes there were right-sided limb twitching and adversive head posturing (case 1); vacant stare (case 2); eye rolling and shaking of all four limbs with facial grimacing, fist clenching, and leg straightening, with an attack-ending scream (case 3); and jaw shaking evolving into whole body shaking with a blank and unresponsive look (case 4).[135] A clear history of stool holding was obtained during initial evaluation in three children and treatment with laxatives resulted in termination of the attacks. Spontaneous recovery in one subject was followed by recurrence 18 months later with anal pain and clear stool holding.[135] EEG recordings in all four children were normal. Anecdotal cases (4–5 year olds) with similar descriptions have also been reported.[136]

Gratification Disorder

Gratification disorder has been previously referred to as infantile masturbation, benign idiopathic infantile dyskinesia, and paroxysmal dystonia, with the term gratification disorder now preferred.[137–141] Masturbation (gratification) is a normal human behavior; however, there is not general awareness that masturbatory behavior occurs in the preadolescent ages and has even been sonographically observed in utero.[142] In the preadolescent age context, this behavior does not conform to the typical manual genital stimulation behavior as in older ages. It is often unrecognized or misidentified as epilepsy, abdominal pain, or another pathological movement disorder such as paroxysmal dystonia/dyskinesia.[137–141] Parents will report observing their child staring into space, rocking with crossed legs, and making grunting vocalizations in seated and prone positions. The most important clinical observation is that the children are easily distracted from engaging in the behavior and appear annoyed when disturbed. Occasionally the child may appear unhappy during the behavior.

A recent report constituting the largest series to date of thirty-one subjects with gratification disorder (eleven boys, twenty girls) identified their median age of onset at 10.5 months (range 3 months to 5 years 5 months). The median frequency of events was seven times per week and the median length 2.5 minutes.[135] Additional common features reviewed in the literature are summarized as (1) onset after the age of 3 months and before 3 years, most commonly; (2) stereotyped episodes of variable duration; (3) vocalizations with quiet grunting; (4) facial flushing with diaphoresis; (5) pressure on the perineum with characteristic posturing of the lower extremities; (6) no alteration of consciousness; (7) cessation with distraction; (8) normal examination; and (9) normal laboratory studies.[135–141]

The behavior may occur in any setting, lying or sitting, at home or elsewhere. Authors have commented upon the difficulty in distinguishing between masturbatory posturing and paroxysmal dystonic choreoathetosis (PDC) because the attacks of PDC can be unilateral or bilateral, short duration without triggers, and begin in infancy.[141, 143, 144] A similar distinction from psychogenic movements can also pose difficulty.[145] Observation in person or on video should allow confirmation of the diagnosis. No further investigation or treatment is needed, although the acknowledgment of the diagnosis by parents may not be immediate. The need is to point out the clinical distinguishing features to them; particularly the ease of distraction from engaging in it may be critical for their acceptance.

Stereotypies/Habit Movements

Stereotypy is a rhythmic, repetitive, patterned, purposeless movement, sometimes complex in nature, engaged in by both normal and neurologically impaired children, with or without autism (Table 7-10).[146–148]

They may be distinguished from other stereotyped behaviors in that the individual can both initiate and suppress the behavior without inner tension. Stereotypies have been referred to under a number of synonyms: motor rhythmias, rhythmic patterns, rhythmic habit patterns, rhythmical stereotypies, habit spasms, mannerisms, and automatisms.[149–152] These are quite common in young children, with a cataloguing of nearly fifty different behaviors previously observed in normal infants.[152] Prominence of these specific behaviors in normal infants escalates over the first 6 months of life, then wanes to resolution (physiologic). The prevalence of some of these behaviors such as head banging, particularly upon recumbency for sleep, has been observed in 5.1%–15.2% of infants and young children, and body rocking and head rolling behaviors noted in 6.3%–19.1% of studied samples (Table 7-11).[153, 154]

Thumb sucking in particular may be nearly universal under the age of 12 months.[155, 156]

Stereotypies may vary in complexity from simple body rocking or foot tapping behavior to more multifaceted movements such as body rocking with hand twirling, repetitive jumping while shaking or flapping, and neck and head thrusting. One hallmark of a stereotypy is the ability to distract the child from

Table 7-10 Causes and Associations of Stereotypies

Physiologically normal children
Stress and anxiety induced
Autism spectrum disorders
Inborn errors of metabolism

- Lesch-Nyan disease
- Neuroacanthocytosis

Mental retardation
Rett syndrome
Tardive dyskinesia
Tourette syndrome
Psychiatric disorders

- Schizophrenia
- Catatonia
- Obsessive-compulsive disorder

Sensory deprivation

- Congenital blindness
- Congenital deafness
- Restraint

Psychogenic

Table 7-11 Approximate Prevalence and Appearance of Common Stereotypies in Normal Children

Stereotypic Behavior	Peak Age	Approximate Prevalence
Body Rocking/Head Rolling	9–17 months	6%–19%
Thumb Sucking/Hand Sucking	<12 months	21%–31%
Nail Biting	NA	12%
Hair Twirling	NA	16%
Head Banging	12–17 months	5%–15%

Source: Modified from References.[149–157]
Note: NA = not available.

the behavior, even if only briefly. Many of the behaviors, particularly in normal children, are precipitated by excitement, anticipation, or being visually engaged or preoccupied (watching TV). The child simply engages in the behavior without apparent conscious thought to do so. Situational stress, such as in a school setting, may promote more "habit movements," such hair twirling, thumb-sucking, nail-biting, lip-picking, etc.[147, 148] These may have a more compulsive quality. Attempts to distract the child or give encouragement to desist may provoke distress and resistance.[157] Nervous habits are more prone in structured settings and associated with negative mood states. The frequency of both stereotypies and habit behaviors may augment with increasing demands placed upon the child to concentrate or perform. In an experiment examining the relationship between rhythmical stereotypies (leg swinging) and heart rate in twelve normal school children, telemetric measurement of heart rate revealed decreased heart rates during leg-swinging behavior in girls to a greater degree than boys. This decrease was more pronounced when school behavior was active rather than when it was passive.[157] The results suggested a calming effect of the stereotypy on the child during stressful tasks in a structured learning environment. Habit reversal and reinforcement of alternative behavior is beneficial in reducing stereotypies in nonautistic children.[158]

Autistic children will often engage in rocking and staring behaviors, particularly gazing at flickering lights, spinning fans, and wheels. They may engage in repetitive touching, smelling, and variations of jumping, pacing, flapping, and finger flicking. These behaviors do not impair function or volitional hand use but may interfere with socialization and educational objectives. Intermittent behavior modification, aversive therapy, and redirection are potential interventions with limited success. Applied behavior analysis techniques employing immediate and consistent reinforcement of behavior modification can have greater benefit. The use of neuroleptic drugs has modest impact. Serotonin reuptake inhibitors (e.g., clomipramine) or opioids antagonists (e.g., naltrexone) have had broader utility but modest benefit.[159]

Another important severe neurodevelopmental disorder often identified by the nature of the stereotypy is Rett's syndrome.[160] The diagnosis is based upon clinical criteria, developed over time, which incorporate apparently normal development and head growth over the first 6 months of life and subsequent head growth deceleration coupled with a loss of purposeful use of the hands, with psychomotor, expressive, and receptive language skill retardation.[161] A characteristic "hand-wringing" stereotypy becomes apparent from 8 months to 3 years of age (97%) and has been a hallmark feature along with a number of other observable behaviors (respiratory stereotypies of hyperventilation, breath holding, and bruxism).[160, 161] The hand stereotypy observed in girls with Rett's syndrome is distinct and in marked contrast to those of autistic children, because these girls lose useful hand function just before (18.5%) or coincident with the onset of this stereotypy (43.3%).[162, 163]

The hypothesis that Rett's syndrome was an X-linked dominant disorder was demonstrated with the identification of mutations in the gene encoding methyl CpG binding protein 2 (MeCP2).[164] In girls less than 10 years of age meeting the diagnostic criteria for Rett's syndrome in whom hand stereotypies without hand gazing are present (or bruxism, or two or more other stereotypies), there was a high likelihood of identifying the MeCP2 mutation.[164] Unfortunately, the knowledge that a loss of function in this gene is present in these girls has not yet allowed an understanding into the pathogenesis of the syndrome nor the cause of the stereotypy, although additional clinical features have been correlated with it.[165] The characteristic "hand wringing" movement at midline, nonetheless, is not amenable to currently available interventions.[166]

Pathologic (persistent) stereotypies are also a common behavior in children with congenital blindness/deafness and in autistic and cognitively impaired children (Table 7-12).[167–169]

Stereotyped behavioral traits were observed in 19/26 (73%) congenitally blind children studied by Fazzi et al.[168] Stereotyped behaviors most frequently observed were body rocking (30.7%), repetitive handling of objects (30.7%), hand and finger movements (26.9%), eye pressing and eye poking (30.7%), lying face downward (22.8%), and jumping (11.4%).[168] A comparative observational study of 400 subjects including 46 with visual impairments, 85 hearing impaired, 29 with infantile autism, and 240 with mental retardation determined that each group had its own characteristic stereotypy.[169] There were marked differences in stereotypy type between the hearing-impaired and visually impaired groups. Whereas autistic children more frequently engaged in

Table 7-12 Common Stereotypies Identified Within Selected Childhood Populations

Autistic Children
Body rocking
Body tensing
Head shaking
Arm/leg flapping
Hand/feet twirling
Hand washing
Hand clapping
Fist clenching
Pacing
Hyperventilating
Breath holding
Head tapping
Tongue protrusion
Bruxism
Hair pulling (trichotillomania)

Congenitally Blind Children
Repetitive handling of objects
Hand and finger flicking
Eye pressing
Eye poking
Lying face downward
Jumping

Mentally Retarded Children
Finger sucking
Hand biting until callus formation
Tongue protrusion
Head banging

Note: Overlap of all types of stereotypies among groups exists.

stereotypies with "bizarre" characteristics, children with blindness and those with autism shared many stereotypies in common. Stereotyped behavior shown by mentally retarded children differed with varying intelligence levels.[169] There was no significant difference in the appearance rate of stereotypies among those with blindness or deafness.[169]

In contrast to children, adult onset stereotypies have a high probability and sufficient distinguishing qualities to be identifiable as tardive stereotypies (dyskinesias) secondary to neuroleptic medication use.[170] In children, especially those with autism, who have been treated with neuroleptics medication, the later determination of stereotypies as tardive and secondary to neuroleptics use is less possible due to significant overlap with premorbid movements.[171] A careful documentation of the baseline movements would be necessary to prospectively determine causes.

Benign Nocturnal Alternating Hemiplegia of Childhood

Benign familial nocturnal alternating hemiplegia of childhood (BNAHC) is a rare paroxysmal syndrome constituting a benign and familial form of the progressive disorder.[172] This is discussed at length in Chapter 4. The plegic events of BNAHC give the appearance of a postictal epileptic paralysis (Todd's paralysis). The child has recurrent attacks of flaccid hemiplegia develop during arousal from sleep without apparent concurrent neurological or cognitive impairment.[172] There has been associated drooling, breathing difficulty, limb ataxia, and dystonic posturing encountered with a positive Babinski sign during attacks.[172] These attacks have a median onset age of 18.5 months with a decreasing frequency of attacks with age. The episodes of hemiplegia last from 5 to 20 minutes, alternate from side-to-side in successive attacks (two children experienced bilateral plegia), begin 20–30 minutes into drowsiness or sleep, and have a variable frequency of 2–12 times per month. A parental (maternal) family history of migraine with or without aura has been noted in four of the families.[172] All investigations thus far fail to reveal an etiology. Treatment responses were only modest with flunarizine and clobazam, and negligible to other anticonvulsants.[172]

Diaphragmatic Flutter

Diaphragmatic flutter (DF) is an infrequent involuntary movement disorder that produces irregular bursts of rhythmic diaphragmatic contractions perceived by the subject as shortness of breath, inspiratory stridor, abdominal wall pain, or epigastric pulsations and may be visibly witnessed as abdominal jerking (the "belly dancer" movement).[173–178] The cervical nerves may in part be involved in the genesis of the motor activity through involvement of accessory muscles of respiration. This sequence was provoked by spinal cord trauma in a child.[173] The first clinical account of diaphragmatic flutter was published by Antony van Leeuwenhoek, the renowned microscopist, in 1723.[174] A surface EMG study done on a child during which time gross abdominal wall tremor was observed identified discrepant and independent muscle activation of the abdominal wall and diaphragm.[175] The authors suggested several possible mechanisms to explain their findings but emphasized two main possibilities: abdominal wall movement as a reaction to increased abdominal pressure due to irregular diaphragmatic movements, or reflex abdominal muscle wall contractions with diaphragm activation.[175] Visualization of the diaphragmatic movements associated with either inspiration or expiration on chest and abdominal fluoroscopy identify an average frequency of 4–6 Hz.[175, 176] DF is thought to be distinguishable from diaphragmatic myoclonus because this later entity has a continuous quality, has slower frequency, is often persistent in sleep, and occurs concurrent with palatal myoclonus.[177] The medulla is felt to be the generator of DF, but peripheral causes have also been posited.[175] Most recent EMG investigations have demonstrated that the abdominal movements resulted from isolated, rhythmic, diaphragmatic contractions with variable EMG burst duration that is suppressible with breath holding and distraction.[178] With these data, the suggestion that there is an element of volitional control can be made.[178] The entity can occur in neonates and has been noted transiently in infants with bronchopulmonary dysplasia after respiratory syncytial virus bronchiolitis.[179, 180] Thus, there may well be a spectrum whereby at one end there are synchronous movements of the diaphragm and accessory muscles of respiration that produce respiratory compromise and abdominal wall movement (diaphragmatic flutter/myoclonus), and at the other end there are those individuals with some voluntary control of diaphragmatic and abdominal wall movement with no respiratory compromise at all (isolated diaphragmatic tremor).[177]

Fever-Precipitated Myoclonus, Ballismus, and Tremor with Effects on Stereotypies

Fever is an expected consequence of childhood illnesses. Although fever is associated with most infectious, connective tissue, collagen-vascular, autoimmune, and neoplastic processes, these underlying etiologies can themselves adversely affect CNS function and produce involuntary movements. However, fever alone may produce these movements as well. The body produces a wide array of pyrogenic cytokines such as interleukins (IL-1, IL-6), interferon, and tumor necrosis factor in response to a pyrogenic stimulus.[181] Both the induction and result of these responses may promote the additional development of autoantibodies. These autoantibodies in turn play a role in the induction of additional CNS morbidity.

Involuntary movements associated with these febrile responses may most often be attributable to CNS-targeted autoantibodies. Notably there has been the appreciation of anti-basal ganglia autoantibodies in children with Syndenham's chorea in the context of acute rheumatic fever conforming to the Jones criteria.[182] This disorder is characterized by chorea, additional motor, and neuropsychiatric manifestations as a delayed result of infection with group A β-hemolytic streptococcal infection.[183] Anti-basal ganglia antibodies identified in the sera of affected children using ELISA and Western immunoblotting have been found to be both sensitive (95%) and specific (93%) in this context.[183] The identification of these autoantibodies has prompted the search for similar or identical antibodies in other subjects with movement disorders, such as adolescents and adults with atypical dystonias and tic disorders. There is now a report with positive findings for similar autoantibodies in 65% of a selected sample of sixty-five subjects presenting with these disorders.[184] Similarly, there have been autoantibodies detected in the sera of patients with opsoclonus-myoclonus-ataxia syndrome.[185] These autoantibodies are directed against intracellular proteins, such as anti-Hu, alpha-enolase, and KHSRP (K homology splicing regulatory protein).[185] There have been additional autoantibodies shown to bind to the surface of neuroblastoma cells and cerebellar granular neurons. These may impart antiproliferative and pro-apoptotic effects on neuroblastoma cell lines.[185] Concurrent febrile illness may provoke relapse of symptoms in patients harboring these specific autoantibodies.[186] Whether this resurgence of symptoms is due to an increase in pyrogenic factors or upregulated antibody production or some other mechanism is unknown. Similarly, the debate and discovery of scientific evidence for the existence (or not) of an immune-mediated mechanism underlying tic disorders continues as well. Ascertainment of a body of credible data to support the hypothesis that Tourette's syndrome and obsessive-compulsive disorder are also a result of an autoimmune response to infection with group A β-hemolytic streptococcal infection, so-called PANDAS (pediatric autoimmune neuropsychiatric disorders associated with streptococcal infection), continues but as yet remain unfulfilled.[187]

There are a few reports, nonetheless, of children affected solely by fever with the development of an identifiable transient movement disorder along a spectrum of severity ranging from mild to more severe quality. Dooley reported three benign examples.[188] These children experienced fever-induced myoclonus characterized by frequent, brief generalized migratory jerks, which resolved over a period of hours to day after the resolution of fever.[188] The generalized nature of the movement suggests a subcortical origin. There is an earlier report of two children with reference to a third, all of whom had dyskinetic cerebral palsy, who exhibited markedly increased severe choreiform and ballistic movements with the development of febrile illnesses.[189] The symptoms only slowly waned when the febrile component of their illness subsided. The accentuation of the underlying ballistic movement disorder was described as "severe" in one child with extreme elevations of serum creatine kinase (30,517 U/L) that required multiple high doses of neuroleptics, sedatives, and antispasticity agents with little benefit until the addition of phenytoin to extreme serum concentrations (70–80 μL/L). The ballistic movements resolved completely over 4 weeks.[189] The consideration to an unusual status epilepticus was considered; however, EEG recording revealed no epileptiform activity in either subject.[189]

There is a more recent report of eleven children (8 months to 11 years old) who suffered generalized myoclonus in response to fever.[190] The myoclonus had durations of 30 minutes to longer than 2 hours. Two children had prior febrile convulsions and one had febrile delirium. EEG was recorded in eight subjects. Eight of the patients (73%) showed some change in mood manifest as fear, surprise, and shouting.[190] Although the EEG was abnormally slow in four patients and spike discharges found in two patients, the myoclonic jerks were non-epileptic. The follow-up course in ten subjects over 2 years revealed no development of epilepsy.[190]

An interesting report pertaining to the beneficial effects of fever on the stereotypies and select symptoms of autistic spectrum disorder in thirty children has been published.[191] In a prospective study of thirty children (aged 2–18 years) with autism spectrum disorders, parent responses to the Aberrant Behavior Checklist (ABC) were collected during a febrile period (body temperature $\geq 38.0°C/100.4°F$) and when the child had been fever-free for 7 days.[191] Data were compared with responses collected from parents of thirty age-, gender-, and language skills-matched afebrile children with autism spectrum disorders during similar time intervals.[191] Fewer aberrant behaviors were recorded for febrile subjects on the ABC subscales of irritability, hyperactivity, stereotypy, and inappropriate speech compared with control subjects. All improvements were transient, however.[191] The authors questioned whether these symptom improvements represented fever-specific effects induced by an undetermined biological mechanism.

Children and Adolescents

Transient Tics

Tics are the most common movement disorder identified in childhood. They are typically not confused with epilepsy especially because these are not associated with loss of consciousness and rarely present as "status." As noted previously, population surveys have identified tics in up to 12%–24% of school-aged children.[13,39,40] A chronic tic disorder or Tourette's syndrome (TS) is estimated in 0.5%–6%, with an overall population prevalence of TS at 1–10 per 1000.[13,40–43] Transient tics are by definition short lived and paroxysmal in character. Transient motor tics generally involve a single muscle group. Preschool and school-aged children 3–10 years of age are most commonly affected.

The diagnosis of tics is clinical. There is no specific laboratory test to aid in confirmation.[13,39] Diagnostic criteria for transient tic disorder, chronic tic disorder, and TS are provided in Table 7-13.[192]

The criteria were developed and adopted in order to facilitate homogeneity in research categorization as well as to aid in diagnosis. As a matter of practicality, tic disorders form a continuum. Annotating whether the tic has been witnessed by a reliable observer (definite) or not (historical) has been adopted by the TS Classification Study Group of the American Tourette's Association.[193] In practice, transient tics and the onset of chronic tic disorders are generally surprising to parents. The rather sudden notation of a rapid, recurrent, non-rhythmic, stereotyped motor movement or vocalization (definition of a tic) will usually generate great anxiety and a desire to investigate. Observation or

Table 7-13 Diagnostic Criteria for Tic Disorders (DSM-IV-TR)

Tourette Syndrome (307.23)

- Both multiple motor and one or more vocal tics have been present at some time during the illness, although not necessarily concurrently.
- The tics occur many times a day (usually in bouts) nearly every day, or intermittently throughout a period of more than a year; during this period there was never a tic-free period of more than 3 consecutive months.
- Onset before the age of 18 years.
- The disturbance is not due to the direct physiological effects of a substance (e.g., stimulants) or a general medical condition (e.g., Huntington's chorea or post-viral encephalitis).

Chronic Motor or Vocal Tic Disorder (307.22)

- Single or multiple motor or vocal tics, but not both, have been present at some time during the illness.
- The tics occur many times a day, nearly every day, or intermittently throughout a period of more than 1 year; during this period there was never a tic-free period of more than 3 consecutive months.
- Onset before the age of 18 years.
- The disturbance is not due to the direct physiological effects of a substance (e.g., stimulants) or a general medical condition (e.g., Huntington's chorea or post-viral encephalitis).
- Criteria have never been met for Tourette's disorder.

Transient Tic Disorder (307.21)

- Single or multiple motor or vocal tics.
- The tics occur many times a day, nearly every day for at least 4 weeks, but for no longer than 12 consecutive months.
- Onset before the age of 18 years.
- The disturbance is not due to the direct physiological effects of a substance (e.g., stimulants) or a general medical condition (e.g., Huntington's chorea or post-viral encephalitis).
- Criteria have never been met for Tourette disorder or chronic motor or vocal tic disorder.

Tic Disorder Not Otherwise Specified (307.20)

- This category is for disorders characterized by tics that do not meet criteria for a specific tic disorder. Examples include tics lasting less than 4 weeks, or tics with an onset after age 18 years.

Source: Modified from Reference.[192]

careful description should suffice to make an appropriate diagnosis. There are, however, specific tic behaviors that may confuse parents, teachers, and clinicians alike and result in unnecessary testing for epilepsy. In particular, when the eyes are involved, especially with rolling movements or repetitive blinking (blepharospasm), an immediate consideration of childhood absence seizures or oculogyric crises may be made. Importantly, even though the motor behavior may repetitively persist over several seconds or longer, there is no alteration in the child's consciousness or perception and the behavior can be voluntarily suppressed or distracted from. These qualities should allow differentiation from other considerations. Tics affecting the eyeballs are, nonetheless, unusual and tend to occur in the context of additional tics. Blepharospasm is the most common unitary ophthalmologic manifestation of a tic disorder when TS populations are evaluated.[194, 195] In a referral population of seventeen children (18 months to 10 years old) to a specialty ophthalmologic hospital for the evaluation of excessive eye blinking of 1 week to 4 months duration with otherwise normal examination, all spontaneously resolved.[196] The resolution occurred within 5 months from examination with only one child experiencing a transient recurrence within that time frame.[196] The authors considered the diagnosis to be "functional" (stress related, psychosomatic); however, a transient tic may have been a consideration, given current criteria for the diagnosis. The differentiation of tics from pseudo-tics or somatization disorder can be a challenge. A few case reports in children have commented on this. The psychogenic tic can occur in isolation or in addition to the tics of a previously diagnosed tic disorder.[197, 198]

Transient tics of childhood cannot be predicted to remit based upon the presentation. Although these most commonly involve the eyelids in the form of blinking, the limbs, trunk, and vocalizations can be the tic presentation. By definition, transient tics have duration of less than 1 year but frequently terminate within 3–6 months from presentation.

Non-Epileptic Head Drops

Head drops are recognized as a manifestation of generalized epileptic seizures.[199] However, a careful clinical description of the head movement may allow distinction between epileptic and non-epileptic types. In a study of 24 children ranging in age from 4 months to 16 years (mean 5 years old) referred for video-telemetry evaluation of seizures, 351 head nodding episodes were recorded and characterized.[199] Children with loss of trunk tone as part of atypical absence seizures were excluded. Subjects were divided into two groups, epileptic and non-epileptic head nod groups, based upon epileptiform activity on EEG during the nodding behavior.[199] There were no differences between groups with respect to gender, age, the presence of mental retardation or abnormal neurological examination findings.[199] Non-epileptic head nods (29% cohort) were characterized by an equivalent rapid drop and rapid recovery to upright in distinction to the rapid drop and slow recovery to upright of epileptic head nods (71% cohort).[199] In addition, only non-epileptic head nods were accompanied by repetitive nodding (head bobs).[199] The frequency of accompanying eye blinks was not significantly different between groups.[199] Epileptic head nods also had subtle extremity myoclonus and a change in facial expression exhibited, whereas non-epileptic head nods did not.[199]

Head Tremor

Head shaking refers to the rotatory oscillation of the head around the cervical axis, whereas nodding is an oscillation within the vertical plane.[200] Each is a form of head tremor when the behavior is sustained and not paroxysmal.

Each is unusual in children. Head shaking/nodding can be noted as a maneuver in compensation for ocular misalignment (strabismus) and nystagmus.[94,95] In this circumstance, surgical correction of the strabismus produces resolution of the movement.[200]

In a unique report of four children (three girls, one boy) with head tremor followed longitudinally over 1–8 years, each demonstrated onset of head tremor between the ages of 5 and 10 months.[89] In each case the head tremor was characterized by a predominant vertical nod ("yes-yes") or axial rotation movement ("no-no") of the head. Two children had a slightly skewed movement with the chin toward the shoulder. Oscillations were at a frequency rate of about 1–2 Hz, accentuated when sitting upright without head support, increased at times of movement, and dissipated while lying flat or sleeping. The children were unable to voluntarily suppress the action and did not experience any sensation of movement. Three of the children had shuddering spells prior to onset of head tremor. Two children have developed mild dystonic posturing of the legs when intently concentrating. No child had strabismus or nystagmus. A family history of tremor was present in two children and infantile shuddering occurred in the father of one child. One child responded well to both timolol and trihexaphenidyl. A second child responded moderately to primidone. Two had head tremor spontaneously remit.[89]

A prospective summary of 120 consecutive essential tremor (ET) patients evaluated in an Asian movement disorders clinic found a 15.5% (19/120) frequency of childhood onset ET patients, with 73.6% of these (14/19) men.[201] Head tremor was observed in only 2/19 (10.5%). The mean age of onset was 10.8 ± 4.1 years. This was a relatively high frequency (15.5%) of childhood ET in this Asian cohort.[201] In contrast, a U.S. pediatric movement disease clinic found only nineteen pediatric ET cases (mean age 12.7 years).[202] The majority (68.4%) were male, and only one had head tremor.[202]

Bobble-Head Doll Syndrome

Although not necessarily benign, this head movement, known as bobble-head doll syndrome (BHDS), deserves mention here for its unique identification in childhood.[203] This is so named for its clinical resemblance to the movements observed on ceramic dolls with weighted detachable heads suspended at the neck with a coiled spring, popularized as rear dashboard ornaments in the 1950s and 1960s. Benton et al. in 1966 first described it in children who had third ventricular cysts.[203] The head movement occurs in paroxysms of slow rhythmic (1–4 Hz) frequency, predominantly vertical ("yes-yes") in direction, when the child is upright.[204] Adjacent shoulder, trunk, and upper limb and hand tremor can be seen in conjunction with the head tremor.[205] The head movements may be voluntarily suppressible with various repositioning attitudes of the head, visual concentration, and with sleep.

The BHDS is clinically manifest in macrocephalic children typically before 10 years of age (mean age 3 years 3 months).[204] Two adult onset cases have been reported at 18 and 21 years of age.[204,206] Although BHDS is associated with hydrocephalus from various causes, the hydrocephalus may be arrested or progressively increasing. The head movement is caused by distension of the third ventricle. This can be due to stenosis or compression of the aqueduct of sylvius from suprasellar arachnoid cysts, third ventricular colloid cysts, trapped fourth ventricle and aqueduct, or tumors in the region, such as a choroid plexus papiloma.[203, 204, 206–211] The mechanism has been postulated to be in part a learned behavior to relieve symptoms of CSF flow obstruction.[211] This was supported by observations of the position of an arachnoid cyst compressing the foramen of Monro made with CT metrizamide cisternography.[211] The movement partially relieved the obstruction. However, direct anatomical impingement upon the periventricular structures adjacent to the mesial dorsomedial thalamic nucleus and dentatothalamic tracts has also been inferred as causative.[203, 212] These pathways project from the dorsomedial nucleus of the thalamus to the midbrain tegmentum and red nucleus via the caudate nucleus and the putamen.[203, 212] The crossed and uncrossed descending motor tracts to the cervical spinal cord that innervate the neck muscles are inadvertently stimulated to produce the movement. Fiber tracts more lateral within thalamus innervate upper trunk and shoulder musculature.[203, 212] Shunt surgery to alleviate the obstruction will also eliminate the head movement.[205] Delayed treatment beyond 6 years from the onset of bobbing will result in persistent head movement despite intervention.[204, 211]

Essential Palatal Tremor

Essential palatal tremor (EPT), also referred to as palatal myoclonus, oculopalatal myoclonus, and palatal nystagmus, is a rare entity composed of rhythmic twitching of the soft palate, pharynx, and larynx with an associated perceived auditory "clicking" sound.[213] This is not likely to be thought of as potentially epileptic, but there have been patients reported with epilepsia partialis continua with palatal tremor associated with perioral twitching and twitching of the floor of the mouth and arm.[214, 215] "Essential" refers to the idiopathic nature of the entity that is seen almost always in children. Although at times incapacitating, no underlying neuroanatomical lesions have been identified and its course may last months to years. Symptomatic palatal tremor (SPT), however, occurs mainly in adults and is secondary to a number of underlying brain lesions (neoplastic, vascular, infectious, degenerative, or traumatic), especially involving the inferior olives within the brainstem or the cerebellum.[216, 217] Rare symptomatic palatal tremor in childhood due to leukodystrophy (Krabbe disease), cerebellar tumor, and encephalitis have been reported.[218–220]

Reviews of childhood palatal tremor (myoclonus), comprising approximately twenty-three reported cases, reveal the age of presentation to fall between 5 and 12 years old, with a mean age of 6 years and the youngest being an infant.[221, 222] All children complained of tinnitus in the form of clicking sounds while awake that diminished with sleep and a few children could transiently suppress it.[221–226] The sound is generally audible enough for parents to hear it (objective tinnitus). The duration of the tinnitus was variable (3 months to 5 years) but often longer than 1 year.[221,222]

The palatal movements in EPT are produced by bilateral contractions of the tensor veli palatini muscle, innervated by the Vth cranial nerve, at a frequency of 40–160 cycles/minute (1–3 Hz), whereas it is the levator veli palatini muscle, innervated by VIIth and IXth cranial nerves, that is activated in SPT.[217] The underlying pathophysiology for EPT is unknown. Subjects studied with EEG, neuroimaging, and SPECT scanning have yielded normal results.[217,221,222]

A report of four children with EPT who took part in a treatment trial using 100–300 mg/kg/d of piracetam (2-oxo-1-pyrrolidine acetamide) showed a prompt (disappeared within 15–30 days) and sustained effectiveness.[222] Remission of the tremor was obtained while on drug and relapse upon withdrawal with remission again induced upon second treatment trial. Other interventions have had only the exceptional responder to sumatriptan, 5-hydroxy-tryptophan (5-HT) agonist, flunarizine, sodium valproate, 5-HT, tetrabenazine, carbamazepine, clonazepam, adenectomy, and botulinum toxin.[227–232]

Additional Unique Childhood Movements Disorders

Hyperekplexia

Hyperekplexia, also referred to as (hereditary) stiff-startle disease, is a rare neurogenetic disorder presenting in the newborn period with exaggerated startle responses, hypertonia, and hyperreflexia in response to an unexpected auditory, somatosensory, or visual stimuli.[233,234] The majority of patients have a dominantly inherited disorder, but sporadic and recessive inheritance patterns have also been recognized. The infants exhibit striking startle responses while being handled or in response to loud noises shortly after birth. Tapping gently on the nose can easily precipitate an attack.[233,234] A positive response to this maneuver (the nose tap sign) should prompt diagnostic consideration. Stimuli from feeding, changing, and cuddling can bring about an excessive startle to the point of tonic posturing with apnea, oropharyngeal obstruction, aspiration, and abdominal tensing resulting in hernias. Early treatment with clonazepam can be life saving when instituted in the neonatal period. Severe apneic episodes as a consequence of a prolonged stiff startle event can be terminated by sudden forced flexion of the head and legs.[235]

The prolonged sustention of a posture against gravity can be an additional clinical hallmark of the disease. Stretching the infant's arm above the face while lying supine and observing the slow and gradual recoil of the limb can provoke this. The startle in both the "major and minor" forms (see below) of hyperekplexia in contrast to normal startles involves the whole body, not just the upper trunk. It produces a large-amplitude movement that poorly habituates. The initial startle is often followed by a more prolonged tonic phase of generalized rigidity that lasts a few seconds. The hypertonia or generalized stiffness and hyperreflexia diminish to normal over the first year of life with a gradual but delayed attainment of motor milestones. After becoming able to independently ambulate, the children experience frequent falls because of the continued exaggerated startle responses and often develop a fear of walking. Walking in close proximity to adjacent walls with one hand in contact with it may compensate for this fear. Over the first several years of life, children experience nocturnal clonic limb jerking of the legs to a greater degree than in the arms. In the major form, the hypertonia and stiffness gradually reemerge in adulthood with hyperreflexia again more evident in the legs. Persons affected with hyperekplexia usually have normal intelligence.

Characterization of Canadian and Dutch families have revealed major and minor forms of the disease.[234] Those individuals with the major form may have additional cognitive impairment and coexistent epilepsy. The minor form exhibits excessive startle and hypnic jerks with periodic leg movements in sleep without the generalized stiffness in adulthood. These later findings are consistent with excessive physiologic startles because genetic studied have failed to demonstrate molecular mutations found in the major clinical form.[234] The disease is transmitted as an autosomal dominant condition with high penetrance and variable expression.[236,237] Sporadic and autosomal recessive familial patterns of inheritance have also been described. Disease-causing mutations have been identified in the inhibitory glycine receptor (GLYR).[234,237,238]

Different mutations in the alpha1 subunit of the inhibitory glycine receptor (GLRA1) gene on chromosome 5q31.2 have been identified in many affected families.[238] Other mutations in the beta subunit of the glycine receptor (GLRB) have been identified in a few additional patients.[239,240] All these mutations, five dominant and four recessive, can result in defective glycine ligand binding and chloride channel function of the inhibitory glycine receptors.[240] This in turn promotes increased excitability in pontomedullary reticular neurons and results in abnormal spinal reciprocal inhibition. Enhancement of the GABA-gated chloride channel can compensate for deficiencies in these inhibitory glycine-gated chloride channels. Clonazepam, a gamma amino butyric acid (GABA) receptor agonist, is highly effective in dampening the excessive startle response presumably through this mechanism in hyperekplexia.[237] Similarly, treatment with clobazam (0.25–0.3 mg/kg/day) has been used successfully in two infants who were severely affected.[241] Valproic acid can also bring about benefit, albeit incomplete.[242]

EMG studies of patients with both the major and minor forms of hyperekplexia have demonstrated that the normal patterns of brainstem motor reflexes are altered.[243] This results in recruitment of cranial nerve innervated muscles in a caudorostral irradiation with very short latencies (<20 ms) after tactile stimuli.[243,244] There is an exaggerated reflex excitation and an attenuated reflex inhibition likely due to defective inhibition mediated by GABAergic and glycinergic brainstem interneurons.

The beta subunit of the glycine receptor binds to a cytoplasmic protein, gephyrin, thereby linking the receptor to the cytoskeleton. Gephyrin is also necessary for the synthesis of molybdenum cofactor (MoCo).[245,246] Molybdenum cofactor deficiency in humans produces severe neurological deficits with hypertonia, myoclonus, and feeding difficulty.[246,247] The co-occurrence of hyperekplexia and molybdenum cofactor deficiency was confirmed in one patient with hypouricemia and in refractoriness to clonazepam, early demise in infancy, and no mutations in the GLRA1 gene.[246,247] This suggests that infants with hyperekplexia who are refractory to treatment with clonazepam and do not have mutations in the GLRA1 gene be evaluated for possible MoCo deficiency due to impaired gephyrin function.

Exaggerated startle responses can also be identified secondary to other causes aside from the hyperekplexias. This can be in association with the Coffin-Lowry syndrome, an X-linked disorder where affected males demonstrate mental retardation, dysmorphic appearance, and puffy thick fingers with tapered ends, hypotonia, and hyperextensible joints.[248,249] These individuals are prone to sudden drop episodes ("cataplexy-like") in response to unexpected tactile and auditory stimuli.[250] EMG studies of these events reveal that in distinction to hyperekplexia the drop attacks of Coffin-Lowry syndrome are associated with a loss of muscle tone and not due to an exaggerated muscle contraction, although this later mechanism may also develop in the same individual over time.[251] However, similar to the hyperekplexias, clonazepam can be beneficial.

Lastly, startle responses and hyperekplexia can be secondary to and associated with other CNS pathology such as posterior fossa and brainstem malformations, and postanoxic and posttraumatic encephalopathy.[252,253]

Infantile Chorea with Severe Bronchopulmonary Dysplasia

An infrequently reported syndrome of generalized chorea has been previously described in seven neonates with severe bronchopulmonary dysplasia. The abnormal movements are observed in the extremities, neck, trunk and orobuccal-lingual regions and consist of a combination of irregular, rapid migratory choreiform-myoclonic jerks superimposed upon a "fidgety" and restless state.[254] These should not ordinarily be confused with epileptic seizures; however, the appearance of the movements occur in the context of neonates with multiple risk factors predisposing to seizures, chronic hypoxia, hypercarbia, poor nutrition, hyperbilirubinemia, and abnormal head ultrasound findings. EEG recordings during the movements are normal or show no correlation to epileptiform activity.[254] The movements appear in the third to fourth postnatal months and are exacerbated with epochs of worsening respiratory distress and attenuated by sleep. The movements, particularly those involving the tongue (tongue thrusting, oro-lingual dyskinesia), interfere with feeding. The movements tended to be static over many months after appearance, although they may both diminish in intensity or resolve 15–30 months after onset.[254] When physically impairing or contributing to the consumption of significant calories, the use of clonazepam has been beneficial.

A single infant has undergone postmortem examination and was found to have neuronal loss and astrogliosis within the caudate, globus pallidus, putamen, thalamus, red nuclei, pontine nuclei, hypothalamus, and inferior olives.[254] These findings came with additional neuronal and myelin loss in the periventricular regions, cerebellar cortex, and hippocampus.[254] This neurological substrate may be attributed to the effects of chronic hypoxemia and glutamine. The concurrent use of theophylline has also been postulated to be an additional inducer.[254]

An EMG study of one affected infant compared to a group of normal infants displaying fidgety movements was described.[255] The EMG muscle activity demonstrated a continuous bursting pattern in contrast to the waxing and waning patterns of normal infant muscle activity.[255] The abnormality has been correlated to the gestational age when normal sleep spindles emerge, and suggested a disturbance in striatal-thalamo-cortical connections.[255]

Cardiac Surgery-Induced Choreoathetosis

First described by Bergouignan, generalized choreoathetosis as a complication of deep hypothermia with and without circulatory arrest for childhood open heart surgery remains a serious and troubling outcome in about 1%–2% of these procedures.[256–261] The movements suddenly appear at 2–12 days after the procedure and involve the face, tongue, and limbs.[262] Beyond the oro-facial dyskinesia, diffuse hypotonia, affective changes, and pseudo bulbar signs are additionally apparent.[263] The identification of the movements while a child is under intermittent sedation may make recognition uncertain and suggest seizures. Electroencephalography and neuroimaging typically fail to detect etiologically significant changes.[257–259,262] A single subject who underwent [18F]fluorodeoxyglucose PET scanning demonstrated patchy hypometabolism.[259] In a minority of children, the movements regress spontaneously within 1–2 months; however, most children who develop the choreoathetosis have it persist for many months, and up to 50%, permanently.[257–259,262] Long-term cognitive assessments of 21/36 (71%) in one series of subjects accrued over a 10-year interval (1986–1995) have revealed a median full-scale IQ measure of 67 (range 40–122).[264] Important additional deficits in memory, attention, and language were also identified.[264]

Originally linked to the degree of deep hypothermia provided (<25°C), its role with the combined effects of pH has also been studied as potentially causative with extended exposure.[259,265] With both the pH-stat (normal pH and hypercapnia at the end of cooling) and alpha-stat (alkalosis and hypocapnia at the end of cooling) strategies, cooling of the patient greatly increases luxury perfusion with a greater flow to metabolism ratio of the cerebral blood flow. However, this luxury perfusion also delivers an increased quantity of micro emboli and is potentially more deleterious.[266] It has been found that hypertensive subjects are at a higher risk for ischemic injury during bypass, and thus perfusion at higher mean perfusion pressures than those for normotensive patients is suggested.[266] No consistently clear associations have been found with age at surgery, aortic cross-clamp time, duration of bypass, arterial pH, and $PaCO_2$ or mean arterial pressure. However, preexisting neurological abnormalities have been consistently associated with a higher risk.[258,259]

In a neuropathological examination of two children who died after acquiring choreoathetosis as a complication of open heart surgery for congenital heart disease, the brains demonstrated neuronal loss, reactive astrocytosis, and degeneration of myelinated fibers primarily of the outer segment of the globus pallidus.[267] The findings were described as both mild and spared other regions more commonly susceptible to hypoxic ischemic injury, implicating disruption of pallidal pathways in the pathogenesis.[267]

Response to therapy has been poor. Haldol and steroids have been administered, with some benefit.[267,268]

Hypoxic ischemic injury, particularly after cardiac arrest, may produce several movement disorders as a consequence. These include myoclonus, dystonia, akinetic-rigid syndromes, tremor, and chorea. Vulnerable regions of the CNS particularly affected by this type of injury and thus pathogenetically responsible for these are the basal ganglia, thalamus, midbrain, and cerebellum.[269]

Myoclonus-Dystonia Syndrome

Myoclonus, as a presenting symptom of neurologic disease, can be both epileptic and non-epileptic in origin. Subcortical myoclonus has several typical features that help to distinguish it from cortical myoclonus (i.e., epilepsy). Subcortical myoclonus is most often (1) generalized in distribution, (2) both proximal and distal in distribution, (3) not associated with an epileptic discharge on EEG, (4) involves co-contraction of agonist and antagonist muscles, and (5) can propagate rostrally up the brainstem.[4,5,8] There are many primary and secondary causes of both myoclonus and dystonia.[4,5,8] Brief mention will be made here of two non-epileptic disorders that have some potential to be confused with epilepsy, the hereditary autosomal-dominant myoclonus-dystonia syndrome and the sporadic opsoclonus-myoclonus-ataxia syndrome. Each of these distinct syndromes has a particular predilection to develop in childhood.

Diagnostic criteria for myoclonus-dystonia (M-D) include (1) onset of myoclonus, usually in the first or second decade of life, with mild dystonic features observed in some affected individuals; (2) myoclonus may rarely be the only manifestation of the disorder; (a) no gender predilection; (b) a benign, often variable, course; (c) autosomal-dominant mode of inheritance with variable severity and incomplete penetrance; (d) absence of dementia, gross ataxia, and other neurologic deficits; and (e) normal EEG, somatosensory evoked potentials, and neuroimaging studies.[270–272] There may be a history of symptom relief with consumption of alcohol and additional psychiatric disturbances.[270–272] A recent report has identified a few individual family members in one pedigree with both EEG abnormalities and epilepsy.[273]

M-D has been linked to mutations in the epsilon-sarcoglycan (SGCE) gene on chromosome 7q21 (DYT11). A new M-D locus has been identified on chromosome 18p11 (DYT15).[274] However, many subjects do not have mutations identified at either genetic loci.[275] It is unknown whether M-D includes patients with "jerky" primary dystonia, benign hereditary chorea, or even Ramsay-Hunt syndrome.[276]

Alpha- , beta- , gamma- , and delta-sarcoglycans (SGs) are transmembrane glycoprotein components of the dystrophin-associated protein (DAP) complex needed to stabilize striated muscle cell membranes.[277] Epsilon-SG, a homologue of alpha-SG, is expressed in striated muscle and various other tissues. The importance of epsilon-SG and its function in the CNS is yet to be fully determined. Two epsilon-SG isoforms coexist within the brain and have been found in neuronal cells.[277] Subcellular fractionation of mouse brain homogenates indicate that epsilon-SG1 and epsilon-SG2 are relatively enriched in post- and pre-synaptic membrane fractions, respectively.[276] These results suggest that the two epsilon-SG isoforms might play different roles in synaptic functions of the CNS.[277]

Grimes et al. studied thirty-one unrelated patients with a typical M-D phenotype to identify clinical factors differentiating M-D patients with and without a mutation in the SGCE gene.[274] Features significantly associated with the presence of an SGCE mutation were, onset in the first two decades of life, onset with myoclonus and dystonia, and a positive family history. The presence of truncal myoclonus and axial dystonia pointed toward a mutation in the SGCE gene.[274] In reviewing published series, forty-six mutation-positive patients (43.8%) showed at least one of the two characteristics (truncal myoclonus and axial dystonia), whereas thirty-three (31.4%) showed truncal myoclonus and sixteen (15.2%) had axial dystonia.[274] Expressivity of symptoms are modified by maternal imprinting.[278] An 8-year-old boy with medically refractory M-D and a mutation in the epsilon-sarcoglycan gene (SGCE) has undergone chronic bilateral stimulation of the globus pallidus internus, which eliminated both myoclonus and dystonia.[279]

Opsoclonus-Myoclonus-Ataxia Syndrome

Opsoclonus-myoclonus-ataxia syndrome (OMA) has been reported under several synonyms, including "dancing eyes dancing feet syndrome," infantile polymyoclonia, acute cerebellar encephalopathy, and Kinsbourne syndrome among them.[186,280–282]

The initial six children reported by Kinsbourne (onset age 9–20 months) were acutely impaired with uncoordinated trunk and limb control, and irregular myoclonic limb and trunk movements, along with chaotic ocular movements.[280] ACTH treatments resulted in improvement in four of the six.[280] Later, the frequent association with sympathetic chain neural tumors was recognized.[282]

The symptoms of OMA most frequently occur in infants between the ages of 16–20 months and often begin within 1 to 2 weeks of a viral illness or immunization.[186,280,283–285] The clinical hallmarks of OMA are the irregular ocular movements, trunkal ataxia, body and limb myoclonus, and associated irritability.[284] Opsoclonus is the chaotic multidirectional saccades of large amplitude and high frequency (10–15 Hz) that are present with fixation, smooth pursuit (tracking), convergence, eye closure, and sleep.[286,287] These differ from ocular flutter in that they are not purely horizontal and distinct from nystagmus in that there is no slow component.[286] Body and limb myoclonus are accompanied by both trunkal ataxia and postural tremor. One can observe that the face, head, trunk, and limbs are consumed by multifocal sudden jolts and changes in body posture. Smaller-scale twitching movements of the eyebrows, eyelids, and lips are superimposed upon an unsteady and lurching trunk. The encephalopathy is characterized by irritability, rage, fretfulness, malaise, and anxiety, without altered consciousness.[284] Significant sleep disturbances are also observed.[284,288] In a report of fifty-one children with OMA, thirty-two (62%) were reported by parents to experience significant sleep problems that were clinically characterized as prolonged sleep latency, fragmented sleep, reduced quantity of sleep, snoring, and nonrestorative sleep. Frequent rage attacks were reported in 25/32 (78%). Trazodone was effective in improving sleep and decreasing rage attacks.[288]

The course of illness in most children is expected to be remitting relapsing, with nonrelapsing disease found in children whose illness was associated with immunization or viral infection.[280,285] The infectious causes reported include coxsackie B3, mumps, Epstein-Barre virus, togavirus, poliomyelitis, Herpes Zoster, lymphocytic choriomeningitis, neurosyphylis, St Louis encephalitis, Salmonella typhi, and H. influenza meningitis.[284] The disease in these instances more often affects older children after age 3 years with relatively short duration of symptoms, varying from 1–2 weeks to several months.[289] A relapsing and prolonged course is typical for the paraneoplastic association with sympathetic chain neural tumors (neuroblastoma and ganglioneuroblastoma/ganglioneuroma) even with effective treatment.[284]

The association of OMA and sympathetic chain neural tumors is now well established.[284,291] Neuroblastoma accounts for approximately 8% of all cancers diagnosed in children less than 15 years of age and for 15% of all cancers in children less than 5 years of age.[290,291] It is the most common extracranial solid tumor of childhood.[290] Of all children who present with neuroblastoma or ganglioneuroblastoma/ganglioneuroma, approximately 2% will develop OMA syndrome.[290,291] Some experts suggest that all children who present with OMA, even if a concurrent viral infection is detected, have either an undetected tumor or one that has undergone spontaneous involution and is no longer present.[284,292] Repeat evaluations for the presence of tumor are required at 3–6 months after an initial OMA presentation and negative tumor evaluation because tumors can have a delayed appearance.[292,293] Of those children in whom a tumor is found, 75%–85% of tumors are neuroblastoma and 15%–25% are ganglioneuroblastoma/ganglioneuroma.[284,290,291] The tumor is found within the thorax more often than in the abdomen.[293] Those patients who have both tumor and OMA have more favorable survival outcomes than patients without OMA.[290,291,294,295] Despite this, tumor survivors with OMA are left with significant and persistent cognitive, neurologic, and behavioral deficits (70%–80%), particularly if the symptoms are recurrent or persistent.[294,295]

Monophasic OMA, however, may still have a benign outcome despite initial severity.

The primary investigations to be undertaken in children identified with OMA are an extensive evaluation for the presence of underlying neuroblastoma or ganglioneuroblastoma/ganglioneuroma. This would include MIBG (metaiodobenzylguanidine) or octreotide scanning, urinary catecholamine determinations, CT scanning, or MRI of the abdomen and mediastinum.[290, 293] Ancillary studies for alternative etiologies should be done in conjunction with a search for those tumors. Brain neuroimaging is typically normal, although in parainfectious causes ponto-cerebellar lesions have been reported in addition to delayed latencies with brainstem auditory evoked potentials that later normalize.[296] A CSF pleocytosis and positive viral antigen studies can be helpful in suspected infectious causes. CSF flow cytometry and immunoglobulin levels can identify clonal expansion of B and T cell populations within the CNS whether or not a neural tumor is identified.[297–299] These clonal expansions may serve as a biomarker for disease activity and response to therapy.[299] EEG is typically normal despite the degree of myoclonus and irritability observed.

Similar to markers found within the CNS, there has been detected autoantibodies in the sera of patients with OMA.[185, 300–302] These autoantibodies are directed against intracellular proteins, such as anti-Hu, alpha-enolase, and KHSRP (K homology splicing regulatory protein).[185] There have also been antineuronal autoantibodies shown to bind to the surface of neuroblastoma cells and cerebellar granular neurons, which may impart antiproliferative and pro-apoptotic effects of these autoantibodies on neuroblastoma cell lines.[185, 301, 302] Few cerebellar biopsy specimens from subjects with OMA with and without identified neural crest tumors have been reported. The findings have been normal or reveal mild demyelination, gliosis, and decreased Purkinje cell numbers.[289, 303] The exact pathophysiologic relationship between the neural crest tumors, immunologic findings, autoantibodies, and OMA are currently better understood. However, the pathophysiologic association among catecholamine excess and other neurotransmitter excretion is less clear. The presence of autoantibodies, antineuronal antibodies, elevated CNS immunoglobulins, and the CNS clonal expansion of activated B- and T-cells, all has relevance. Removal and treatment of an underlying tumor is necessary if identified. Nonetheless, this is usually not sufficient to reduce the neurological symptoms, which may respond, or partially respond, then reappear after resection.[284, 304, 305] Current treatment strategies aimed at reducing a global immune response and preferentially reducing the production of both immunoglobulins and activated B cells that specifically target the CNS have proven beneficial. Corticotropin (ACTH gel, 10–40 IU/d) given via intramuscular injection over weeks to months has been helpful in most instances to improve clinical manifestations.[283, 284, 297] The dose may need adjustment depending upon response and tolerance. Prednisone has been used as an alternative but has been found to be less effective.[283] Relapses often necessitate repetitive treatments.

Hypothesizing that reduction in activated B-cells would reduce CNS clonal expansion and immunoglobulin attack on selective CNS sites, a clinical trial of rituximab, a monoclonal antibody directed against the CD20 surface antigen of mature B cells, has been reported. Rituximab administered in combination with ACTH and pulse intravenous immunoglobulin (IVIg) therapy has been both well tolerated and has shown benefit.[306] In a single-blinded study of sixteen subjects with OMA (50% with neural crest tumors), 81% of OMS had a lower motor severity score, and 44% improved one severity category.[306] Rituximab reduced rage score, nighttime awakenings, and the number of children with opsoclonus, action myoclonus, drooling, gait ataxia, and rage.[306] Relapses were not observed in 9/11 (81%) despite reductions of >50% in ACTH dosage.[306] The percentage of CSF CD19+ (and CD20+) B-cells was lowered in all children (undetectable in six), with a 90% reduction in the group mean ($p = 0.00003$).[306] CSF B-cells were no longer expanded compared with controls. In both blood and CSF, the number of CD19+ B-cells decreased.[306] The serum IgM fell by 69% (below reference range), with no statistically significant change in IgG or IgA levels.[306] This was not a direct comparison to conventional ACTH and IVIg therapy; however, the authors suggest that these results represent a synergism to induce B-cell apoptosis, not realized with conventional therapy alone.[297, 306]

Paroxysmal Dyskinesias

The primary paroxysmal dyskinesias are a group of genetically determined and clinically heterogeneous disorders producing hyperkinetic movements without loss of consciousness manifest by episodic dystonia/chorea/choreo-athetosis (Table 7-14).[307–311]

These are to be distinguished from the sporadic secondary dyskinesias caused by specific underlying diseases (Table 7-15).[2, 143, 325–327, 328]

The fact that these disorders clinically manifest episodically increases the potential confusion with epilepsy. In fact, some of these disorders are combined with an epileptic symptomatology. Surveys of final diagnoses made at EEG telemetry laboratories identify 1%–2% of referred subjects as having one of these disorders.[330–332]

The most discrete and recognizable of these primary disorders include paroxysmal kinesiogenic dyskinesia manifest by choreo-athetosis/dystonia (PKD/PKC, Kertesz-type) localized to chromosome 16q13-q22.1, paroxysmal non-kinesiogenic dyskinesia manifest by dystonic choreo-athetosis (PNKD/PDC, Mount and Reback-type) localized to chromosome 2q33-35, and paroxysmal exercise-induced dystonia (PED, Lance-type) not yet localized to a specific chromosome but linkage to the PNKD locus has been excluded.[144, 307–316] Other primary paroxysmal dyskinesias have been described but are less well characterized. These include paroxysmal hypnogogic nocturnal dyskinesia (PHD) (see Chapter 4), paroxysmal choreo-athetosis, and spasticity (CSE) localized to chromosomes 2q31-36 and 1p; infantile convulsions and paroxysmal choreo-athetosis (ICCA) localized to chromosome

Table 7-14 Paroxysmal Dyskinesias

	Paroxysmal Nonkinesigenic Dyskinesias (PNKD, PDC)	Paroxysmal Kinesigenic Choreoathetosis (PKD, PKC)	Infantile Convulsions and Paroxysmal Choreoathetosis (ICCA)	Paroxysmal Exercise-Induced Dyskinesia (PED)	Choreoathetosis and Spasticity (CSE)
Inheritance	Autosomal dominant	Autosomal dominant	Autosomal dominant	Autosomal Dominant	Autosomal dominant
Gene Locus	2q33-35	16q13-q22.1	16q11-q12	—	2q31-36
Provocations	Alcohol, caffeine, hunger, stress, fatigue	Sudden movement, startle, hyperventilation	Sudden movement, stress, excitement	Prolonged exercise	Exercise, stress, fatigue, and alcohol
Onset Age/Gender	6 months to 16 years M = F	6 months to 16 years M:F = 4:1	Infant to 16 years	2–30 years M:F = 1:4	<20 years
Duration of Attack	Minutes–hours	<5 minutes	<5 minutes	Minutes–hours	15–20 minutes
Frequency	2–3 times/day	Multiple times/day (~100)	Variable time/day	Variable	<5 times/day
Treatment	Benzodiazepines, acetazolamide, gabapentin	Carbamazepine, oxcarbazepine, levetiracetam, levodopa, primidone, valproate phenytoin	Carbamazepine, oxcarbazepine, levetiracetam, primidone, valproate phenytoin	Carbamazepine, trihexaphenidyl, levodopa	?
Associated Conditions	Migraine, dystonia, dysarthria, dysphagia	–	Benign neonatal seizures	–	Spasticity during and between attacks

Source: Modified from References.[2,144,145,307–324]

Table 7-15 Conditions Associated with Secondary Paroxysmal Dyskinesias

Antiepileptic drugs (hydantoins, gabapentin)
Basal ganglia calcification
Cystinuria
Cortical dysgenesis/vascular malformations
Encephalitis (CMV, HIV, syphilis)
Hartnup disease
Head trauma
Hypocalcemia
Hypoglycemia
Hyperglycemia
Hypoparathyroidism
Hypoxic-ischemic encephalopathy
Migraine
Multiple sclerosis
Non-ketotic hyperglycinemia
Peripheral nerve trauma
Postinfectious encephalopathy
Pyruvate decarboxylase deficiency
Stroke
Systemic Lupus Erythematosis
Thalamic infarction
Transient ischemic attacks
Thyrotoxicosis

Source: Modified from References.[2, 325–327, 329]

16p11-q12; and Rolandic epilepsy – paroxysmal exercise-induced dystonia and writer's cramp (RE-PED-WC) localized to chromosome 16q12-11.2.[307, 308] There is considerable overlap among several of these specific disorders with overlapping genetic loci and additional families, with novel genetic loci being investigated currently.

PKD is manifest in children commonly between ages 6 and 16 years (range 6 months to 40 years) by abrupt isolated daily episodes of choreoathetosis/dystonia lasting 1–2 minutes, or in multiple single short epochs over the day.[317, 318] There is a male-to-female predominance of about 4:1.[317, 318] Startle, stress, and sudden movements almost always precipitate attacks. Each attack may initiate with an unusual sensation or paresthesias. Arousal from sleep will precipitate the non-kinesiogenic form (PNKD), which can be helpful in differentiation. The child remains aware and alert but often frustrated or uncomfortable as the disorder produces uncontrolled limb and body movements. These are predominantly manifest as unilateral movements or of alternate sides but can be generalized. Most familial and sporadic cases respond favorably to carbamazepine or phenytoin.[319] Oxcarbazepine and levetiracetam have both recently been shown to be effective as have primidone and sodium valproate.[333–335] The attacks diminish with age. This disorder shares similarity and management approaches to ICCA.[311, 320]

PNKD is manifest by abrupt attacks of combinations of chorea, ballismus, athetosis, and/or dystonic posturing of the limbs, trunk, jaw, and
tongue.[145,310,315] Whole body involvement is not usual, and involvement of the
larynx and throat can evoke dysphagia and dysarthria. These attacks may also
be unilateral, bilateral, or affect alternate sides as seen in PKD. The onset age is
again typically between 6 and 16 years of age (range 2 months to 30 years old).
The attacks of PNKD in contrast to PKD last as long as10 minutes to up to
4 hours, are less often precipitated by sudden movement, but are exacerbated
by alcohol, caffeine, fatigue, and stress.[145,315] Often the attacks are preceded
by paresthesias or uncomfortable sensations. PNKD attacks are much less frequent than in PKD and occur only 2–3 times per day, with many weeks or
months of reprieve. Awakening from sleep can be a trigger in some patients.
Paroxysmal events had their onset in a 3-year-old boy who by age 6 years
had evolved into persistent dystonia.[145] The disorder can be managed with
clonazepam and typically is unresponsive to other anticonvulsants.[144] Treatment with acetazolamide and other benzodiazepines have had some success.[145]
Gabapentin has also been reported as beneficial.[336] PNKD shares clinical similarity to CSE.[321] This later disorder (CSE) has the additional clinical features
of perioral paresthesias, headache, diplopia, and spastic diplegia.[321] Although
subjects with CSE have paroxysmal dystonic attacks similar to PNKD, these
attacks are often precipitated by physical exercise.

Lastly, PED is a sporadic disorder where attacks of dystonia lasting minutes
to 1 hour are precipitated by prolonged exercise.[144,311,312] Common activities
inducing attacks in childhood are bike riding, jogging, or prolonged walking. The dystonia appears a few minutes after the exercise has ceased, with
the legs prominently involved although the arms and face may be included.
Onset age is between 2 and 30 years of age.[144,311,318] Antiepileptic drugs offer
little benefit. Treatment has been modest in a few patients with carbamazepine,
trihexaphenidyl, and levodopa.[322]

Only a few members of an isolated family have been reported with RE-PED-
WC.[323] This comprises subjects experiencing benign partial (Rolandic) seizures
and writers cramp in early childhood. Later in childhood, 3–8 years of age,
dystonia of the trunk and hemidystonia become manifest after exercise.[323] The
least common of the primary dyskinesias is PHD. In PHD the child's sleep is
suddenly interrupted by brief periods (less than 1 minute) of severe dystonic
movements of the limbs, several times each night.[324] They are usually painful
and provoke screaming during the event. Treatment with carbamazepine has
been helpful. At least some of these children have autosomal-dominant frontal
lobe epilepsy (ADFLE).

Benign Hereditary Chorea

Benign hereditary chorea is an autosomal-dominant disorder first described in
1967 by Pincus and Chutorian, and independently that same year by Haerer
et al.[337,338] Autosomal-recessive and X-linked inheritance patterns were also
later described.[339,340] There have been some forty-two families now reported

in the literature, a review of which has been provided by Kleiner-Fishman and Lang.[341] The onset of symptoms can be throughout childhood, with predominance at about 1 year of age or after the attainment of independent walking.[337,338,341] Children are often referred for evaluation of developmental delays in walking or frequent falling.[337,338,341] This is when the choreiform movements become obvious to the point of disrupting normal independent gait.[341] The choreic movements can be quick and myoclonic in quality, mainly involving the trunk, tongue, and proximal limbs.[337,338,341] This quality mimics myoclonic epilepsy; however, there is no definite progression, although there is escalation into adolescence, with improvement in adulthood.[337,338,341] Intention tremor, sensorineural hearing loss, and axial dystonia have been described in individuals.[337,341] There are no additional commonly associated neurological abnormalities on examination. The more important differential diagnostic considerations are Sydenham's chorea, Huntington's disease, torsion dystonia, Wilson's disease, and cerebellar degenerations. The movements are not paroxysmal in description, however, are exacerbated by excitement and stress, and diminish with sleep.

Recent investigations have identified a mutation on chromosome 14, spanning the thyroid transcription factor gene, TITF-1.[341,342] Now, a number of families have been identified with this gene mutation whose members manifest not only chorea but also congenital hypothyroidism and pulmonary dysfunction.[329,342] This has prompted the term "Brain-Thyroid-Lung syndrome" and an expanded clinical phenotype.[329] Neuropathology on two subjects with the TITF-1 gene mutation has been normal.[343,344]

Otitis Media Spells

As with all fields of medicine, new observations are made regularly. Despite the high frequency of visits to the doctor for a complaint of ear pain, the diagnosis of otitis media has only recently been associated with a presentation of seizure-like behavior. Soman et al. reported on a group of eight children aged 8 months to 4 years old who were initially referred for behaviors thought to be seizures. There was some consistency for each child, but not all children shared equivalent features. Nonetheless, there were several characteristic signs among many of the children reported, and these included sudden stare (two) with or without adversive head posturing (one), eye fluttering (one) or eye rolling (four) with or without sudden limp tone (four), and loss of posture.[15] The clinical presentations suggested absence seizures in three subjects; atonic seizures in three other children and five of the children on repeat otitis media infections had behaviors suggestive of intermittent complex partial seizures.[15] Each child had normal neurological examinations and underwent EEG recording during events with normal results. All children had remission of spells after appropriate antibiotic therapy was introduced. The authors speculated that the spells were mediated by the vestibular labyrinth system and/or otolith systems.[15]

In an interesting converse analogy, there is a single report of a 2-year child who was referred for episodic eye fluttering, head nodding, and unresponsiveness.[345] He was confidently diagnosed with absence seizures using EEG video telemetry. Upon treatment of the absence epilepsy with valproate, the seizures abated. However, the child then began to experience sudden onset of paroxysmal tonic upgaze manifest by "eyes-up and chin-down" posturing events.[345] This too was confirmed as non-epileptic upon recording with repeat EEG video telemetry. Discontinuation of the valproate reduced these events, which suggests a possible relationship between GABAergic systems and the production of this eye-gaze disorder.[345]

As a final note, there are a number of useful medication interventions available for the various types of movements observed in childhood (Table 7-16).

Table 7-16 Drug Treatment Considerations in Childhood Movement Disorders

Generic Name	Indicated Movement Types	Usual Dosages	Mechanisms of Action
Baclofen	C, D, M, S, T	Dose titration at 7-d intervals to effective dose Child < 2 yrs: 2.5–10 mg PO q8h, max 20–30 mg/d Child 2–7 yrs: 5–20 mg PO q8h, max 30–40 mg/d Child >8 yrs: 5–20 mg PO q8h, max 40–60 mg/d	γ-aminobutyric acid (GABA) agonist that inhibits transmission of reflexes at the spinal cord
Carbamazepine	D, T, PD	Child: initial: 5–10 mg/kg/d ÷ bid Maintenance: 10–25 mg/kg/d ÷ bid, qid Adult: 400–2400 mg/d ÷ bid, qid Initial dose: 100–200 mg hs for 5–7 days then increase by 200 mg/d every 5–7 days	Modulates sodium channels
Clonazepam	C, D, M, T, Tr	0.01–0.3 mg/kg/d ÷ bid or tid	Facilitates the actions of γ-aminobutyric acid (GABA)
Clonidine	S, T	Start at 0.05 mg/d and increase by 0.05 mg every week, to a maximum of 0.3 mg/d ÷ tid	Centrally acting α_2_adrenergic agonist that increases presynaptic inhibition of motoneurons

Clorazepate	Tr	Adult: 7.5 mg PO ÷ bid; increase by 7.5 mg at weekly intervals to maximum of 90 mg/d given in individual doses Child 9–12 yrs: 3.75 mg PO ÷ bid; increase by 3.75 mg at weekly intervals not to exceed 60 mg/d in divided doses	Facilitates the action of γ-aminobutyric acid (GABA)
Dantrolene	S	Adult: 25 mg PO gid; increase q4-7 days to maximum of 400 mg ÷ 4 doses/d Child >5 yrs: 0.5 mg/kg PO ÷ bid; to max of 12 mg/kg ÷ 4 doses/d	Interferes with calcium ion release from sarcoplasmic reticulum of skeletal muscles
Diazepam	S, Tr	Adults: 2–10 mg PO ÷ bid to qid Child: 0.05–0.1 mg/kg PO ÷ bid to qid (maximum of 0.8 mg/kg/d)	Facilitates the actions of γ-aminobutyric acid (GABA)
Fluphenzaine	C, T	0.25–1 mg/d PO and increase by 1 mg each week Usual maintenance dose is 4–6 mg (max 10 mg/d)	Dopamine receptor-D_2 antagonist
Gabapentin	PD, M, T	Adult: 900–3600 mg PO ÷ tid to qid Child: up to 60 mg/kg/d ÷ tid to qid	Unknown
Guanfacine	T	Child: 0.25–0.5 mg/d PO increase to maintenance of 0.5–3 mg/d ÷ bid, tid	Centrally acting α_2-adrenergic agonist
Haloperidol	C, T	Start at 0.5 mg PO qhs and increase by 0.5 mg each week; maximum dose is 0.15 mg/kg/d ÷ bid, tid	Dopamine receptor-D_2 antagonist
Levetiracetam	M, PD	25 mg/k/d PO ÷ bid, tid escalate to 50–75 mg/kg/d	Modifies the synaptic release of glutamate and γ-aminobutyric acid (GABA) via vesicular function
Levodopa/ Carbidopa	D	1–2 tablets PO bid, qid	Dopamine precursor, indirect receptor agonist

continued

Table 7-16 continued

Generic Name	Indicated Movement Types	Usual Dosages	Mechanisms of Action
Lorazepam	D, M, Tr	Adult: 1–10 mg/d PO ÷ bid, qid Child: 0.01–0.1 mg/kg/d PO ÷ bid, qid	Benzodiazepine receptor agonist
Phenytoin	PD	Adult: 100–400 mg/d PO ÷ bid, qd Child: 2–5 mg/k/d PO ÷ bid, qd	Alters Na^+, K^+, and Ca^{2+} conductance, membrane potentials, and the concentrations of norepinepherine, acetylcholine, and γ-aminobutyric acid (GABA).
Pimozide	C, T	Start at 1 mg/d PO and increase by 1 mg each week; maintenance dose is 2–4 mg/d ÷ bid, tid; maximum dose is 10 mg/d	Dopamine receptor-D_2 antagonist
Piracetam (unavailable in the United States)	M, Tr	Dose range is 4.8–24 mg/d PO ÷ tid	Unknown but modifies the synaptic release of glutamate and γ-aminobutyric acid (GABA) via vesicular function
Primidone	M, Tr	Child: <8 yrs, initial, 50 mg PO at bedtime for 3 days, increase dose by 50 mg/day (divided doses) every 3 days to reach a dose of 125–250 mg (10–25 mg/kg) 3 times a day	Enhancement of γ-aminobutyric acid (GABA)
Propranolol	M, Tr	Start at 0.5–1 mg/kg/d PO ÷ tid; increase every 5 days to a maintenance dose of 2–6 mg/kg/d or ≤35 kg: 10–20 mg 3/d ÷ tid; >35 kg: 20–40 mg 3d ÷ tid	B-Blocker
Reserpine	C, D, T	0.1–3 mg/d PO ÷ bid	Presynaptic depletion of catecholamine

Risperidone	T	0.25 mg/d PO escalate to 1–3 mg/d PO ÷ bid, tid	Dopamine receptor-D_2 antagonist
Tetrabenazine	C, D, M, T	12.5–100 mg/d	Irreversible catecholamine granular storage depletor and dopamine receptor blocker
Tiagabine	S	Adult: 32–56 mg/d PO ÷ bid to qid (start with 4 mg PO qid, adjust weekly) Child: 0.1 mg/kg/d PO; increase to 0.5 mg/kg/d	Inhibits neuronal and glial uptake of GABA
Tizanidine	S	Adult: initial dosing is 1 mg PO q8h prn; may increase to maximum of 36 mg/d Child: initial dosing 1 mg PO qhs for <10 yrs, 2 mg PO qhs for >10 yrs with maintenance at 0.3–0.5 mg/kg/d ÷ qid	Centrally acting α_{2-} adrenergic agonist that increases presynaptic inhibition of motoneurons
Trihexphenidyl	D, M	Initial dose is 2–2.5 mg/d PO; increase by 2–2.5 mg every other week to a maximal dose as high as 60 mg/d	Anticholinergic
Valproate	C, M	Initial: 5–10 mg/kg/d PO (÷ bid to qid) Maintenance: 15–60 mg/kg/d (750–4000 mg/d) ÷ bid to qid)	Enhances action of GABA
Zonisamide	M	Initial: 2–4 mg/kg/d PO (÷ qd to bid) Maintenance: 4–12 mg/kg/d (÷ qd to bid)	Multiple mechanisms of action

Source: Modified from References.[2, 89, 91, 237, 242, 307–310, 335, 344, 346, 347]
Notes: PO = orally, mg = milligram, d = day, kg = kilogram, qHS = at hour of sleep, qd = each day, bid = twice a day, tid = three times a day, qid = four times a day, GABA = gaba-aminobutyric acid, prn = as needed, S = spasticity, D = dystonia/athetosis, PD = paroxysmal dyskinesia, T = tics, Tr = tremor, C = chorea, M = myoclonus.
This table is not all-inclusive but offers a compilation from a number of sources.[346, 347]

REFERENCES

1. DiMario FJ. The nervous system. In *Rudolph's Fundamentals of Pediatrics*. Eds: AM Rudolph, RK Kamei, KJ Overby. 3rd edition, New York, Mcgraw Hill, 2002; 796–846.
2. Fernandez-Alverez E, Aicardi J. *Movement Disorders in Children*. Int Rev Child Neurol Series, London England: Mac Kieth Press, 2001.
3. Glaze DG, Frost JD, Jankovic J. Sleep in Giles de la Tourette syndrome: a disorder of arousal. Neurology 1983; 3; 586–592.
4. Tarsay D, Simon DK. Dystonia. N Engl J Med 2006; 355; 818–829.
5. Fahn S, Jankovic J. *Principles and Practice of Movement Disorders*. Philadelphia, PA: Chuchill-Livingstone Elseiver, 2007.
6. Delgado MR, Albright L. Movement disorders in children: definitions, classifications, and grading systems. J Child Neurol 2003; 18; S1–S8.
7. Pearl PL, Taylor JL, Trzcinski S, et al. The pediatric neurotransmitter disorders. J Child Neurol 2007; 22; 606–616.
8. Sanger T. Pathophysiology of pediatric movement disorders. J Child Neurol 2003; 18; S9–S24.
9. Fernandez-Alvarez E. Transient movement disorders in children. J Neurol 1998; 245; 1–5.
10. DiMario FJ. Paroxysmal non-epileptic events of childhood. Semin Pediatr Neurol 2006; 13(4); 208–221.
11. Rodnitzky RL. Drug-induced movement disorders in children. Semin Pediatr Neurol 2003; 10(1); 80–87.
12. Rajput A. Cetirizine-induced dystonic movements. Neurology 2006; 66; 143–144.
13. Dooley JM. Tic disorders in childhood. Semin Pediatr Neurol 2006; 13(4); 231–242.
14. Denoyelle F, Garabedian EN, Roger G, et al. Laryngeal dyskinesia as a cause of stridor in infants. Arch Otolaryngol Head Neck Surg 1996; 122; 612–616.
15. Soman TB, Krishnamoorthy KS. Paroxysmal non-epileptic events resembling seizures in children with otitis media. Clin Pediatr (Phila) 2005; 44; 437–441.
16. Singer H, Movement disorders in children. In *Parkinson's Disease and Movement Disorders*. Eds: JJ Jankovic, E Tolosa. 4th edition. Philadelphia, PA, Lippincott Williams & Wilkins, 2002; 451–472.
17. Lee EJ, Choi JY, Lee SH, et al. Hemichorea-hemiballism in primary diabetic patients: MR correlation. J Comp Assist Tom 2002; 26(6); 905–911.
18. Chang CV, Felicio AC, Godeiro Cde O, et al. Chorea-ballism as a manifestation of decompensated type 2 diabetes mellitus. Am J Med Sci 2007; 333(3); 175–177.
19. Finelli P, DiMario FJ. Diagnostic approach in patients with symmetric imaging lesions of the deep gray nuclei. Neurologist 2003; 9; 250–261.
20. Kotagal P, Costa M, Wyllie E, et al. Paroxysmal non-epileptic events in children and adolescents. Pediatrics 2002, 110(4); e46–e51. http://www.pediatrics.org/cgi/content/full/110/4/e46.
21. Bye AM, Kok DJ, Ferenschild FT, et al. Paroxysmal non-epileptic events in children: a retrospective study over a period of 10 years. J Paediatr Child Health 2000; 36(3); 244–248.
22. Donat JF, Wright FS. Episodic symptoms mistaken for seizures in the neurologically impaired child. Neurology 1990; 40(1); 156–157.

23. Gibbs J, Appleton RE. False diagnosis of epilepsy in children. Seizure 1992;1; 15–18.
24. Stroink H, van Donselaar CA, Geerts AT, et al. The accuracy of the diagnosis of paroxysmal events in children. Neurology 2003; 60; 979–982.
25. Uldall P, Alving J, Hansen LK, et al. The misdiagnosis of epilepsy in children admitted to a tertiary epilepsy centre with paroxysmal events. Arch Dis Child 2006; 91; 219–221.
26. Beach R, Reading R. The importance of acknowledging clinical uncertainty in the diagnosis of epilepsy and non-epileptic events. Arch Dis Child 2005; 90; 1219–1222.
27. Hindley D, Ali A, Robson C. Diagnoses made in a secondary care "fits, faints, funny turns" clinic. Arch Dis Child 2006; 91; 214–218.
28. Desai P, Talwar D. Nonepileptic events in normal and neurologically handicapped children: A video-EEG study. Pediatr Neurol 1992; 8; 127–129.
29. Holmes G, McKeever M, Russman B. Abnormal behavior or epilepsy? Use of long-term EEG and video monitoring with severely to profoundly mentally retarded patients with seizures. Am J Ment Ret 1983; 87(4); 456–458.
30. Neill JC, Alvarez N. Differential diagnosis of epileptic versus pseudoepileptic seizures in developmentally disabled persons. Appl Res Ment Ret 1986; 7(3); 285–298.
31. Winter S, Autry A, Boyle C, Yeargin-Allsopp M. Trends in the prevalence of cerebral palsy in a population-based study. Pediatrics 2002; 110(6); 1220–1225.
32. Stanley F, Blair E, Alberman E. *Cerebral Palsies: Epidemiology and Causal Pathways.* 1st edition. London, United Kingdom: Mac Keith Press, 2000.
33. Hagberg B, Hagberg G, Olow I. The changing panorama of cerebral palsy in Sweden. VI. Prevalence and origin during the birth year period 1983–1986. Acta Paediatr 1993; 82; 387–393.
34. Pharoah PO, Cooke T, Rosenbloom I, et al. Trends in birth prevalence of cerebral palsy Arch Dis Child 1987; 62; 379–384.
35. Stanley FJ, Watson L. The cerebral palsies in Western Australia: trends, 1968 to 1981 Am J Obstet Gynecol 1988; 158; 89–93.
36. Stanley FJ, Watson L. Trends in perinatal mortality and cerebral palsy in Western Australia, 1967 to 1985 BMJ 1992; 304; 1658–1663.
37. Hagberg B, Hagberg G, Olow I, et al. The changing panorama of cerebral palsy in Sweden. VII. Prevalence and origin in the birth year period 1987–90. Acta Paediatr1996; 85; 954–960.
38. Aicardi J, Bax M. Cerebral palsy. In *Diseases of the Nervous System in Childhood.* Ed: Aicardi J. 2nd edition. London, England, MacKieth Press, 1998; 210–239.
39. Jancovic J. Tourette's syndrome. N Engl J Med 2001; 345; 1184–1192.
40. Scahill L, Tanner C, Dure L. The epidemiology of tics and Tourette syndrome in children and adolescents. Adv Neurol 2001; 85; 261–271.
41. Snider LA, Seligman LD, Ketchen BR, et al. Tics and problem behaviors in schoolchildren: prevalence, characterization, and association. Pediatrics 2002; 110; 331–336.
42. Kurlan R, McDermott MP, Deeley C, et al. Prevalence of tics in schoolchildren and association with placement in special education. Neurology 2001; 57; 1383–1388.
43. Khalifa N, von Knorring AL. Prevalence of tics disorders and Tourette syndrome in a Sweedish school population. Dev Med Child Neurol 2003; 45(5); 315–319.
44. Krauss JK, Jankovic J. Head injury and post-traumatic movement disorders. Neurosurgery 2002; 50; 927–940.

45. Costeff H, Gorswasser Z, Goldstein R. Long-term follow-up review of 31 children with severe closed head trauma. J Neurosurg 1990; 73; 684–687.
46. Johnson SL, Hall DM, Post-traumatic tremor in head injured children. Arch Dis Child 1992; 67; 227–228.
47. Szelozynaska K, Znamirowski R. Extrapyramidal syndrome in posttraumatic hemiparesis in children. Neurol Neurochir Pol 1974; 8; 167–170.
48. Afifi AK. The basal ganglia: a neural network with more than motor function. Semin Pediatr Neurol 2003; 10(1); 3–10.
49. Mink JW. The basal ganglia and involuntary movements: impaired inhibition of competing motor patterns. Arch Neurol 2003; 60; 1365–1368.
50. Centonze D, Bernardi G, Koch G. Mechanisms of disease: basic–research-driven investigations in humans–the case of hyperkinetic disorders. Nat Clin Prac Neurol 2007; 3(10); 572–580.
51. Alexander GE, Crutcher MD. Functional architecture of basal ganglia circuits: neural substrates of parallel processing. Trends in Neurosci 1990; 13; 266–271.
52. Bar-Gad I, Morris G, Bergman H. Information processing, dimensionality reduction and reinforcement learning in the basal ganglia. Prog Neurobiol 2003; 71; 439–473.
53. Wichmann T, Delong MR. Functional neuroanatomy of the basal ganglia in Parkinson's disease. Adv Neurol 2003; 91; 9–18.
54. Wichmann T, Delong MR. Pathophysiology of Parkinson's disease: the MPTP primate model of the human disorder. Ann NY Acad Sci 2003; 991; 199–213.
55. Mink JW. The basal ganglia: focused selection and inhibition of competing motor programs. Prog Neurobiol 1996; 50; 381–425.
56. Bhatia KP, Marsden CD. The behavioral and motor consequences of focal lesions of the basal ganglia in man. Brain 1994; 117; 859–876.
57. Heidenreich R, Natowicz M, Hainline BE, et al. Acute extrapyramidal syndrome in methylmalonic acidemia: metabolic stroke involving the globus pallidus. J Pediatr 1988; 113; 1022–1027.
58. Calne DB, de la Fuente-Fernandez R, Kishore A. Contributions of positron emission tomography to elucidating the pathogenesis of idiopathic parkinsonism and dopa responsive dystonia. J Neural Transm Suppl 1997; 50; 47–52.
59. Hikosaka O, Wurtz RH. Modification of saccadic eye movements by GABA-related substances. II. Effects of muscimol in monkey substancia nigra pars reticulata. J Neurophysiol 1985; 53; 292–308.
60. Shuper A, Zalzberg J, Weitz R, et al. Jitteriness beyond the neonatal period: a benign pattern of movement in infancy. J Child Neurol 1991; 6; 243–245.
61. Parker S, Zuckerman B, Bauchner H, et al. Jitteriness in full-term neonates: prevalence and correlates. Pediatrics 1990; 85(1); 17–23.
62. Ozkan H, Anal O, Turan A, et al. Maternal preeclampsia and jitteriness in preterm infants. Pediatr Int 1999; 41(5); 557–560.
63. Kramer U, Nevo Y, Harel S. Jittery babies: a short-term follow-up. Brain Devel 1994; 16; 112–114.
64. Zeskind PS, Stephens LE. Maternal selective serotonin reuptake inhibitor use during pregnancy and newborn neurobehavior. Pediatrics 2004; 113(2); 368–375.
65. Volpe JJ. Neonatal seizures. *Neurology of the Newborn*. 3rd edition. Philadelphia, PA: WB Saunders Co, 1995, 172–207.
66. Chasnoff IJ. Drug use in pregnancy: parameters of risk. Pediatr Clin North Am 1988; 35(6); 1403–1412.

67. Massaro D. Ventisei casi di geniospasmo attraverso cinque geneazioni: contributo clinico allo studio dell'eredita fisiopatologica. I Pisani (Palermo) 1894; 1; 47–56.
68. Massaro D. Ving-six cas de genio'-spasme en cinq generations. Rev Neurol 1894; 2; 534.
69. Chalaupka FD, Bartholini F, Mandich G, et al. Two families with hereditary essential chin myoclonus: clinical features, neurophysioloical findings and treatment. Neurol Sci 2006; 27; 97–103.
70. Destee A, Cassim F, Defebvre L, Guieu JD. Hereditary chin trembling or hereditary chin myoclonus? J Neurol Neurosurg Psychiatr 1997; 63(6); 804–807.
71. Jarman PR, Wood NW, Davis MT, et al. Hereditary geniospasm: linkage to chromosome 9q13-q21 and evidence for genetic heterogeneity. Am J Hum Genet 1997; 61; 928–933.
72. Grimes DA, Han F, Bulman D, et al. Hereditary chin trembling: a new family with exclusion of the chromosome 9q13-q21 locus. Mov Disord 2002; 17(6); 1390–1392.
73. Ouvrier RA, Billson F. Benign paroxysmal tonic upgaze of childhood. J Child Neurol 1988; 3; 177–180.
74. Deonna TH, Roulet E, Meyer HU. Benign paroxysmal tonic upgaze of childhood. A new syndrome. Neuropediatrics 1990; 21; 213–214.
75. Ahn JC, Hoyt WF, Hoyt CS. Tonic upgaze in infancy. Arch Ophthalmol 1989; 107; 57–58.
76. Echenne B, Rivier F. Benign paroxysmal tonic upward gaze. Pediatr Neurol 1992; 8; 154–155.
77. Mets M. Tonic upgaze in infancy. Arch Ophthalmol 1990; 108; 482–483.
78. Sugie H, Sugie Y, Ito M, et al. A case of paroxysmal tonic upgaze associated with psychomotor retardation. Dev Med Child Neurol 1995; 37; 362–369.
79. Campistol J, Prats JM, Garaizar C. Benign paroxysmal tonic upgaze of childhood with ataxia. A neuroophthalmological syndrome of familial origin? Dev Med Child Neurol 1993; 35; 436–439.
80. Kleiman MD, DiMario FJ, Leconche DA, et al. Benign transient downward gaze in preterm infants. Pediatr Neurol 1994; 10; 313–316.
81. Hoyt CS. Nystagmus and other abnormal ocular movements in children. Ed: Martyn LJ. Pediatric Clinics of North America, Philadelphia, PA: WB Saunders, 1987; 34; 1415–1423.
82. Hoyt CS, Mousel DK, Weber AA. Transient supranuclear disturbances of gaze in healthy neonates. Am J Ophthalmol 1980; 89; 708–713.
83. Yokochi K. Paroxysmal ocular downward deviation in neurologically impaired infants. Pediatr Neurol 1991; 7; 426–428.
84. Yoshikawa H. Benign "setting sun" phenomenon in full-term infants. J Child Neurol 2003; 18(6); 424–425.
85. Vanasse M, Bedard P, Andermann F. Shuddering attacks in children: an early clinical manifestation of essential tremor. Neurology 1976; 26; 1027–1030.
86. Findley LJ, Koller WC. Essential tremor: a review. Neurology 1987; 37; 1194–1197.
87. Holmes GL, Russman BS. Shuddering attacks. Am J Dis Child 1986; 140; 72–73.
88. Kanazawa O. Shuddering attacks: report of four children. Pediatr Neurology 2000; 23(5); 421–424.
89. DiMario FJ. Childhood head tremor. J Child Neurol 2000; 15; 22–25.
90. Bucher SF, Seelos KC, Dodel RC, et al. Activation mapping in essential tremor with functional magnetic resonance imaging. Ann Neurol 1997; 41; 32–40.

91. Barron TF, Younkin DP. Propranolol therapy for shuddering attacks. Neurology 1992; 42; 258–259.

92. Onofrj M, Thomas A, Paci C, et al. Gabapentin in orthostatic tremor: results of a double-blind crossover with placebo in four patients. Neurology 1998; 51; 880–882.

93. Glass GA, Ahlskog JE, Matsumoto JY. Orthostatic myoclonus. Neurology 2007; 68; 1826–1830.

94. Gresty MA, Leech J, Sanders M, et al. A study of head and eye movement in spasmus nutans. Br J Ophthalmol 1976; 60; 652–654.

95. Gottlob I, Zubkov AA, Wizov SS, et al. Head nodding is compensatory in spasmus nutans. Ophthalmol 1992; 99(7); 1024–1031.

96. Gottlob I, Zubkov AA, Catalano RA, et al. Signs distinguishing spasmus nutans (with and without central nervous system lesions) from infantile nystagmus. Ophthalmol 1990; 97(9); 1166–1175.

97. Shawkat FS, Kriss A, Russel-Eggitt I, et al. Diagnosing children presenting with asymmetric pendular nystagmus. Dev Med Child Neurol 2001; 43(9); 622–627.

98. Klibinger GD, Wallace BS, Hines M, et al. Spasmus nutans-like nystagmus is often associated with underlying ocular, intracranial, or systemic abnormalities. J Neuro-Ophthalmol 2007; 27(2); 118–122.

99. Kim JS, Park S-H, Lee K-W. Spasmus nutans and congenital motor apraxia with cerebellar vermian hypoplasia. Arch Neurol 2003; 60(11); 1621–1624.

100. Arnoldi KA, Tychsen L. The presence of intracranial lesions in children initially diagnosed with dysconjugate nystagmus. J Pediatr Ophthalmol Strabismus 1995; 32(5); 296–301.

101. McLean R, Proudlock F, Thomas S, et al. Congenital nystagmus: Randomized, controlled, double-masked trial of memantine/gabapentin. Ann Neurol 2007; 61; 130–138.

102. Lombroso CT, Fejerman N. Benign myoclonus of early infancy. Ann Neurol 1977; 1; 138–143.

103. Pachatz C, Fusco L, Vigevano F. Benign myoclonus of early infancy. Epilep Dis 1999; 1(1); 57–61.

104. Maydell BV, Berenson F, Rothner AD, et al. Benign myoclonus of early infancy: An imitator of West's syndrome. J Child Neurol 2001; 16; 109–112.

105. Vigevano F, Lispi ML. Tonic reflex seizures of early infancy: an age-related non-epileptic paroxysmal disorder. Epilep Dis 2002; 3; 133–136.

106. Vigevano F, Tonic reflex seizures of early infancy: an undescribed non-epileptic paroxysmal disorder. Epilepsia 1996; 37(Suppl 4); 87.

107. Snyder CH. Benign paroxysmal torticollis in infancy. A possible form of labyrynthitis. Am J Dis Child 1969; 117; 458–460.

108. Deonna T, Martin D. Benign paroxysmal torticollis in infancy. Arch Dis Child 1981; 56; 956–958.

109. Hanukoglu A, Somekh E, Fried D. Benign paroxysmal torticollis of infancy. Clin Pediatr 1984; 23; 272–274.

110. Cataltepe SU, Barron TF. Benign paroxysmal torticollis presenting as "seizures" in infancy. Clin Pediatr 1993; 32; 564–565.

111. Roulet E, Deonna T. Benign paroxysmal torticollis in infancy. Dev Med Child Neurol 1988; 30; 409–410.

112. Andermann F, Ohtahara S, Andermann E, et al. Infantile hypotonia and paroxysmal dystonia – a variant of alternating hemiplegia of childhood. Mov Disord 1994; 9; 227–229.

113. Dunn DW, Snyder CH. Benign paroxysmal vertigo of childhood. Am J Dis Child 1976; 130;1099–1100.

114. Sanner G, Bergstrom B. Benign paroxysmal torticollis in infancy. Acta Paediatr Scan 1979; 68; 219–223.

115. Kimura S, Nezu A. Electromyographic study in an infant with benign paroxysmal torticollis. Pediatr Neurol 1998; 19; 236–238.

116. Ducros A, Denier C, Joutel A, et al. The clinical spectrum of familial hemiplegic migraine associated with mutations in a neuronal calcium channel. N Engl J Med 2001; 345; 17–24.

117. Giffin NJ, Benton S, Goadsby PJ. Benign paroxysmal torticollis of infancy: four new cases and linkage to CACN1A mutation. Dev Med Child Neurol 2002; 44; 490–493.

118. Sommerfelt K, Pedersen P, Ellertsen B, et al. Transient dystonia in non-handicapped low-birthweight infants and later neurodevelopment. Acta Paediatr 1996; 85; 1445–1449.

119. de Groot L, Van der Hoek AM, Hopkins B, et al. Development of the relationship between active and passive muscle power in preterms after term age. Neuropediatrics 1992; 23; 298–305.

120. de Groot L, Van der Hoek AM, Hopkins B, et al. Development of muscle power in preterm infants: individual trajectories after term age. Neuropediatrics 1993; 24; 68–74.

121. Drillien CM. Abnormal neurological signs in the first year of life in low birthweight infants: possible prognostic significance. Dev Med Child Neurol 1972; 14; 575–584.

122. van der Fits I, Hadders-Algra M. Development of postural adjustments during reaching in preterm infants. Pediatr Res 1999; 46; 1–7.

123. Willemse J. Benign idiopathic dystonia in the first year of life. Dev Med Child Neurol 1986; 28; 355–363.

124. Deonna T, Ziegler AL, Nielson J. Transient idiopathic dystonia in infancy. Neuropediatrics 1991; 22; 220–224.

125. Angelini L, Lamperti E, Nardocci N. Transient paroxysmal dystonia in infancy. Neuropediatrics 1988; 19; 171–174.

126. Kinsbourne M. Hiatus hernia with contortions of the neck. Lancet 1964; i; 1058–1061.

127. Mandel H, Tirosh E, Berant M. Sandifer syndrome reconsidered. Acta Paediatr Scand 1989; 78; 797–799.

128. Sutclife J. Torsion spasm and abnormal postures in children with hiatus hernia Sandifer's syndrome. Prog Pediatr Radiol 1969; 2; 190–197.

129. Gellis SS, Feingold M. Syndrome of hiatus hernia with torsion spasms and abnormal posturing. Am J Dis Child 1971; 121; 43–54.

130. Puntis JWL, Smith HL, Buick RG, et al. Effect of dystonic movements on oesophageal peristalsis in Sandifer's syndrome. Arch Dis Child 1989; 64; 1311–1313.

131. Wyllie E, Wyllie R, Rothner AD, et al. Diffuse esophageal spasm: A cause of paroxysmal posturing and irritability in infants and mentally retarded children. J Pediatr 1989; 115(2); 261–263.

132. Wenzl TG, Pfeifer UW, Uelter M, et al, German Pediatric Impedance Group. Bolus-induced reflux dystonia (BIRDy)—a new entity. J Pediatr Gastroent Nutr 2006; 42(5); Abstr E55–E56.

133. Corrado G, Cavaliere M, D'Eufemia P, et al. Sandifer's syndrome in a breast-fed infant. Am J Perinatol 2000; 17(3); 147–150.

134. Patterson R, Schatz M, Horton M. Munchausen's stridor: a nonorganic laryngeal obstruction. Clin Allergy 1974; 4; 307–310.

135. Cohn A. Stool withholding presenting as a cause of non-epileptic seizures. Devel Med Child Neurol 2005; 47; 703–705.

136. Loddenkemper T, Wyllie E, Kaplan B, et al. Stoolwithholding activity mimicking epilepsy. Neurology 2003; 61; 1454–1455.

137. Nechay A, Ross LM, Stephenson JBP, et al. Gratification disorder ("infantile masturbation"): a review. Arch of Dis Child 2004; 89; 225–226.

138. Wulff CH, Livingston S, Berman W, et al. Masturbation simulating epilepsy. Clin Pediatr 1975; 14; 232–234.

139. Fleisher DR, Morrison A. Masturbation mimicking abdominal pain or seizures in young girls. J Pediatr 1990; 116; 810–814.

140. Couper RT, Huynh H. Female masturbation masquerading as abdominal pain. J Pediatr Child Health 2002; 38; 199–200.

141. Mink JW, Neil JJ. Masturbation mimicking paroxysmal dystonia or dyskinesia in a youg girl. Mov Disord 1995; 10; 518–520.

142. Meizner I. Sonographic observation of in utero fetal "masturbation". J Ultrasound Med 1987; 6; 111.

143. Lotze T, Jankovic J. Paroxysmal kinesiogenic dyskinesias. Semin Pediatr Neurol 2003; 10(1); 68–79.

144. Lance JW. Familial paroxysmal dystonic choreoathetosis and its differentiation from related syndromes. Ann Neurol 1977; 2; 285–293.

145. Bressman SB, Fahn S, Burke RE. Paroxysmal non-kinesiogenic dystonia. Adv Neurol 1988; 50; 403–413.

146. Smith EA, Van Houten R. A comparison of the characteristics of self-stimulatory behaviors in "normal" children and children with developmental delays. Res Dev Disabil 1996; 17; 253–268.

147. Tan A, Salgado M, Fahn S. The characterization and outcome of stereotypical movements in nonautistic children. Mov Disord 1997; 12; 47–52.

148. Foster LG. Nervous habits and stereotyped behaviors in preschool children. J Am Acad Child Adol Psychiatry 1998; 37(7); 711–717.

149. Backwin H, Backwin RM. *Behavior Disorders in Children*. Philadelphia, PA: WB Saunders, 1972.

150. Lourie RS. The role of rhythmic patterns in childhood. Am J Psychiatr 1949; 105; 653–660.

151. Kravitz H, Bohem J. Rhythmic habit patterns in infancy: their sequence, age of onset, and frequency. Child Devel 1971; 42; 399–413.

152. Thelen E. Rhythmical behaviors in infancy: an ethological perspective. Dev Psychol 1981; 17; 237–257.

153. de Lissovoy V. Head banging in early childhood. J Pediatr 1961; 58; 803–805.

154. Sallustro F, Artwell C. Body rocking, head banging, and head rolling in normal children. J Pediatr 1978; 93; 704–708.

155. Werry J, Carlielle J, Fitzpatrick J. Rhythmic motor activities (stereotypies) in children under five: etiology and prevalence. J Am Acad Child Psychiatr 1983; 22; 329–336.

156. Troster H. Prevalence and functions of stereotyped behaviors in non-handicapped children in residential care. J Abnorm Child Psychol 1994; 22; 79–97.

157. Soussigan R, Koch P. Rhythmical stereotypies (leg-swinging) associated with reductions in heart-rate in normal school children. Biol Psychol 1985; 21; 161–167.

158. Miller JM, Singer HS, Bridges DD, et al. Behavioral therapy for treatment of stereotypic movements in nonautistic children. J Child Neurol 2006; 21; 119–125.

159. Rapp JT, Vollmer TR. Stereotypy II: a review of neurobiological interpretations and suggestions for an integration with behavioral methods. Res Devel Disabil 2005; 26(6); 548–564.

160. Hagberg B, Aicardi J, Dias K, et al. A progressive syndrome of autism, dementia, ataxia and loss of purposeful hand use in girls: Rett's Syndrome: Report of 35 cases. Ann Neurol 1983; 14; 471–479.

161. The Rett Syndrome Diagnostic Criteria Work Group. Diagnostic criteria for Rett syndrome. Ann Neurol 1988; 23; 425–428.

162. Temudo T, Oliveira P, Santos M, et al. Stereotypies in Rett syndrome. Analysis of 83 patients with and without deteted MECP2 mutations. Neurology 2007; 68; 1183–1187.

163. Temudo T, Maciel P, Sequeiros J. Abnormal movements in Rett syndrome are present before the regression period: a case study. Mov Disord 2007; 22(15); 2284–2287.

164. Amir RE, Van den Veyver IB, Wan M, et al. Rett syndrome is caused by mutations in X-linked MECP2, encoding methyl-CpG-binding protein 2. Nature Genet 1999; 23; 185–188.

165. Amir RE, Zoghbi HY. Rett syndrome: methyl-CpG-binding protein 2 mutations and phenotype-genotype correlations. Am J Med Genet 2000; 97; 147–152.

166. Nomura Y, Segawa M. Characteristics of motor disturbances of the Rett syndrome. Brain Dev 1990; 12(1); 27–30.

167. Brown R, Hobson RP, Lee A, et al. Are there "autistic-like" features in congenitally blind children? J Child Psychol Psychiatr 1997; 38(6); 693–703.

168. Fazzi E, Lanners J, Danova S, et al. Stereotyped behaviours in blind children Brain Dev 1999; 21(8); 522–528.

169. Sakuma M. A comparative study by the behavioral observation for stereotypy in the exceptional children. Folia Psychiatr Neurol Japon 1975; 29(4); 371–391.

170. Stacy M, Cardoso F, Jankovic J. Tardive stereotypy and other movement disorders in tardive dyskinesias. Neurology 1993; 43(5); 937–941.

171. Meiselas KD, Spencer EK, Oberfield R, et al. Campbell M. Differentiation of stereotypies from neuroleptic-related dyskinesias in autistic children. J Clin Psychopharm 1989; 9(3); 207–209.

172. Chaves-Vischer V, Picard F, Andermann E, et al. Benign nocturnal alternating hemiplegia of childhood: Six patients and long term follow-up. Neurology 2001; 57; 1491–1493.

173. Iriarte J, Narbona J, Garcia del Barrio L, et al. Diaphragmatic flutter after spinal cord trauma in a child. Neurol 2005; 65(1); 1839.

174. Larner AJ. Antony van Leeuwenhoek and the description of diaphragmatic flutter (respiratory myoclonus). Mov Disord 2005; 20(8); 917–918.

175. Rigatto H, Correa CEC. Diaphragmatic flutter with an electromyographic study. J Pediatr 1968; 73(5); 757–759.

176. Illiceto G, Thompson PD, Day BL, et al. Diaphragmatic flutter, the moving umbilicus syndrome, and "bell dancer's" dyskinesia. Mov Disord 1990; 5(1); 15–22.

177. Chen R, Remtulla H, Bolton CF. Electrophysiological study of diaphragmatic myoclonus. J Neurol Neurosurg Psych 1995; 58; 480–483.

178. Espay AJ, Fox SH, Marras C, et al. Isolated diaphragmatic tremor. Is there a spectrum in "respiratory myoclonus"? Neurology 2007; 69; 689–692.

179. Riordan LL, Eavey RD, Strieder DJ. Neonatal diaphragmatic flutter. Pediatr Pulmonol 1990; 8(3); 209–211.

180. Adams JA, Zabaleta IA, Sackner MA. Diaphragmatic flutter in three babies with bronchopulmonary dysplasia and respiratory syncytial virus bronchiolitis. Pediatr Pulmonol 1995; 19(5); 312–316.

181. Biddle C. The neurobiology of the human febrile response. AANA J 2006; 74(2); 145–150.

182. Special Writing Group of the Committee of Rheumatic Fever, Endocarditis, and Kawasaki Disease of the Council on Cardiovascular Disease of the Young of the American Heart Association. Guidelines for the diagnosis of rheumatic fever. JAMA 1992; 268; 2069–2073.

183. Church AJ, Cardoso F, Dale RC, et al. Anti-basal ganglia antibodies in acute and persistent Syndenham's chorea. Neurology 2002; 59; 227–231.

184. Edwards MJ, Trikouli E, Martino D, et al. Anti-basal ganglia antibodies in patients with atypical dystonia and tics. Neurology 2004; 63; 156–158.

185. Kirsten A, Beck S, Fuhlhuber V, et al. New autoantibodies in pediatric opsoclonus myoclonus syndrome. Annal New York Acad Sci 2007; 1110; 256–260.

186. Boltshauser E, Deonna T, Hirt HR. Myoclonic encephalopathy of infants or "dancing eyes syndrome". Helv Paediat Acta 1979; 34; 119–133.

187. Harris K, Singer HS. Tic disorders: Neural circuits, neurochemistry, and neuroimmunology. J Child Neurol 2006; 21; 678–689.

188. Dooley JM, Hayden JD. Benign febrile myoclonus in childhood. Can J Neurol Sci 2004; 31(4); 504–505.

189. Harbord MG, Kobayashi JS. Fever producing ballismus in patients with choreoathetosis. J Child Neurol 1991; 6; 49–52.

190. Onoe S, Nishigaki T. A clinical study of febrile myoclonus in children. Brain Dev 2004; 26(5); 321–325.

191. Curran LK, Newschaffer CJ, Lee Li-C, et al. Behaviors associated with fever in children with autism spectrum disorders. Pediatrics 2007; 120(6); e1386–e1392.

192. *Diagnostic and Statistical Manual of Mental Disorders (DSM-IV-TR)*, 4th edition, text revision, Washington, DC: American Psychological Association, 2000.

193. Tourette Syndrome Classification Group. Definitions and classification of tic disorders. Arch Neurol 1993; 50; 1013–1016.

194. Frankel M, Cummings JL. Neuro-ophthalmic abnormalities in Tourette's syndrome: functional and anatomic implications. Neurology 1984; 34(3); 359–361.

195. Tatlipinar S, Iener EC, Ilhan B, et al. Ophthalmic manifestations of gilles de la Tourette syndrome. Eur J Ophthal 2001; 11(3); 223–226.

196. Vrabec TR, Levin AV, Nelson LB. Functional blinking in childhood. Pediatrics 1989; 83; 967–970.

197. Kurlan R, Deeley C, Como PG. Psychogenic movement disorder (pseudo-tics) in a patient with Tourette's syndrome. J Neuropsych Clin Neurosci 1992; 4(3); 347–348.

198. Dooley JM, Stokes A, Gordon KE. Pseudo-tics in Tourette syndrome. J Child Neurol 1994; 9(1); 50–51.

199. Brunquell P, McKeever M, Russman BS. Differentiation of epileptic from non-epileptic head drops in children. Epilepsia 1990; 31; 401–405.

200. Brodsky MC, Wright KW. Infantile esotropia with nystagmus: a treatable cause of oscillatory head movements in children. Arch Ophthal 2007; 125(8); 1079–1081.

201. Tan EK, Lum SY, Prakash KM. Clinical features of childhood onset essential tremor. Eur J Neurol 2006; 13(12); 1302–1305.

202. Louis ED, Dure LS 4th, Pullman S. Essential tremor in childhood: a series of nineteen cases. Mov Disord 2001; 16(5); 921–923.

203. Benton JW, Nellhaus G, Huttenlocher PR, et al. The bobble-head doll syndrome. Report of a unique truncal tremor associated with third ventricular cyst and hydrocephalus in children. Neurology 1966; 16; 725–729.

204. Mussell HG, Dure LS, Percy AK, et al. Bobble-head doll syndrome: report of a case and review of the literature. Mov Disord 1997 12(5); 810–814.

205. Russman B, Tucker SH, Schut L. Slow tremor and macrocephaly: expanded version of the bobble-head doll syndrome. J Pediatr 1975; 87(1); 63–66.

206. Desai KI, Nadkarni TD, Muzumdar D, et al. Suprasellar arachnoid cyst presenting with bobble-head doll movements: A report of 3 cases. Neurol India 2003; 51; 407–409.

207. Pollack IF, Schor NF, Martinez AJ, et al. Bobble-head doll syndrome and drop attacks in a child with a cystic choroids plexus papilloma of the third ventricle. J Neurosurg 1995; 83; 729–732.

208. Turgut M, Ozcan OE. Suprasellar arachnoid cyst as a cause of precocious puberty and bobble-head doll phenomenon. Eur J Pediatr 1992; 151; 76.

209. Dell S. Further observations on the "Bobble-head doll syndrome". J Neurol Neurosurg Psychiatr 1981; 44; 1046–1049.

210. Coker S. Bobbel-head doll syndrome due to trapped fourth ventricle and aqueduct. Pediatr Neurol 1986; 2; 115–116.

211. Wiese JA, Gentry LR, Menezes AH. Bobble-head doll syndrome. Review of the pathophysiology and CSF dynamics. Pediatr Neurol 1985; 1; 361–366.

212. Russo RH, Kindt GW. A neuroanatomical basis for the bobble-head doll syndrome. J Neurosurg 1974; 41; 720–723.

213. Herrmann C, Brown JW. Palatal myoclonus: a reappraisal. J Neurol Sci 1967; 5; 473–492.

214. Tatum WO, Sperling MR, Jacobstein JG. Epileptic palatal myoclonus. Neurology 1991; 41; 1305–1306.

215. Noatchar S, Ebner A, Witte OW, et al. Palatal tremor of cortical origin presenting as epilepsia partialis continua. Epilepsia 1995; 36; 207–209.

216. Lapresle J. Rhythmic palatal myoclonus and the dentato-olivary pathway. J Neurol 1979; 220; 223–230.

217. Deuschl G, Toro C, Hallett M. Symptomatic and essential palatal tremor. Differences of palatal movements. Mov Disord 1994; 9; 676–678.

218. Yamanouchi H, Kasai H, Sakuragawa N, et al. Palatal myoclonus in Krabbe disease. Brain Dev 1991; 13; 355–358.

219. Nathanson M. Palatal myoclonus. Further clinical and pathological observations. Arch Neurol Psychiatr 1956; 75; 285–296.

220. Baram TZ, Parke JT, Mahoney DH. Palatal myoclonus in a child: Herald of acute encephalitis. Neurology 1986; 36; 302–303.

221. MacDonald JT. Objective tinnitus due to essential palatal tremor in a 5-year-old. Pediatr Neurol 2007; 36; 175–176.

222. Campistol-Plana J, Majumdar A, Fernandez-Alvarez E. Palatal tremor in childhood: clinical and therapeutic considerations. Devel Med Child Neurol 2006; 48; 982–984.

223. Yokota T, Hirashima F, Ito Y, et al. Idiopathic palatal myoclonus. Acta Neurol Scand 1990; 81; 239–242.
224. de CamposCC, Campos CAH, Rosemberg S. Tinitus objective e mioclonias velopalatinas na crianca. Una analise de quarto casos. Rev Bras Neurol 1986; 22; 165–167. (In Portugese)
225. Jacobs L, Newman RP, Bozian D. Disappearing palatal myoclonus. Neurology 1981; 31; 748–751.
226. Boulloche J, Aicardi. Syndrome de myoclonies du voile du palais spontanement regressif chez l'enfant. Arch Fren Pediatr 1984; 41; 645–647. (In French)
227. Cakmur R, Idiman E, Idiman F, et al. Essential palatal tremor successfully treated with flunarizine 1997; 38; 133–134.
228. Scott BL, Evans RW, Jancovic J. Treatment of palatal myoclonus with sumatriptan 1996; Mov Disord 1996; 11; 748–751.
229. Sakai T, Shiraishi S, Murakami S. Palatal myoclonus responding to Carbamazepine. Ann Neurol 1981; 9; 199–200.
230. Borggreve F, Hageman G. A case of idiopathic palatal myoclonus: treatment with sodium valproate. Eur Neurol 1991; 31; 403–404.
231. Deuschl G, Lohle E, Heinen F, et al. Ear click in palatal tremor: its origin and treatment with botulinum toxin. Neurology 1991; 41; 1677–1679.
232. Cho JW, Chu K, Jeon BS. Case of essential palatal tremor: atypical features and remarkable benefit from botulinum toxin injection. Mov Disord 2001; 16; 779–782.
233. Gordon N. Startle disease or hyperekplexia. Dev Med Child Neurol 1993; 35(11); 1015–1018.
234. Tijssen MAJ, Vergouwe MN, Gert van Dijk J, et al. Major and minor form of hereditary hyperekplexia. Mov Disord 2002; 17(4); 826–830.
235. Vigevano F, di Capua M, Dalla Bernardia B. Startle disease: an avoidable cause of sudden infant death. Lancet 1989; 1; 216.
236. Ryan SG, Dixon MJ, Nigro MA, et al. Genetic and radiation hybrid mapping of the hyperekplexia region on chromosome 5q. Am J Hum Genet 1992; 51(6); 1334–1343.
237. Ryan SG, Sherman SL, Terry JC, et al. Startle disease, or hyperekplexia: response to clonazepam and assignment of the gene (STHE) to chromosome 5q by linkage analysis. Ann Neurol 1992; 31(6); 663–668.
238. Shiang R, Ryan SG, Zhu YZ, et al. Mutations in the alpha 1 subunit of the inhibitory glycine receptor cause the dominant neurological disorder, hyperekplexia. Nat Genet 1993; 5(4); 351–358.
239. Rees MI, Lewis TM, Kwok JBJ, et al. Hyperekplexia associated with compound heterozygote mutations in the beta-subunit of the human inhibitory glycine receptor (GLRB). Hum Mol Genet 2002; 11; 853–860.
240. Khasani S, Beker K, Meinck HM. Hyperekplexia and stiff-man syndrome: abnormal brainstem reflexes suggest a physiological relationship. J Neurol Neurosurg Psychiatry 2004; 75; 1265–1269.
241. Stewart WA, Wood EP, Gordon KE, et al. Successful treatment of severe infantile hyperekplexia with low-dose clobazam. J Child Neurol 2002; 17; 154–156.
242. Dooley JM, Andermann F. Startle disease or hyperekplexia: adolescent onset and response to valproate. Pediatr Neurol 1989; 55(2); 126–127.
243. Brown P. Neurophysiology of the startle syndrome and Hyperekplexia. In *Myoclonus and Paroxysmal Dyskinesias. Advances of Neurology.* Ed: S Fahn. Philadelphia, PA, Lippincott Williams & Wilkins, 2002; 89; 153–159.

244. Zhou L, Chillag KL, Nigro MA. Hyperekplexia: a treatable neurogenetic disease. Brain Dev 2002; 24; 669–674.

245. Feng G, Tintrup H, Kirsch J, et al. Dual requirement for gephyrin in glycine receptor clustering and molybdenzyme activity. Science 1998; 282(5392); 1321–1324.

246. Macaya A, Brunso L, Fernandez-Castillo N, et al. Molybdenum cofactor deficiency presenting as neonatal hyperekplexia: a clinical, biochemical and genetic study Neuropediatrics 2005; 36(6); 389–394.

247. Singer H, Movement disorders in children, In *Parkinson's Disease and Movement Disorders*, Eds: JJ Jankovic, E Tolosa. 4th edition. Philadelphia, PA, Lippincott Williams & Wilkins, 2002; 451–472.

248. Coffin GS, Siris E, Wegienka LC. Mental retardation with osteocartilaginous anomalies. Am J Dis Child 1966; 112; 205–213.

249. Lowry B, Miller JR, Frazer FC. A new dominant gene mental retardation syndrome. Am J Dis Child 1971; 121; 496–500.

250. Stephenson JBP. More than "cataplexy" in Coffin-Lowry syndrome: tonic as well as atonic semiology in sound-startle collapse. Dev Med Child Neurol 1999; 41(Suppl 82); 28–30.

251. Nelson GB, Hahn JS. Stimulus-induced drop episodes in Coffin-Lowry syndrome. Pediatrics 2003; 111(3); e197–e202.

252. Brown P, Rothwell JC, Thompson PD, et al. The hyperekplexias and their relationship to the normal startle reflex. Brain 1991; 114; 1903–1928.

253. Goraya JS, Shah D, Poddar B. Hyperekplexia in a girl with posterior fossa malformations. J Child Neurol 2002; 17; 147–149.

254. Perlman JM, Volpe JJ. Movement disorder of premature infants with severe bronchopulmonary dysplasia: a new syndrome. Pediatrics 1989; 84; 215–218.

255. Hadders-Algra M, Bos AF, Martijn A, et al. Infantile chorea in an infant with severe bronchopulmony dysplasia: an EMG study. Dev Med Child Neurol 1994; 36; 173–182.

256. Bergouignan M, Fontan F, Trarieux M, et al. Syndromes choreiformes de l'enfant au decours d'interventions cardiochirurgicales profonde. Rev Neurol 1961; 105; 48–60.

257. Brunberg JA, Doty DB, Reilly EL. Choreoathetosis in infants following cardiac surgery with deep hypothermia and circulatory arrest. J Pediatr 1974; 84; 232–235.

258. DeLeon SY, Ilbawi M, Archilla R, et al. Choreoathetosis after deep hypothermia without circulatory arrest. Ann Thorac Surg 1990; 50; 714–719.

259. Medlock MD, Cruse RS, Winek SJ, et al. A 10-year experience with postpump chorea. Ann Neurol 1993; 34; 820–826.

260. Ferry PC. Neurologic sequelae of open-heart surgery in children. An "irritating question". Am J Dis Child 1990; 144; 369–373.

261. Robinson RO, Samuels M, Pohl KRE. Choreic syndrome after cardiac surgery. Arch Dis Child 1988; 63; 1466–1469.

262. Gherpelli JL, Azeka E, Riso A, et al. Choeroathetosis after cardiac surgery with hypothermia and extracorporeal circulation. Pediatr Neurol 1998; 19(2); 113–118.

263. Wical BS, Tomasi LG. A distinctive neurologic syndrome after induced profound hypothermia. Pediatr Neurol 1990; 6; 202–205.

264. du Plessis AJ, Bellinger DC, Gauvreau K, et al. Neurologic outcome of choreoathetoid encephalopathy after cardiac surgery. Pediatr Neurol 2002; 27(1); 9–17.

265. Levin DA, Seay AR, Fullerton DA, et al. Profound hypothermia with alpha-stat pH management during open heart surgery is associated with choreoathetosis. Pediatr Cardiol 2005; 26; 34–38.

266. Taylor KM. Central nervous system effects of cardiopulmonary bypass. Ann Thorac Surg 1998; 66(5 Suppl); S20-24.

267. Kupsky WJ, Drozd MA, Barlow CF. Selective injury of the globus pallidus in children with post-cardiac surgery chorea. Dev Med Child Neurol 1995; 37(2); 135–144.

268. Blunt SB, Brooks DJ, Kennard C. Steroid-responsive chorea in childhood following cardiac transplantation. Mov Disord 1994; 9; 112–114.

269. Venkatesan A, Frucht S. Movement disorders after resuscitation from cardiac arrest. Neurol Clin 2006; 24(1); 123–132.

270. Klein C. Myoclonus and myoclonic dystonias. In:*Genetics of Movement Disorders*. Ed: Pulst SM. New York, Academic Press, 2003; 451–471.

271. Nygaard TG, Raymond D, Chen C, et al. Localization of a gene for myoclonus dystonia to chromosome 7q21-31. Ann Neurol 1999; 46; 794–798.

272. Zimprich A, Grabowski M, Asmus F, et al. Mutations in the gene encoding epsilon-sarcoglycan cause myoclonus-dystonia syndrome. Nat Genet 2001; 29; 66–69.

273. O'Riordan S, Ozelius LJ, de Carvalho Aguiar P, et al. Inherited myoclonus-dystonia and epilepsy: further evidence of an association? Mov Disord 2004; 19(12); 1456–1459.

274. Grimes DA, Han F, Lang AE, et al. A novel locus for inherited myoclonus dystonia on 18p11. Neurology 2002; 59; 1183–1186.

275. Gerrits MCF, Foncke EMJ, de Haan R, et al. Phenotype-genotype correlation in Dutch patients with myoclonus-dystonia. Neurology 2006; 66; 759–761.

276. Valente EM, Edwards MJ, Mir P, et al. The epsilon-sarcoglycan gene in myoclonic syndromes. Neurology 2005; 64(4); 737–739.

277. Nishiyama A, Endo T, Takeda S, et al. Identification and characterization of epsilon-sarcoglycans in the central nervous system. Brain Res Mol Brain Res 2004; 125(1–2); 1–12.

278. Müller B, Hedrich K, Kock N, et al. Evidence that paternal expression of the epsilon-sarcoglycan gene accounts for reduced penetrance in myoclonus-dystonia. Am J Hum Genet 2002; 71; 1303–1311.

279. Cif L, Valente EM, Hemm S, et al. Deep brain stimulation in myoclonus-dystonia syndrome. Mov Disord 2004; 19(6); 724–727.

280. Kinsbourne M. Myoclonic encephalopathy of infants. J Neurol Neurosurg Psychiatr 1962; 25; 271–276.

281. Dyken P, Kolar O. Dancing eyes, dancing feet: infantile polymyoclonia. Brain 1968; 91; 305–320.

282. Bray PF, Ziter FA, Lahey ME, et al. The coincidence of neuroblastoma and acute cerbellar encephalopathy. J Pediatr 1969; 75; 983–990.

283. Hammer MS, Larsen MB, Stack CV. Outcome of children with Opsoclonus-myoclonus regardless of etiology. Pediatr Neurol 1995; 13; 21–24.

284. Pranzatelli MR. The neurobiology of the Opsoclonus-myoclonus syndrome. Clin Neuropharm 1992; 15(3); 186–228.

285. McCallister RM. Neuroblastoma: a viral etiology? J Pediatr Surg 1968; 3; 138.

286. Wong A. An update on Opsoclonus. Curr Opin Neurol 2007; 20; 25–31.

287. Alabduljalil T, Behbehani R. Paraneoplastic syndromes in neuro-ophthalmology. Curr Opin Ophthalmol 2007; 18; 463–469.

288. Pranzatelli MR, Tate ED, Dukart WS, et al. Sleep disturbance and rage attacks in opsoclonus-myoclonus syndrome: response to trazodone. J Pediatr 2005; 147(3); 372–378.

289. Tuchman RF, Alvarez LA, Kantrowitz AB, et al. Opsoclonus-myoclonus syndrome: correlation of radiographic and pathological observations. Neuroradiology 1989; 31(3); 250–252.

290. Brodeur GM, Castleberry RP. Neuroblastoma. In: *Principles and Practices of Pediatric Oncology*. Eds: Pizzo PA, Poplack DG. 3rd edition. Philadelphia, PA, Lippencott-Raven, 1997; 761–797.

291. SEER Cancer statistics review, 1975–1995. Retrieved on February 7, 2008 from the World Wide Web: http://www-seer.cancer.gov/publications/childhood/sympathetic.pdf.

292. Carlsen NLT. Neuroblastoma: epidemiology and pattern of regression. Problems in interpreting results of mass screening. J Pediatr Hemat Oncol 1992; 14; 103–110.

293. Farrelly C, Daneman A, Chan HSL, et al. Occult neuroblastoma presenting with opsomyoclonus: utility of computed tomography. AJR 1984; 142; 807–810.

294. Koh PS, Raffensberger JG, Berry S, et al. Long-term outcome in children with opsocolonus-myoclonus and ataxia and coincident neuroblastoma. J Pediatr 1994; 125; 712–716.

295. Pohl E, Pritchard J, Wilson J. Neurological sequelae of the dancing eye syndrome. Neuropediatr 1996; 155; 237–244.

296. Kalmanchey R, Veres E. Dancing eyes syndrome. Brain acoustic evoked potential approach. Neuropediatrics 1988; 19; 193–196.

297. Sun JB. Autoreactive T and B cells in nervous system diseases. Acta Neurol Scand 1993; 142(Suppl); 1–56.

298. Thomas RS, Beuche W, Felgenhauer K. The proliferation rate of T and B lymphocytes in cerebrospinal fluid. J Neurol 1991; 238; 27–30.

299. Pranzatelli MR, Travelstead AL, Tate ED, et al. CSF B-cell expansion in opsoclonus-myoclonus syndrome: a biomarker of disease activity. Mov Disord 2004; 19; 770–777.

300. Pranzatelli MR. Travelstead AL. Tate ED, et al. B- and T-cell markers in opsoclonus-myoclonus syndrome: immunophenotyping of CSF lymphocytes. Neurology 2004; 62(9); 1526–1532.

301. Antunes NL, Khakoo Y, Mattay KK, et al. Antineuronal antibodies in patients with neuroblastoma and paraneoplastic opsoclonus-myoclonus. J Pediatr Hematol Oncol 2000; 22; 315–320.

302. Blaes F, Fühlhuber V, Korfei M, et al. Surface-binding autoantibodies to cerebellar neurons in opsoclonus syndrome. Ann Neurol 2005; 58; 313–317.

303. Ziter FA, Bray PF, Cancilla PA. Neuropathologic findings in a patient with neuroblastoma and myoclonic encephalopathy. Arch Neurol 1979; 36; 51–55.

304. Martin ES, Griffith JF. Myoclonic encephalopathy and neuroblastoma. Am J Dis Child 1971; 122; 257–258.

305. Moe PG, Neilhaus G. Infantile polymyoclonia-opsoclonus syndrome and neural crest tumors. Neurol 1970; 20; 756–764.

306. Pranzatelli MR, Tate ED, Travelstead AL, et al. Rituximab (anti-CD20) Adjunctive Therapy for Opsoclonus-Myoclonus Syndrome. J Pediatr Heme Onc 2006; 28(9); 585–593.

307. Bhatia KP. The paroxysmal dyskinesias. J Neurol 1999; 246; 149–155.

308. Bhatia KP. Familial (idiopathic) paroxysmal dyskinesias: an update. Sem Neurol 2001; 21(1); 69–74.

309. Zori G, Conti C, Erba A, et al. Paroxysmal dyskinesias in childhood. Pediatr Neurol 2003; 28(3); 168–172.

310. Vidailhet M. Paroxysmal dyskinesias as a paradigm of paroxysmal movement disorders. Curr Opin Neurol 2000; 13: 457–462.

311. Bruno MK, Hallett M, Gwinn-Hardy K, et al. Clinical evaluation of idiopathic paroxysmal kinesigenic dyskinesia: new diagnostic criteria. Neurology 2004; 63; 2280–2287.

312. Kertesz A. Paroxysmal kinesiogenic choreoathetosis. Neurology 1967; 17; 680–690.

313. Mount LA, Reback S. Familial paroxysmal choreoathetosis: preliminary report on a hitherto undescribed clinical syndrome. Arch Neurol Psychiatr 1940; 44; 841–847.

314. Bruno MK, Lee H-Y, Auburger GWJ, et al. Genotype-phenotype correlation of paroxysmal nonkinesiogenic dyskinesia. Neurology 2007; 68; 1782–1789.

315. Barnnett LB, Roach ES, Bowcock AM. A locus for paroxysmal kinesiogenic dyskinesia maps to human chromosome 16. Neurology 2000; 54(1); 125–136.

316. Fink JK, Hedera P, Mathay JG, et al. Paroxysmal dystonic choreoathetosis linked to chromosome 2q: Clinical analysis and proposed pathophysiology. Neurology 1997; 49; 177–183.

317. Li Z, Turner RP, Smith G. Childhood paroxysmal kinesiogenic dyskinesia: Report of seven cases with onset at an early age. Epilep Behav 2005; 6; 435–439.

318. Demkirkiran M, Jankovic J. Paroxysmal dyskinesias: Clinical features and classification. Ann Neurol 1995; 38; 571–579.

319. Hwang WJ, Lu CS, Tsai JJ. Clincal manifestations of 20 Taiwanese patients with paroxysmal kinesiogenic dyskinesia. Acta Neurol Scand 1998; 98; 340–345.

320. Szepetowski P, Rochette J, Berquin P, Familial infantile convulsions and paroxysmal choreoathetosis: A new neurological syndrome linked to the pericentromeric region of human chromosome 16. Am J Hum Genet 1997; 61; 889–898.

321. Auburger G, Ratzlaff T, Lunkes A, et al. A gene for autosomal dominant paroxysmal choreoathetosis/spasticity (CSE) maps to the vicinity of a potassium channel gene cluster on chromosome 1P, probably within 2cM between D15443 and D15197. Genomics 1996; 31; 90–94.

322. Bhatia KP, Soland VL, Bhatt VH, et al. Paroxysmal exercise-induced dystonia: Eight new cases and a review of the literature. Mov Disord 1997; 12; 1007–1012.

323. Guerrini R, Bonanni P, Nardocci N, et al. Autosomal recessive Rolandic epilepsy with paroxysmal exercise-induced dystonia and writer's cramp: Delineation of the syndrome and gene mapping to chromosome 16p12-11.2. Ann Neurol 1999; 45; 344–352.

324. Godbout R, Montplaisir J, Rouleau I. Hypnogognic paroxysmal dystonia: epilepsy or sleep disorder? Clin Electroencephalogr 1985; 16; 136–142.

325. Schmidt BJ, Pillay N. Paroxysmal dyskinesia associated with hypoglycemia. Can J Neurol Sci 1993; 20; 151–153.

326. Mores CA, Dire DJ. Movement disorders as a manifestation of nonketotic hyperglycemia. J Emerg Med 1989; 7; 359–364.

327. Tabae-Zadeh MJ, Frame B, Kapphahn K. Kinesiogenic choreoathetosis and idiopathic hypoparathyroidism. N Engl J Med 1972; 286; 762–763.

328. Blakely J, Jankovic J. Secondary paroxysmal dyskinesias. Mov Disord 2002; 17(4); 726–734.

329. Willemsen MA, Breedveld GJ, Wouda S, et al. Brain-Thyroid-Lung syndrome: a patient with a severe multi-system disorder due to a de novo mutation in the thyroid transcription factor 1 gene. Eur J Pediatr 2005; 164; 28–30.

330. Bye AM, Kok DJ, Ferenschild FT, et al. Paroxysmal non-epileptic events in children: a retrospective study over a period of 10 years. J Paediatr Child Health 2000; 36(3); 244–248.

331. Gibbs J, Appleton RE. False diagnosis of epilepsy in children. Seizure 1992; 1; 15–18.

332. Uldall P, Alving J, Hansen LK, et al. The misdiagnosis of epilepsy in children admitted to a tertiary epilepsy centre with paroxysmal events. Arch Dis Child 2006; 91; 219–221.

333. Gokcay A, Gokcay F. Oxcarbazepine therapy in paroxysmal kinesiogenic choreoathetosis. Acta Neurol Scand 2000; 101; 344–345.

334. Chattergee A, Louis ED, Frucht S. Levetiracetam in the treatment of paroxysmal kinesiogenic choreoathetosis. Mov Disord 2002; 17(3); 614–615.

335. Suber DA, Riley TL. Valproic acid and normal computerized scan in kinesiogenic paroxysmal choreoathetosis. Arch Neurol 1980; 37; 327.

336. Chudnow RS, Mimbela RA, Owen DB, et al. Gabapentin for familial paroxysmal dystonic choreoathetosis. Neurology 1997; 49; 1441–1442.

337. Pincus JH, Chutorian A. Familial benign chorea with intention tremor: a clinical entity. J Pediatr 1967; 70(5); 724–729.

338. Haerer AF, Currier RD, Jackson JF. Hereditary nonprogressive chorea of early onset. N Engl J Med 1967; 276; 1220–1224.

339. Chun RW, Daly RF, Mansheim BJ, et al. Benign familial chorea with onset in childhood. JAMA 1973; 225; 1603–1607.

340. Schrag A, Quinn NP, Bhatia KP, et al. Benign hereditary chorea: Entity or syndrome? Mov Disord 2000; 15; 280–288.

341. Kleiner-Fishman G, Lang AE. Benign hereditary chorea revisited: a journey to understanding. Mov Disord 2007; 22(16); 2297–2305.

342. Breedveld GJ, van Dongen JW, Danesino C, et al. Mutations in TITF-1 are associated with benign hereditary chorea. Hum Mol Genet 2002; 11; 971–979.

343. Asmus F, Horber V, Pohlenz J, et al. A novel TITF-1 mutation causes benign hereditary chorea with response to levodopa. Neurology 2005; 64(11); 1952–1954.

344. Kleiner-Fisman G, Rogaeva E, Halliday W, et al. Benign hereditary chorea: clinical, genetic, and pathological findings. Ann Neurol 2003; 54(2); 244–247.

345. Luat AF, Asano E, Chugani HT. Paroxysmal tonic upgaze of childhood with co-existent absence epilepsy. Epilep Dis 2007; 9(3); 332336.

346. Johannessen LC. Antiepileptic drugs in non-epilepsy disorders: relations between mechanisms of action and clinical efficacy. CNS Drugs 2008; 22(1); 27–47.

347. Edgar TS. Oral pharmacotherapy of childhood movement disorders. J Child Neurol 2003; 18(Suppl); S40–S49.

8

Headache Syndromes

INTRODUCTION TO HEADACHE SYNDROMES

Epileptic seizures, particularly those of focal onset, often initiate with an aura. These may be sudden, short-lived alterations in visual, psychic, somatosensory, and other sensory experiences. Although auras can precede both simple and complex partial seizures with or without secondary generalized motor convulsions, they, too, may terminate without further evolution. In either case subsequent headache may be experienced after the motor phenomena has terminated. Many partial onset motor seizures may further resolve with a postictal transient residual motor paresis or neurological deficit. Headache syndromes in children include migraine, complicated migraine, and a number of so-called periodic syndromes unique to childhood. Each of these specific categories of headache syndrome may have specific sensory auras and transient neurological deficits peculiar to the unique syndrome at hand. Visual scotomas, gastrointestinal upset, a confused sensorium, and transient motor paresis may each accompany certain of the migraine syndromes encountered in childhood. Epileptic seizures and migraine syndromes, in particular, additionally share similar pathophysiological mechanisms. Consequently, confusion in diagnosis can be anticipated. Parallels in treatments often reinforce this confusion rather than offer clarity. The following chapter will articulate those elements of clinical and physiological distinction that allow for greater precision in diagnosis.

THE CLINICAL PROBLEM AND EPIDEMIOLOGY

The most common paroxysmal phenomenon experienced by children are headaches.[1,2] This symptom can be an accompaniment to systemic disease or psychological stress or produced by local factors within and around the head and neck or as a primary neurological disorder. The definition of migraine and the clinical diagnosis of migraine in children have been the focus of more sophisticated study.[3-7] Important clinical approaches to the evaluation of headaches in childhood are offered in Table 8-1.

Early definitions of migraine have evolved into an internationally derived and generally accepted classification schema and set of diagnostic criteria with special considerations for children (Tables 8-2, 8-3, and 8-4).[7-9]

Table 8-1 Clinical Approach to History

Key Clinical Components of History

- Is there more than one type of headache?
- What is the quality of the headache—intermittent (repetitive), continuous (without stopping), episodic (paroxysmal), or sustained?
- What is the headache pain described as (throb, pound, squeeze, ache, tight, etc.)?
- How long do the headaches last?
- Where is the headache pain located?
- What makes the headaches better and worse?
- Are there any specific precipitants (food, drugs, exercise, infection, etc.) or palliatives (rest/sleep, food)?
- Does it occur with wakefulness, at sleep, or both?
- Is there a sensory component or warning before the headache begins?
- Are there or have there been any associated neurological and/or systemic abnormalities?
- Is there a familial pattern to the headache?
- Were there any significant perinatal, natal, or postnatal complications or findings?
- Have there been periods of encephalopathy, hemiplegia, ocular abnormalities, or vomiting?
- What was the age of onset?
- Does the character of the headache evolve over a period of time (minutes, hours, day–night)?
- Has the character of the headache evolved over a lifetime?
- What do you do during the headache?
- Is the headache interfering with functioning?
- Is there a secondary gain for the child because of the headache?
- Are the symptoms gone completely between headache attacks?

Key Clinical Components of Examination

- Careful general examination
- Examine, palpate, and percuss the neck, scalp, and spine
- Carefully directed observation of all limb, face, ocular, and trunk movements
- Direct the child to move limbs toward a target, write/draw, run, climb, and ambulate on toes/heels/and in tandem
- Careful funduscopic examination of visual acuity
- Assess the child's demeanor, affect, and interaction with the parents and examiner
- Standard neurological examination

Elements of these definitions are sometimes made difficult to ascertain because of the relative lack of awareness of these symptoms in children, the difficulty in abstracting careful descriptions from children about their headaches, and the variability of symptoms experienced by children from attack to attack. Epidemiologic studies depend upon a commonly accepted set of diagnostic criteria and for this reason earlier epidemiologic data vary owing to differences in case definition and ascertainment methods used.

Table 8-2 2004 International Classification of Headache Disorders

1. Migraine
   1.1 Migraine without aura
   1.2 Migraine with aura
       1.2.1 Typical aura with migraine headache
       1.2.2 Typical aura with non-migraine headache
       1.2.3 Typical aura without headache
       1.2.4 Familial hemiplegic migraine (FHM)
       1.2.5 Sporadic hemiplegic migraine
       1.2.6 Basilar-type migraine
   1.3 Childhood periodic syndromes that are commonly precursors of migraine
       1.3.1 Cyclical vomiting
       1.3.2 Abdominal migraine
       1.3.3 Benign paroxysmal vertigo of childhood
       1.3.4 Alternating hemiplegia of childhood
       1.3.5 Benign paroxysmal torticollis
   1.4 Retinal migraine
   1.5 Complications of migraine
       1.5.1 Chronic migraine
       1.5.2 Status migrainosus
       1.5.3 Persistent aura without infarction
       1.5.4 Migrainous infarction
       1.5.5 Migraine-triggered seizure

Source: Modified from Reference.[8]

Table 8-3 2004 International Headache Society Criteria for Pediatric Migraine Without Aura 1.1

Diagnostic Criteria

1. At least five attacks fulfilling criteria 2–4
2. Headache attacks lasting 1–72 hours
3. Headache has at least two of the following characteristics:
   (a) Unilateral location, may be bilateral, frontotemporal (not occipital)
   (b) Pulsing quality
   (c) Moderate or severe pain intensity
   (d) Aggravation by or causing avoidance of routine physical activity (e.g., walking or climbing stairs)
4. During the headache, at least one of the following:
   (a) Nausea and/or vomiting
   (b) Photophobia and phonophobia, which may be inferred from behavior.
5. Not attributed to another disorder.

Source: Modified from Reference.[8]

**Table 8-4 2004 International Classification of Headache Disorders Criteria
for Diagnosis of Typical Aura with Migraine Headache 1.2**

Diagnostic Criteria

1. At least two attacks fulfilling criteria 2–5.
2. Fully reversible visual, sensory, or speech symptoms, but no motor weakness.
3. At least two out of the following:
   a. Homonymous visual symptoms including positive features (i.e., flickering lights, spots, or lines) and/or negative features (i.e., loss of vision) and/or unilateral sensory symptoms including positive features (i.e., pins and needles) and/or negative features (i.e., numbness).
   b. At least one symptom develops gradually over 55 minutes, and/or different symptoms occur in succession.
   c. Each symptom lasts for 5–60 minutes.
4. Headache that meets criteria 2–4 for migraine without aura (1.1) begins during the aura or follows aura within 60 minutes.
5. Not attributed to another disorder.

Source: Modified from Reference.[8]

Initial population prevalence figures suggested that approximately 3%–8% of children have experienced a headache by the age of 3 years.[10,11] These figures increase to 37%–51.5% of children by age 7 years of age and up to 57%–82% of children aged 15 years.[4,10–13] This headache prevalence appears to be equal for both boys and girls and stable until 14 years of age, when there is then a decline in prevalence for boys after age 14 years with a concomitant increase in prevalence for girls.[12,14] Migraine headaches, defined more strictly in clinic-based populations, were experienced by 1.5%–3.2% of 7-year-olds, 4%–11% of 7- to 11-year olds, and anywhere from 8% to 23% of children over the age of 11 years.[4,10–12] However, with the adoption of the International Headache Society (IHS) classification of headaches diagnostic criteria (ICHD-I) and its subsequent revision (ICHD-II), further examination into the prevalence of childhood migraine has yielded comparable and less varied findings.[6,8] Migraine diagnoses in school-based population studies using the ICHD-I criteria reveal that about 6%–10.6% of school children aged 5–15 years satisfy the definition.[14–19] That prevalence figure increases to 28% (19% without aura and 9% with aura) in older adolescents.[19,20] These figures are based upon survey results from over 20,000 subjects and have been found to be similar across many different international school and population-based cohorts within the United Kingdom, Italy, Taiwan, Saudi Arabia, Norway, and Poland. Similar-prevalence data using the ICHD-II criteria have been few. Karli et al. reported that 14.5% of Turkish children from a survey of over 2300 secondary school students had migraine based upon the most recently revised criteria.[21]

Despite the revisions in diagnostic criteria provided in the 2004 ICHD-II, difficulties continue to exist in their application for young children.[22] Lima and colleagues compared the sensitivity and specificity of the criteria in a retrospectively studied clinic population of 496 adolescents using the 1988 ICHD-I and 2004 ICHD-II compared to a "gold standard" clinical diagnosis.[22] When ICHD I-1988 was used, the sensitivity of migraine without and with aura was 21% and 27%, respectively, whereas when applying the ICHD II-2004 it changed to 53% and 71% without affecting specificity.[22] The authors concluded that although the current criteria are an improvement in specificity over the 1988 criteria, they remain insensitive.[22] Indeed, the current criteria now carries footnotes to acknowledge the shorter duration of migraine, the bilateral location, and the parental observations that imply the presence of photophobia and phonophobia appreciated in children. Hershey and colleagues tested these allowances in a study of 260 patients, 18 years of age and under, with clinically diagnosed migraine.[23] Data analysis applying the ICHD-I and ICHD-II criteria in comparison with clinical impression for the diagnosis of migraine determined that 183/260 patients (70.4%) met ICHD-I criteria and 161/260 patients (61.9%) met the ICHD-II criteria.[23] When allowance for shorter duration of headache was made (ICHD-II allows 2 hours), 187/260 patients (71.9%) met the criteria, which improved to 192/260 patients (73.9%) with a 1-hour duration. If duration was excluded, 210/260 patients (80.8%) met the criteria on the basis of focal head pain.[23] Sensitivity approached 85% if either bilateral or unilateral location, shortened duration, and modified associated symptoms were considered.[23]

Longitudinal studies on migraine outcomes in children are sparse. From a sample of 9000 school children followed for up to 37 years, Bille noted prolonged remissions in migraine attacks of up to 2 years.[4,24] However, even after 30 years, only 40% remained migraine free.[24] Long-term remissions and cessation of migraines in 35% of boys and 21% of girls were reported by Hockaday in a longitudinal study of subjects followed for 8–25 years.[25] Similarly, Congdon and Forsythe reported their experience with three hundred 5- to 14-year-olds who were followed over a 10-year interval.[26] They found that, overall, 29% of the cohort experienced an 8-year remission and 34% had a 10-year remission.[26] This frequency of remission was further emphasized in an 8-year follow-up study of one hundred subjects followed in a headache center, which reported an overall remission rate of 34%.[25] Remission rates in relation to age of onset has revealed interesting data as well. In a cohort of 2921 school children, migraineurs with onset prior to age 7 years old had total remission rates of 26% in boys and 19% in girls 15 years after diagnosis compared to 22% in boys and 27% in girls with onset between the ages of eight and fourteen. About one-third (37%) of both boys and girls in the early onset group had a partial remission.[10,11]

Taken in composite, migraine affects up to 3% of children younger than age seven with boys more often affected than girls. The prevalence increases with age such that by age eleven almost 11%, equal numbers of boys and girls, suffer with migraine. However, by age fifteen girls with migraine far outnumber boys, contributing to a prevalence approaching 25% in this age group. It is clear that early-onset migraine, especially in girls, is less likely to remit over the long term. Nonetheless, a substantial proportion of childhood migraineurs may be expected to experience improvement into adulthood.

OVERVIEW OF PATHOPHYSIOLOGY AND MECHANISMS

Headache pain and the migraine experience constitute the result of a complex integration of a genetic predisposition, the anatomic structure, physiologic functioning of specific neurovascular circuits, the cumulative expression of inflammatory and pain-mediator substances, the processing of pain-mediated sensory signaling, and the individual's response to the culmination of these events.[27]

In-depth reviews of genetic contributions to the development of migraine have concluded that migraine without aura is a multifactor disorder with combinations of effects from both genetic and environmental factors.[27, 28] By comparison, migraine with aura has strong genetic influences, with additional environmental factors at play. These inferences are additionally supported by studies of population-based twin pair registries. An in-depth analysis of sixteen twin-pair registry reports of migraine without aura and seven additional twin-pair registry reports of migraine with aura were summarized and expanded upon by Russell.[28] His data analysis and tabulations reached the same conclusions.[28]

The most convincing new data in regard to the genetic component of migraine with aura can be gleaned from genetic analyses of subjects with familial hemiplegic migraine (FHM) syndrome. A number of these families have been studied and identified as carrying one of at least three different genetic mutations now known to cause the syndrome. These mutations have been identified in genes that code for proteins involved in the structure of several subunit components of three different ion channels. Mutations in the *CACN1A* gene on chromosome 19p13, encoding for the subunit alpha-1A of the voltage-dependent P/Q-type calcium channel, is associated with FHM type 1 and found in over 50% of affected families.[27, 29–32] Mutations in the *ATP1A2* gene on chromosome 1q, encoding for the sodium/potassium-transporting ATPase alpha-2, is associated with FHM type 2.[27, 34, 35] An additional FHM type 3 syndrome is associated with mutations in the *SCN1A* gene on chromosome 2q, which encodes for the sodium channel protein type 1 alpha subunit.[36] These same genetic mutations have been likewise associated with other neurological presentations (e.g., episodic ataxia syndromes, several specific epilepsy syndromes, and a number of periodic paralyses and muscle myotonia disorders).[37] FHM type 1 families can have pure hemiplegia, coma, or combinations of hemiplegia, with several cerebellar signs (e.g., ataxia, nystagmus), depending on the specific mutation of the *CACN1A* gene identified.[31] These combination clinical syndromes and the genetic mutations associated with them herald a greater understanding of the underlying pathophysiology of not only migraine but also these other paroxysmal disorders. The concept of phenotypic heterogeneity allows for different clinical presentations despite having the same genetic mutation, in this case, a specific channel disturbance, or channelopathy. In the same manner, different genetic mutations may, in turn, produce the same clinical disorder (i.e., genetic heterogeneity). Other genetic loci and associations with migraine aura are yet to be confirmed.[37,38]

The migraine attack is characterized by a sequence of clinical phases associated with specific neurovascular changes, enhanced and promulgated by several neurophysiologic mechanisms. These phases are identified in sequence as the premonitory phase, the aura, the headache phase, and the postdrome (Table 8-5). The central role of ion channels has particular relevance here because these are intimately involved in cell excitability, and thereby can contribute to the induction of physiologic events that ultimately lead to the genesis of migraine.[27] This cortical hyperexcitability may be directly or indirectly related to an alteration in dopaminergic and serotoninergic systems. The constitutional symptoms of the prodrome reflect these neurotransmitter alterations. The underlying neurovascular anatomy relates specific pain-sensitive structures and pain processing pathways (Table 8-6).

Table 8-5 Migraine Phases

Phase	Clinical Characterization	Timing
Premonitory	Physiologic: depression, irritability, fatigue, muscle tenderness, restlessness	Hours to days before the attack
	Neurological: hypersomnia, photophobia, phonophobia, sonophobia, inattention, acuity of all senses	
	Constitutional: thirst, anorexia, food cravings, yawning, sluggishness	
	Autonomic: mottling, cold sensations, diaphoresis	
Aura	Positive or negative symptoms of visual, somatosensory, motor, brainstem dysfunction	Evolve 5–20 minutes prior to the migraine and last up to 60 minutes
Headache	Bilateral or unilateral throbbing quality, aggravated by movement or physical activity	Gradual onset usual, with typical headache lasting 1–4 hours in children
Postdrome	Tired feeling, with diminished energy, malaise, and decreased concentration, often with residual scalp tenderness	May last hours to days

Source: Modified from References.[38,42,45]

Table 8-6 Neuroanatomical Structures and Humoral Factors Involved with Headache Genesis

Structure	Innervation/Relays	Receptors and Neuroactive/Vasoactive Substances
Intracranial vessels Dura and pia mater Venous sinuses	$V_{1,2,3}$ branches of the trigeminal nerve via trigeminal ganglion (trigeminal nucleus caudalis) C1 & C2 nerve roots Nucleus tractus solitarius Dorsal vagal complex Pons (locus coeruleus, superior salivatory nucleus) Midbrain (periaqueductal grey, dorsal raphe nucleus) Thalamus/Hypothalamus (intralaminar complex, ventrobasal complex, ventroposteromedial) Cortex (frontal, cingulate)	$5HT_{1A}$, $5HT_{1B}$, $5HT_{1D}$, $5HT_{1F}$. $5HT_2$ B-adrenoceptors Substance P Mast cell degranulation Calcitonin gene-related peptide Vasoactive intestinal peptide Catecholamines Excitatory amino acids GABA-$_A$ receptors

Source: Modified from References.[43,45,46,84]
Notes: V_1 = ophthalmic branch; V_2 = maxillary branch; V_3 = mandibular branch; C= cervical; 5HT = 5-hydroxytryptophan (serotonin) receptor subtypes; GABA = γ-aminobutyric acid

Nerve fibers from the ophthalmic division of the trigeminal ganglion and upper cervical nerve roots innervate large intracerebral vessels, pial vessels, venous sinuses, and the meninges. Nociceptive signals carried via these fibers are modulated within the midbrain, pons, and diencephalon before relay to the cortex. A number of individually recognized and often poorly characterized triggers (trauma, sleep deprivation, hormones, foods, stress, noise, weather, etc.) initiate what has been identified as a spreading wave (2–6 mm/minute) of cortical depression.[45] This wave of depolarization and consequent hyperemia is associated initially with positive migraine aura symptoms followed by a phase of hyperpolarization and oligemia associated with transient neurological deficits.[27,42,45,46] This cortical spreading depression (CSD) is postulated to induce both neurogenic plasma extravasations (sterile inflammation) and direct stimulation of the trigeminal neurons predominantly via the ophthalmic branch (V_1).[27,46] The migraneur who harbors any of the known and likely additional ion channel gene mutations to be identified in the future is predisposed to an enhanced neuronal susceptibility of the production and perpetualization of CSD by a reduction in the threshold at which CSD is both initiated and maintained. In FHM type 1 the voltage-dependent P/Q-type calcium channels are coupled to neurotransmitter release. Mutations allow for enhanced calcium channel current through gain of function, and augmented neurotransmission with reduced threshold and increased velocity of CSD. This enhanced susceptibility accounts for prompt and sustained severe migraine auras (i.e., hemiplegia and additional transient neurological deficits).[27,42,46] In FHM type 2, mutation in the sodium/potassium-transporting ATPase pump leads to decreased pump activity and lower clearance of potassium and glutamate. This in turn allows for greater susceptibility of CSD.[27,42,46] Finally, in FHM type 3, the affected voltage-gated sodium channels suffer a reduction in fast channel inactivation with a resultant enhancement of glutamate release and an elevation of extracellular potassium that enhances the initiation of CSD.[27,42,43]

Several coincident biochemical changes occur with CSD, among which is the release of a number of vasoactive peptides by trigeminal neurons. These substances additionally diffuse through the extracellular space and in turn further stimulate the trigeminovascular fibers to activate additional peripheral and central relay nuclei. Sites of treatment intervention at this stage of the migraine cascade involve the potential activation of serotonin receptors, which in turn serve to dampen further neurotransmission by thalamic neurons.[43] It has been demonstrated that the site of a high concentration of $5HT_{1D}$ receptors are located along nerve fibers within the dura.[43] They are also found within the cornea and within the lumbar dorsal root ganglia but not cervical ganglia.[44] These later locations suggest that mere anatomic location of the receptors cannot fully account for preferential analgesic effects of triptan activation upon migraine pain and that additional factors may be relevant.[43,44] Furthermore, there may be a potential for triptan use for other pain syndromes and more widespread analgesic effects. Additional experimental evidence in rats treated with chronic migraine prophylaxis agents (topiramate, amitriptyline, valproate, methysergide, DL-propranolol) has also been demonstrated to effectively suppress CSD.[42,47] Whether or not there are additional stimuli from mast cell aggregation and degranulation of vasoactive substances remains under study but are potentially important.[48]

Trigeminovascular fibers transmit nociceptive information into the brainstem, triggering the locus coeruleus and associated parasympathetic nuclei before relaying signal on toward the cortex.[49] This autonomic activation enhances further meningeal vasodilatation, photophobia, phonophobia, and the production of additional autonomic effects that are then symptomatically experienced (e.g., nasal congestion, tearing, nausea, vomiting, etc). Further sensory input extending from the trigeminal nucleus caudalis to the upper cervical spinal cord dorsal root zones extend the perceived pain field to the territory of the upper cervical nerves. It has been postulated and experimentally demonstrated that after the initial and early (<1 hour) activity-dependent inflammatory mediators diffuse within the dura, an activity independent and prolonged (>4 hours) V1 and central dorsal horn spinal cord neuronal firing occurs.[50,51] This peripheral nociceptive signaling can lead to peripheral sensitization of these dural nociceptors to additional intracranial mechanical stimulation, increased central sensitization to extracranial mechanical and thermal stimuli, and enhanced cardiovascular responses consistent with that evoked by pain.[50,51] It has been hypothesized that this peripheral stimulation induces the throbbing quality of migraine and that central pain sensitivity accounts for the experience of allodynia.[50,51] This central sensitization theory of migraine integrates the genesis of CSD and the early trigeminovascular components of clinical migraine and our evolving understanding of the concurrent neuronal dysfunction accompanying it. It further serves to accommodate the concept of transformed migraine.

Recent neuroimaging studies utilizing MRI, functional MRI, SPECT, and PET scanning techniques corroborate several important principals in migraine pathophysiology.[49,52–57] In summary, these include the following findings: (1) the visual aura is associated with decreased occipital blood flow and decreased occipital lobe activation on SPECT, perfusion-weighted fMRI, and BOLD (blood oxygen level-dependent) imaging without changes in apparent diffusion coefficient maps; (2) the migraine headache phase is associated with increased blood flow in the rostral pons and midbrain (periaqueductal gray, dorsal raphe nucleus, locus coeruleus), anterior cingulate cortex, posterior cingulated cortex, cerebellum, thalamus, insular, prefrontal cortex, posterior hypothalamus and temporal lobes on PET, fMRI, and increased cortical T2 intensity signal contralateral to hemiplegia on MRI; and finally (3) post-migraine anatomic findings of increased white matter T2 intensity signal and small cerebellar infarcts on MRI may be identified.[49,52–57] The identification of specific dorsolateral pontine and midbrain locations for activation during migraine may help to explain the laterality of symptoms in the absence of vascular mechanisms. Migraine therefore should be viewed as a primary neuronal disorder. Calcitonin gene-regulated peptide (CGRP) may have particular relevance in this regard since projections from these regions involve rich networks of aminergic neuronal projections that may be amenable to CGRP receptor blockade.

The migraine aura deserves particular mention here. Visual auras are the most commonly identified, but other sensory and dysphasic events may also occur. Although visual auras have a limited documentation and investigation in children, these have been noted in the literature since the 1800s.[58,59] The evolution of scintillating scotomas during a typical migraine was first analytically illustrated and studied by Lashley as he documented visual aura of his own migraine.[60] It was from examining his own scotoma evolution that he was able to deduce that there was a spreading wave of cortical involvement approximating 3 mm/minute.[60] This velocity of evolution corresponds well to that of observed CSD reported by Leao.[45] Lashley's and other illustrations of zigzag lines and shimmering appearance of fortification spectra remain remarkably similar from individual to individual over the published history of visual aura depictions as reviewed by Schott.[61] Young children, however, describe more elemental changes such as colored blobs, lights that sparkle, or image distortions such as micropsia and macropsia without inducing fear.[9,62–64] In a unique study of visual auras, 100 children who experienced them from a cohort of 244 with migraine were identified, accounting for an incidence of 41%.[65]

Sixty-seven of these children, assisted by a medical artist, were able to describe and draw what they visualized during their attacks. Three typical patterns of visual aura were identified: binocular impairment with scotoma (77%), visual distortions (16%), and monocular impairment and scotoma (7%).[65] These specific patterns of visual aura were attributed to disturbances in the territories of the basilar, middle cerebral, and ophthalmic arteries, respectively.[65] Confusion with amnesia, aphasia, brainstem disturbances with vertigo, tinnitus, hyperacusis, paresthesias, and motor paresis are additional auras identified in this age group.[9,65–70]

An important aspect of migraine auras are their relationships to epileptic auras. Recent theories of migraine and converging lines of evidence support the view that similar, if not same, pathophysiologic mechanisms underlie each clinical entity migraine and epilepsy.[40] Thus, it is now becoming more usual to identify both entities within the same individual or at least within the same family with individual members manifesting one or the other.[71–73] This is particularly true in the childhood benign epilepsies.[71–73] As the genetic identification of causative mutations emerge, the influence of environment and modifying genes will take on greater prominence as trigger mechanisms.[33,37,40] Recent family studies have revealed that visual aura as a manifestation of occipital-temporal lobe epilepsy or migraine occurred as separate attacks in all but one member of a large twenty-one-member Belgian family.[74] Furthermore, a novel linkage to chromosome 9q was revealed, which supports the likelihood of monogenic gene defects underlying the pathophysiologic causes common to each disorder. In a population-based case-control study of Icelandic children aged 5–15 years, at first unprovoked seizure, investigators evaluated the relative contribution of migraine with aura and without aura to incident epilepsy.[75] The investigators found that migraine with aura was associated with a four-fold increased risk for developing epilepsy but not migraine without aura.[75] This increased risk extended across all seizure types, causes, and both genders, suggesting that migraine with and without aura are separate disease entities.[75]

The use of neurophysiologic tools to study the evolution of migraine aura in children is limited, but there exists some concurrent EEG, transcranial Doppler (TCD), and brain SPECT scanning reports of children with migraine and aura. In four children studied with SPECT imaging during attacks of the Alice in Wonderland symptomatology (visual hallucinations with perceptual distortions of size, form, and color), decreased perfusion of the visual cortex extending into the temporal lobes was found.[76] Eleven children (ages 8–15 years) from a series of twenty-five with aura lasting a minimum of 5 hours were studied using a combination of neurophysiologic techniques with concurrent brain EEG, TCD, and SPECT.[77] Nine children had visual aura, four had hemiparesis and numbness, three had aphasia, and five had diminished levels of consciousness.[77] EEG abnormalities consisting of slow waves in the temporal-occipital regions or diffusely were apparent between 1–3 hours into the aura.[77] These slow waves were only identified in the occipital regions by

12–24 hours later. On the first day of study, each subject demonstrated hypoperfusion on SPECT within the same regions demonstrating slow waves on EEG and a subsequent hyperperfusion measured over the subsequent 12–24 hours.[77] TCD studies of all patients showed a decrease of mean velocity within the middle cerebral artery of the migrainous hemisphere compared to the nonmigrainous side (50 cm/sec vs. 61 cm/sec $p = 0.04$).[77] Structural imaging studies using MRI and CT scanning in nonprogressive headache syndromes conforming to ICHD diagnostic criteria in children with normal examinations have not identified etiologically significant lesions in the vast number of series. A recent retrospective review of 302 subjects (6–18 years old) with ICHD-coded headache syndromes found that of 107 with uncomplicated migraine and 30 with chronic daily headache all had normal examinations.[78] Of these subjects, 64/137 underwent neuroimaging, and abnormalities were identified in 3.7% of migraineurs and 16.6% of chronic daily headache subjects. No abnormality required intervention and none were associated with headache presentation.[78] A meta-analysis of the reported literature in children has been reviewed and practice guidelines issued from the Quality Standards Subcommittee of the American Academy of Neurology and the Practice Committee of the Child Neurology Society.[79] Based upon the analysis of 605 subjects who underwent imaging for recurrent headaches, the committee suggested that obtaining a neuroimaging procedure on a routine basis is not indicated.[79] The frequency of incidental findings or unrelated lesions varies (0%–16%), and only 3% (14/605) had a lesion that was surgically treatable or required medical intervention.[79] Importantly, in all the subjects with lesions considered surgically treatable, there were significant abnormalities identified on neurological examination.[78]

THE CLINICAL CONDITIONS AND TREATMENTS

Migraine

Migraine with and without aura are well described in children, and recent modifications to the ICHD-II code of headache syndromes account for additional diagnostic nuances encountered in this age group (see Tables 8-2, 8-3, 8-4, 8-7, 8-8).[8]

As discussed in the previous sections, complete acceptance by clinicians of the diagnostic criteria may require further evolution of the definitions; however, they have acquired greater precision and applicability.[22,23] In a study conducted in Serbia, from a population of over 2 million, a multi-staged stratified clustered sampling procedure was carried out in twenty-three preschools and forty-two grade schools within nine different cities using a semi-structured headache questionnaire.[80] The first-stage questionnaire identified 30,636 children aged 3–17 years (mean 9.2 years, 49.6% girls) with recurrent headaches based upon the most recent ICHD-revised headache

Table 8-7 2004 International Classification of Headache Disorders Criteria for Familial Hemiplegic Migraine 1.2.4 and Non-Familial Hemiplegic Migraine 1.2.5

Familial Hemiplegic Migraine 1.2.4
Description

Migraine with aura including motor weakness and at least one first- or second-degree relative who has migraine aura including motor weakness.
Diagnostic criteria:

1. At least two attacks fulfilling criteria 2 and 3
2. Aura consisting of fully reversible motor weakness and at least one of the following:
   a. fully reversible visual symptoms including positive features (e.g., flickering lights, spots, or lines) and/or negative features (i.e., loss of vision)
   b. fully reversible sensory symptoms including positive features (i.e., pins and needles) and/or negative features (i.e., numbness)
   c. fully reversible dysphasic speech disturbance
3. At least two of the following:
   a. at least one aura symptom develops gradually over ≥5 minutes and/or different aura symptoms occur in succession over ≥5 minutes
   b. each aura symptom lasts ≥5 minutes and <24 hours
   c. headache-fulfilling criteria 2–4 for 1.1 migraine without aura begins during the aura or follows onset of aura within 60 minutes.
4. At least one first- or second-degree relative has had attacks fulfilling these criteria 1–5
5. Not attributed to another disorder

1.2.5 Sporadic Hemiplegic Migraine 1.2.5
Description

Migraine with aura including motor weakness but no first- or second-degree relative has aura including motor weakness.
Diagnostic criteria:

1. At least 2 attacks fulfilling criteria 2 and 3
2. Aura consisting of fully reversible motor weakness and at least one of the following:
   a. fully reversible visual symptoms including positive features (e.g., flickering lights, spots, or lines) and/or negative features (i.e., loss of vision)
   b. fully reversible sensory symptoms including positive features (i.e., pins and needles) and/or negative features (i.e., numbness)
   c. fully reversible dysphasic speech disturbance
3. At least two of the following:
   a. at least one aura symptom develops gradually over ≥5 minutes and/or different aura symptoms occur in succession over ≥5 minutes
   b. each aura symptom lasts ≥5 minutes and <24 hours
   c. headache fulfilling criteria 2–4 for 1.1 migraine without aura begins during the aura or follows onset of aura within 60 minutes
4. No first- or second-degree relative has had attacks fulfilling these criteria 1–5
5. Not attributed to another disorder

Source: Modified from Reference.[8]

Table 8-8 2004 International Classification of Headache Disorders for Basilar-Type Migraine 1.2.6

Description

Migraine with aura symptoms clearly originating from the brainstem and/or from both hemispheres simultaneously affected, but no motor weakness.

Diagnostic criteria:

1. At least two attacks fulfilling criteria 2–4
2. Aura consisting of at least two of the following fully reversible symptoms, but no motor weakness:
    a. dysarthria
    b. vertigo
    c. tinnitus
    d. hypacusia
    e. diplopia
    f. visual symptoms simultaneously in both temporal and nasal fields of both eyes
    g. ataxia
    h. decreased level of consciousness
    i. simultaneously bilateral paraesthesias
3. At least one of the following:
    a. at least one aura symptom develops gradually over >5 minutes and/or different aura symptoms occur in succession over >5 minutes
    b. each aura symptom lasts >5 and <60 minutes.
4. Headache fulfilling criteria 2–4 for 1.1 migraine without aura begins during the aura or follows aura within 60 minutes
5. Not attributed to another disorder

Source: Modified from Reference.[8]

diagnostic criteria. A second-stage face-to-face interview of those with recurrent headaches gathered data from this sample and classified 5812 (18.97%) with primary non-migraine recurrent headaches and 2644 (8.63%) migraine headaches.[80] The onset age of typical migraine was at a mean of 5.14 years (range 2.8–14 years) and followed an identical recurrent pattern in nearly 95% of affected children.[80] The migraine events occurred monthly in 78% and were relieved by sleep in the vast majority (76.7%). They occurred in the morning hours for most (58.5%) and lasted several hours in 45.1% of those affected.[80] Discriminate analysis identified statistically significant (discriminant coefficient >0.3) distinguishing features of migraine from non-migraine as follows: vomiting impulse or retching (0.945), relief after sleep (0.945), photophobia (0.523), nausea (0.379), and phonophobia (0.354).[80] The most highly correlated symptoms of migraine in children were nausea and phonophobia (0.75).[80] Important corollaries of the study were that of the children who did not experience either nausea or vomiting only 0.7% had migraine headaches and that almost 75% of the children in the study reported recurrent abdominal pain during their migraine attacks.[80]

Migraine aggregating in families has been well established. The inheritance pattern has been complex and multifactorial, with up to 50%–90% of relatives of children with migraine being identified as having migraine headaches as well.[28,29,81-83] Recent face-to-face population surveys have identified strong evidence for familial aggregation with higher relative risk (RR = 1.88) compared to controls. Furthermore, the earlier the onset and the greater the severity of migraine in the probands, the higher the levels of familial aggregation compared to controls.[83] The RR for familial aggregation was 2.50 compared to controls when migraine in the proband was prior to age 16 years.[84] Similarly, the RR of familial aggregation was 2.38 compared to controls in those probands with the most severe pain levels (9–10 on a scale 0–10).[84] This has also been equated with greater functional disability (e.g., missing school or work).[85] These subjects are also more apt to have persistent headache disorders such that the earlier the onset of headaches the longer the duration of the disease.[84] Dominant inheritance of a specific migraine syndrome, familial hemiplegic migraine, has been clearly demonstrated. Several genetic mutations have now been identified, and further characterization of the underlying mechanisms for this disorder has been under study.[31-36,38]

Migraine without aura is the most prevalent form of childhood migraine. An estimated 60%–85% of childhood migraineurs suffer from migraine without aura. Data from a large pharmaceutical treatment trial database identified 1932 adolescents aged 12–17 years (54% female) with ICHD-II-defined migraine, 67% (1121/1932) of whom had migraine without aura.[87] This would be consistent with long-term outcome studies of adolescent migraine in that migraine without aura is more likely to persist into adulthood (frequency range 23.6%–56.2%), or convert into tension-type headache (20%–62.9%).[87-91] Migraine with aura may be more likely to remit (13.5%–28.1%).[87-91] However, familial predisposition (familial migraine with aura) confers a more unfavorable outcome.[88-91] Overall remission rates from adolescence into adulthood for all migraine types, however, show rates of 14.7%–44.5%.[88-91]

Migraine without aura

Migraine without aura is not associated with neurological deficits (Table 8-3). There are unique migraine syndromes in childhood where transient neurological dysfunctions not ascribed as an aura do occur. Reference to these as "complex migraine" can be found in the literature. **Confusional migraine** is one such syndrome noted in childhood where an acute encephalopathy develops concurrent with or following headache symptoms, although headache may not always be apparent. A positive family history for migraine is commonly elicited. This type of migraine has been estimated to be present in <7% of childhood migraine populations.[67,92-94] Early references to children who became disoriented and confused during a migraine event were first reported on by Lance and Anthony in 1966.[92] The term confusional migraine was first coined by Gascon and Barlow in 1970 and used to imply a combination of symptoms that included agitation, aphasia, visual hallucinations, and impaired attention and memory.[93] Other descriptions have followed, but little additional insight has developed beyond the clinical phenomenology, epidemiologic recognition, and suggestion of vasoconstrictive mechanism.[93–95] There may be a period of apprehension followed by escalating combativeness, which can make diagnostic evaluation impossible without sedation.[96] Whether or not this action is taken, further laboratory evaluation is necessary to exclude toxic/metabolic, CNS infectious/inflammatory, and epileptic causes. Confusional migraine is most often recognized in children 5–16 years old and can be the initial migraine event for the subject. This migraine presentation can make definitive diagnosis one of exclusion even if a family history of migraine is evident. The duration of the attacks are usually several hours to a day, although periods as brief as <30 minutes have been observed.[92–94] The clinical phenomenon has been likened to that of the adult syndrome of transient global amnesia, in that children will appear to have memory disturbances and amnesia for the event afterwards.[96, 97] There is often (30%–40%) a history of minor head trauma precipitating the event.[93, 94, 98] The attacks bear resemblance to the "type 2" attacks of somnolence, irritability, and vomiting described in 14/50 attacks in 25 adult subjects reported by Haas et al.[98] Electroencephalography typically demonstrates frontal intermittent rhythmic delta activity (FIRDA) during episodes.[94, 99] Immediately after the episode, some patients' EEGs show global slowing, with a return to normal within 1–3 days.[99]

Migraine with aura

Migraine with aura has a number of specific neurological symptoms described and diagnostic criteria identified (Table 8-4). Auras in these migraine types include visual, sensory, and speech disturbances but no motor weakness. Visual auras concerning children have been described in the preceding sections. An additional element of visual aura interpreted from artistic depictions from migraineurs is that of the "out-of-body experience." As a result of sponsored art competitions, Boehringer Ingelheim UK Limited had collected 562 pieces of art depicting an individual's migraine experience.[100, 101] Podoll and Robinson reported a study of this collection, which revealed that 1.2% (7/562) pieces portray an "out-of-body experience."[102] These subjects were evaluated in interviews subsequently and data were combined with ten additional cases reported in the literature.[102, 103] They found that most often the experiences began in childhood preceding or shortly after the onset of the subjects' migraine disorder.[102] They occurred repeatedly over several decades and were generally stereotyped in description, lasting seconds to up to 10 minutes.[102] Most were in combination with headache, but several subjects reported the experiences without headache as well.[102] Subjects described and depicted macro- and microsomatognosia, out-of-body experiences with autoscopy, and reduplication phenomena. Other complex visual illusions (dysmetropsia, metamorphopsia, oblique and inverted vision, visual allesthesia, diplopia, polyopia) were combined with varieties of the typical zigzag fortification spectra.[101, 102] Many of the descriptions and interpretations of the artwork are not only reminiscent of the illusionary experiences described in what is known as **the "Alice in Wonderland" syndrome** but have been interpreted as such.[9, 62–65] This peculiar syndrome of visual and interpretive distortions of body and environmental surroundings is well recognized in children but can be also identified in adults.[64, 102–104] The descriptive name, "Alice in Wonderland" syndrome, was first applied by Lippman in 1952 in his descriptions of adult migraine auras recognized as similar to the unusual experiences of Lewis Carroll's Alice when she enters the looking glass.[103] The visual disturbances can be accompanied by somatic and speech disturbances less frequently. Young children can additionally perceive what is a difficult-to-describe sense of altered time. They may explain that "things are going too fast" or "too slow" in an effort to impart their aberrant perceptions of time and motion. This type of aura evolves over 15–20 minutes and then is usually followed by throbbing headache. The headache may be contralateral to visual illusions when the appearance is unilateral but bilateral and frontal in most young children.

A logical digression from the foregoing discussion is to include at this juncture a discussion on **the basilar artery migraine syndrome (BAM)**. This unique headache syndrome is characterized by the experience of symptoms referable to alterations in function of structures nourished within the basilar artery territory. Bickerstaff and Birm first suggested this as a discrete headache entity.[105] The frequency with which it is experienced in children has been variably reported from 3%–19% in both pediatric and adult headache populations.[9, 66, 67, 105–109] The diagnosis has been reported in children as young as 7 months.[110] The hallmark symptoms as listed in the ICHD criteria are heavily represented by ataxia, vertigo, and cranial nerve disturbances in young children (Table 8-8).[110] Children may demonstrate diminished levels of alertness, visual symptoms, dysarthria, and bilateral paresthesias.

The aura in BAM has been quantified to last a mean of 60 minutes (range 2 minutes to 72 hours) in a study of thirty-eight subjects.[66] In a concurrent family study, these thirty-eight BAM subjects were equally distributed among families with and without migraine and typical aura, and when tested were found to have no genetic mutations consistent with familial hemiplegic migraine.[66] A full 79% of the BAM subjects also had episodes of aura without headache, and overall 95% of these also had migraine with typical aura at other times.[66] The authors suggested that BAM may not be an independent disorder distinct from migraine with typical aura.[66] Nonetheless, there are data reporting the anatomic effects of the syndrome when physiologic and neuroimaging investigations of the anatomic region involved have been undertaken. In a study evaluating brainstem functioning in twenty subjects with BAM (age range 9–48 years), electronystagmography disclosed abnormal eye tracking in six subjects (30%), and abnormal optokinetic nystagmus and absent or delayed vestibular evoked myogenic potentials in nine subjects (45%); caloric testing revealed canal paresis in seven patients (35%) and directional preponderance in four patients (20%).[111] The findings were interpreted to be a result of hypoperfusion in the territory of the basilar artery affecting the descending pathway from the saccule through the brainstem to cranial nerve XI, which normalized over 3 months in the absence of headache symptoms.[111] Other evidence for vascular effects have been sought after using neuroimaging. Transient and reversible noncontrast-enhancing T2 high signal lesions visualized with MRI have been reported in BAM in a 17-year-old.[112] Shifting lesions of probable cytotoxic edema within alternating areas of the occipital cortices were imaged on serial studies, which normalized over time.[112, 113] No irreversible abnormalities were noted. The lack of contrast enhancement, the confinement of abnormalities to the gray matter of the cortex, and the lack of persistent lesions, all suggests a mechanism of cytotoxic edema and not ischemia. The reversibility of this mechanism is also reflected in the few EEG studies reported in childhood BAM.

The EEG findings of four children with BAM (11–13.5 years old) during acute attack showed diffuse polymorphic delta activity within 4 hours of attack onset and delta-theta activity predominant over the occipital regions performed 16 hours after onset.[114] All abnormalities resolved at follow-up within a period of 4–18 days.[114] In another study, the long-term follow-up outcomes of seven children with BAM and demonstrated occipital spike-wave complexes were studied over a period of 8–16 years and reported by De Romanis et al.[115] The authors found that when BAM resolved the EEG findings also normalized in all subjects.[115] Older literature can be found that also identified benign focal epileptiform discharges in childhood migraine in about 9% of migraineurs ("common, classic, basilar").[116] This frequency compares to 1.9% identification in the normal population.[116] In a recent review it has been suggested that when either epilepsy, basilar migraine, migraine with prolonged aura, or alternating hemiplegia is suspected, an EEG should be performed.[117] The presence of epileptiform activity will usually suggest epilepsy even in subjects with BAM, such as the childhood epilepsy with occipital paroxysms syndrome.[117] However, not only may both disorders occur concurrently, but also the EEG evolution may demonstrate evolution to normal over time in each, and thus an ultimate diagnosis will remain a clinical determination and not one solely dependent upon EEG findings.[115–117]

The advent of genetic testing offers the potential to provide clarity in circumstances with diagnostic ambiguity. There has been a recent genetic analysis of an Italian family with a 17-year-old proband diagnosed with a 2-year history of BAM reported.[118] Ten members of the pedigree, including the proband, were analyzed and shown not to carry the CACNA1A gene mutation of FMH-1, but three first-degree relatives and the proband, all with BAM, did carry a novel ATP1A2 mutation of the FHM-2 gene.[118] None of the family members have clinical symptoms of hemiplegic migraine. The term "familial basilar migraine" had been proposed to describe this family. Similarly, the clinical association of occipital-temporal lobe epilepsy and migraine with visual aura has been conclusively shown to have linkage to a single locus on chromosome 9q21-q22, suggesting a common monogenic gene defect.[75] Population studies from a Danish headache registry identified 362 probands with familial nonhemiplegic migraine with visual aura ($n = 35$, 10% of the cohort with BAM) according to the ICHD-II criteria who underwent a semi-structured interview process.[119] There were several clinical features of familial nonhemiplegic migraine with aura that differed from nonfamilial migraine with aura in the general population; the age of onset was earlier, with a mean of 21 years (range 5–77 years); the age at remission was older and not influenced by age of onset; the auras were more severe and included some migraine events with visual aura in 99%, sensory aura in 54%, and aphasia in 32% of family members; and, finally, the occurrence of migraine aura without headache was substantially more frequent than in nonfamilial migraine subjects.[119] This "unfavorable outcome" for familial migraine has been previously identified in long-term outcome studies of adolescent migraine.[88–91] Newer intriguing data has revealed a potential genetic association between a functional polymorphism (short and long alleles) in the 5-HTT (serotonin transporter) gene and migraine with aura.[120] The authors suggested that this polymorphism has functional relevance in migraine with aura as it was present in a higher frequency when compared to a control population and with patients with migraine without aura. They postulated the likely mechanism by which the short allele exerts effect to be through the 5-HT (serotonin) content of serotonergic neurons and platelets and by affecting the overall serotonergic neurotransmission. Similar findings have been reported by Borroni et al.[121] However, these findings could not be replicated in a larger sample, and thus remain in question as to their significance.[122] Numerous other biomarkers are currently under study in the quest to better understand migraine pathogenesis.[123]

Familial (FHM) and sporadic (SHM) hemiplegic migraines are subtypes of and distinguished from other migraines with aura by the presence of motor weakness in addition to other aura symptoms (Table 8-7).[8] The familial form is characterized by a dominant inheritance pattern with affected first- and/or second-degree relatives experiencing the same clinical migraine syndrome, whereas subjects with the sporadic form do not. This syndrome is uncommon and a true prevalence is difficult to ascertain. The results of a nationwide epidemiologic survey of the entire Danish population of 5.2 million inhabitants estimated the prevalence of FHM to be 0.005%.[124] The clinical presentation is in childhood or adolescence with a strokelike quality, resulting in variable degrees of hemiparesis and other symptoms. The awareness of prodromal features or other concurrent aura symptoms may escape detection in children when initially being evaluated but should be specifically sought out during the ictus or at least in retrospect. Recent reviews describe the mean progression time of the motor, sensory, and visual aura symptoms as gradually developing over 27, 32, and 16 minutes, respectively. In addition to these three main aura symptoms, 55%–69% of the patients have BAM symptoms.[31,124] Hemi-sensory deficits; aphasia, or complex visual symptoms are required to be present in addition to the motor weakness.[31,124,125] All symptoms are reversible, however, and evolve over minutes to 24 hours but can rarely last longer.[31,124,125] The headache concurrently develops within 60 minutes of symptom onset and is but not invariably contralateral to the motor deficit. If the diagnosis is not known within the family or is presenting in the proband for the first time, clinical investigations to exclude other underlying etiologies must be undertaken.[9,31,125] Particular attention to etiology needs to be undertaken when there exists no family history of similar migraine events, with specific investigation for vascular anomalies and mitochondrial disorders.

A significant percentage of subjects (40%) will experience atypical and severe symptoms of prolonged hemiplegia or coma, occasionally associated with fever, meningismus, and epileptic seizures.[124–126] Persistent cerebellar deficits, nystagmus and prolonged diminished levels of consciousness, aphasia, and motor apraxia have been identified.[125,126] In one report of an adult with known FHM who had a severe attack with seizures, diminished consciousness, hemiparesis, and hemianopsia, he displayed persistent aphasia and motor apraxia at 2 years status post ictus.[126] Serial neuroimaging demonstrated persistent left hemisphere glucose hypometabolism on PET and reduced cerebral blood flow on SPECT-imaging without evidence of infarction.[126,127] Similar findings have been noted in less lengthy (10 days) durations of neurological deficit.[127] MR perfusion imaging in an 8-year-old child during a hemiplegic migraine event showed transient unilateral cerebral hyperperfusion associated with dilatation of the middle and posterior cerebral artery branches on the side contralateral to the aura during the headache phase.[128] Two additional reports of children under age 10 years presenting with prolonged periods of hemiplegia identified their respective family members to carry mutations (A606T, N717K, R1002Q) in the *ATP1A2* gene consistent with FHM type-2.[129,130] In one report, three children (two girls and one boy, ages 9, 10, and 7 years) were described with dense hemiplegic episodes lasting up to a week. In two of these subjects this was their first episode.[129] One child had accompanying global aphasia and a second child experienced a concurrent epileptic seizure. The dense hemiplegia in all three children resolved within 5–10 days; however, complete recovery required an additional several days to 6 weeks.[129] The child with global aphasia needed 7 weeks for language to return to normal. EEG recordings done in all three children demonstrated background slowing contralateral to the hemiplegia, which normalized at repeat recording several weeks later.[129] The child who experienced a seizure had a diffusion-weighted MRI that revealed increased signal intensity and corresponding decreased signal intensity on apparent diffusion coefficient mapping of the parietal region sparing the cortex.[129] This child had had prior episodes of hemiplegic migraine precipitated by minor head trauma in the past. MRI examinations in the other two children were normal.[129] There is a separate report of a 9-year-old girl along with several family members later diagnosed with FHM type-2 (G615R *ATP1A2* gene mutation). This subject experienced two separate events of transient cortical blindness, gaze deviation, restlessness, and fever at 2 years of age, with normal MRI each time, and two subsequent hemiplegic events with concurrent epileptic seizures and somnolence at ages 4 and 7 years.[130] All events were precipitated by mild head trauma and EEG showed diffuse polymorphic delta slowing. An MRI 2 weeks after her third event demonstrated swelling and hyperintensity on fluid-attenuated inversion recovery (FLAIR) sequences of the cortex contralateral to the hemiplegia without contrast enhancement.[130] These MRI abnormalities later resolved. Importantly, the child exhibited cognitive and behavioral regression after the initial presentations with incomplete recovery thereafter. Wechsler Intelligence Scale for Children-Revised IQ score measured 70 at 8 years of age.[130] Treatment with acetazolamide over 2 years has continued without migraine events recurring.[130] The child's father and paternal uncle and aunt each carried the same mutation and had experienced similar migraine events without sequelae. This family is reminiscent of another autosomal-dominant condition described in a family with transient cortical blindness after mild head trauma associated with childhood epilepsy and familial hemiplegic migraine called "elicited repetitive daily blindness" (ERDB).[131] This familial disorder has had genetic linkage to the FHM type-1 gene excluded but has not had the *ATP1A2* gene evaluated.[131]

In a study of fifteen FHM subjects (ages 16–63 years old) carrying the *CACN1A* gene mutation (FHM type-1) from three families, MR spectroscopy [(^{1}H) MRS] results were obtained and compared to controls.[132] Each subject had cerebellar deficits on neurological examination graded for severity and correlated with (^{1}H) MRS findings. The findings demonstrated significantly decreased NAA (N-acetyl aspartate), elevated mI (myoinositol), and decreased Glu (glutamate) concentrations in the superior cerebellar vermis compared to controls.[132] No other regions of brain (visual and parietal cortices) demonstrated abnormality. Although there were no persisting correlations with clinical function grading after repeated testing, initial analysis showed that a worse ataxia grade correlated with more atrophy and diminished NAA levels in the superior cerebellar vermis.[132]

Histopathologic findings in one neuropathologic autopsy specimen from an FHM type-1 subject disclosed Purkinje cell loss within the cerebellar vermis.[133] There is another report of neuropathological findings from a 19-year-old, whose sister and mother had FHM attacks.[134] The subject was not recognized to have had hemiplegic migraines, but did have mild mental retardation, cerebellar ataxia, and MRI-identified cerebellar atrophy. Among other findings, chronic degenerative changes within the cerebellar vermis and glial bundles within the cranial nerves were identified.[134] Striking Purkinje cell aberrations were noted and included; dendritic expansions, asteroid bodies, somatic sprouts, and torpedoes, as can be seen in other metabolic encephalopathies (e.g., Menkes disease, Tay-Sachs disease, mitochodropathies, and organic mercury intoxication).[134] How relevant these findings are to the pathophysiology of FHM remains speculative.

Disease-causing genetic mutations in three different genes, the *CACNA1A* (FHM type 1) gene, the *ATP1A2* (FHM type 2) gene, and the *SCN1A* (FHM type 3) gene, have been identified to date. These have been studied in both in vitro and in vivo animal models. Mutations in the *CACN1A* gene on chromosome 19p13, encoding for the subunit alpha-1A of the voltage-dependent P/Q-type calcium channel is found in over 50% of affected FHM type 1 families.[27,29–32,124] The defective channel function allows for a gain of function resulting in neurotransmitter release from cortical neurons and facilitation of CSD.[27,29–32,124] These are also the major calcium channels in Purkinje cells. Mutations in the *ATP1A2* gene on chromosome 1q, encoding for the sodium/potassium-transporting ATPase alpha-2, is associated with FHM type 2.[27,34,35,124] This channel defect produces a loss in function and results in disturbed neuronal function.[27,34,35,124] An additional FHM type 3 syndrome is associated with mutations in the *SCN1A* gene on chromosome 2q, which encodes for the sodium channel protein type 1 alpha subunit.[36,124] This mutation results in a gain of function and an accelerated recovery from fast inactivation of Nav1.5/Nav1.1 channels.[36,124] Each mutation contributes to the increase in extracellular synaptic concentrations of glutamate and potassium, thereby enhancing individual susceptibility to CSD. These same genetic mutations have been likewise associated with other neurological presentations (e.g., episodic ataxia syndromes, several specific epilepsy syndromes, and a number of periodic paralysis) and muscle myotonia disorders.[37]

The SHM prevalence is estimated to be 0.005%, and patients have clinical symptoms identical to patients with FHM, have no increased risk of migraine without aura, but have a higher risk of typical migraine with aura when compared to the general population.[135,136] In SHM there are very few subjects who carry any of the previously noted disease-causing genetic mutations. However, combined reports disclose that four of thirty subjects with SHM were found to harbor *CACN1A* gene mutations.[31,137–139] There has been recent report of a 5-year-old girl who suffered prolonged coma and hemiplegia requiring mechanical ventilation for 24 days, with nearly three additional months of encephalopathy, in response to minor head trauma.[140] No family member had migraines or exhibited similar clinical events. The child was found to have the S218L mutation of the *CACN1A* gene.[140] Neither parent had the mutation. An additional pediatric subject (boy) with an illness defined by episodes of ataxia, alternating hemiplegic migraine, and epileptic seizures initiating at age 6 months of age has also been described.[141] Episodes of transient hypotonia/hemiplegia were documented at ages 6 months, 12 months, 18 months, 3 years, and 6 years with comparative MRI images showing swelling and hyperintensity on fluid-attenuated inversion recovery (FLAIR) sequences of the cortex contralateral to the hemiplegia without contrast enhancement.[141] The child experienced aphasia, hemifield visual distortion, slurred speech, and worsening ataxia of varied degrees with individual attacks. EEG demonstrated epileptiform activity over the ipsilateral cortex and slowing over the contralateral cortex to the hemiplegia during two attacks.[141] By the age of 10 years, his neurological examination showed only mild truncal ataxia and hyperreflexia. Weschler Intelligence Scale for Children-III performance IQ score measured 72 and verbal IQ of 89 at 10 years of age.[141] Treatment with antiepileptic drugs and verapamil were discontinued and substitution to flunarazine has continued. A mutation was found in the *SLC1A3* gene, which encodes for the excitatory amino acid transporter 1 (EAAT1), which in turn is critical for the clearance of glutamate from the synaptic clefts.[141] This mutation was shown to cause drastically reduced glutamate uptake in mutant transporter transfected cells.[141] This proposed disturbance in glutamate clearance might serve as an additional mechanism, producing the hemiplegic migraine plus syndromes described especially in subjects without ion channel defects.[141] An additional interesting clinical question arises as to whether this child may actually have alternating hemiplegia syndrome rather than hemiplegic migraine (see below).

CHILDHOOD PERIODIC SYNDROMES

Childhood periodic syndromes are an important subset of migraine syndromes in children. Although these are categorized as "migraine equivalents," headache is not actually a prominent feature of the events. Autonomic symptoms and behavioral alterations are the principal features, associated with other discrete signs such as vomiting, nystagmus, hemiplegia, and torticollis, among others (Table 8-2). The prevalence of these syndromes is not well known (range 3.1%–10.5%) and is dependent upon the nature of the referral setting. In a recent survey of all migraineurs who were evaluated in an ambulatory general pediatric neurology practice, 1106 migraine subjects from 5848 patients over an 8-year time interval were identied.[67] From this cohort of 108 subjects (1.8% of total), 9.8% of all migraineurs had experienced childhood periodic syndromes.[67] The reported data from a smaller selected population of children with headaches referred for exclusion of intracranial lesions by transcranial ultrasound study, 202 migraine subjects were identified with only 10 subjects (4.7%) who were identified with a childhood periodic syndrome.[142] Similarly, 3.1% (38/4237) of all EEG telemetry referrals were identified with periodic syndromes compared to 10.5% (25/380) of all children referred for evaluation of non-epileptic events (see Chapter 1, Table 1-6).

Cyclic Vomiting Syndrome

Cyclic vomiting syndrome (CVS) is a self-limited episodic condition of childhood, with intense and rapidly sequential episodes of vomiting, accompanied by nausea and lethargy, interspersed among periods of complete normality (Table 8-9). The vomiting epochs are stereotyped for the individual and may last for up to five consecutive days with repetitive emesis periods over hours at a time. The first published description of the syndrome is attributed to Samuel Gee of St Bartholomew's Hospital, London, in 1882.[143] His description is as apt now as it was then: "These cases seem to be all of the same kind, there being fits

Table 8-9 2004 International Classification of Headache Disorders Criteria for Cyclical Vomiting 1.3.1

Description

1. Recurrent episodic attacks, usually stereotypical in the individual patient, of vomiting and intense nausea.
2. Attacks are associated with pallor and lethargy.
3. There is complete resolution of symptoms between attacks.

Diagnostic criteria:

(1) At least five attacks fulfilling criteria 2 and 3
(2) Episodic attacks, stereotypical in the individual patient, of intense nausea and vomiting, lasting 1 hour to 5 days
(3) Vomiting during attacks occurs at least four times/hour for at least 1 hour
(4) Symptom-free between attacks
(5) Not attributed to another disorder; history and physical examination do not show signs of gastrointestinal disease.

Source: Modified from Reference.[8]

of vomiting which recur after intervals of uncertain length. The intervals themselves are free from signs of disease. The vomiting continues for a few hours or days. When it has been severe, the patients are left much exhausted."[143]

By criteria, there must be at least five episodes of emesis per hour for at least 1 hour to satisfy the definition of an attack for 1 day. The onset is usually in preschool-aged children, but can begin in early infancy or as late as adulthood. The average frequency of vomiting bouts has been reported as monthly events over several years.[144] Each child may fall into an individual and somewhat predictable pattern of attacks. Earlier prevalence studies estimated that 1.9%–2.3% of all school-aged children may be affected.[145, 146] However, these estimates incorporate many mildly affected children and are likely an overestimate of the more severe part of the spectrum. Some authors have found that up to 68% of subjects may self-identify triggers of their CVS, including infections (41%) and psychological stresses (34%), but no definitive trigger is most common.[147] Even more remarkable is the absence of a diagnostic laboratory, radiological, or endoscopic finding. Early identification depends upon the exclusion of potential confounding organic illnesses before satisfying the diagnostic criteria. An average onset age is about 4–5 years, with a gradual induction of remission by age 10 years. Curiously, headache is not typically a feature of the syndrome in childhood but becomes more evident in adolescence.

Identification of significant findings from investigations of the underlying pathogenesis has been limited. Fourteen subjects with CVS, ages 3–16 years, eleven of whom had a family history of migraine, underwent analysis of autonomic regulation by To and colleagues.[148] The investigators used power spectral analysis of the beat-to-beat heart rate variability signal and found that

CVS subjects had an elevated sympathetic tone represented by the low frequency/high frequency ratio (1.45 ± 0.42 in CVS subjects compared to 0.89 ± 0.29 in healthy control subjects, $p < 0.001$).[148] Additional evidence provided by autonomic investigations conducted and compared in five groups are as follows: 41 normal pediatric controls, 12 pediatric subjects with chronic vomiting, 15 subjects with CVS, 21 adults subjects with migraine headaches, and 40 normal adult controls.[149] Sympathetic and cholinergic functions were assessed by vasoconstriction to cold, postural adjustment ratio (30:15), Valsalva ratio, ECG R-R interval measures, and a total autonomic score. The most pronounced abnormality after intergroup comparison was in the measurement of a low postural adjustment ratio of extremity capillary flow as measured by infrared photoplethysmography in both CVS and migraine groups ($p < 0.05$), pointing to a similar adrenergic autonomic abnormality in both these groups not identified in the others.[149] In an additional study of autonomic function in six subjects with CVS, each with a personal or family history of migraine headaches, all were found to have normal cardiovascular responses to deep breathing and to the Valsalva maneuver.[150] However, all six had a significant increase in heart rate (>30 beats per minute) with tilt testing; 2/3 subjects had a vasodepressor tendency, who described abdominal pain or had syncope with blood pressure nadir.[150] All six subjects also had abnormal sudomotor test results.[151] The combined results in CVS subjects indicate autonomic dysfunction affecting mainly sympathetic vasomotor and sudomotor functions and suggest that an alteration in autonomic regulation could play a role in the genesis of CVS, although its cause is not known.

Given the natural evolution of the syndrome, one might postulate a maturational dysregulation that becomes more balanced over time. Additional support for a neuro-gastroenterological connection exists with the findings of a hypothalamic-pituitary-adrenal axis disturbance. Sato et al. found elevated levels of corticotrophin, cortisol, vasopressin, prostaglandin E_2, and catecholamines in two children with CVS and profound lethargy and hypertension.[151] Further postulation of the CNS and the central role of the neuroendocrine system in the mediation of CVS were suggested as attacks appear to be precipitated by stimuli or states associated with stimulation of corticitropin releasing factor (CRF) release (i.e., the "stress response") and CRF effects.[152] These include similar endocrine, autonomic, and visceral changes as those clinically observed and identified through investigation.[153]

Clinical experience of severe CVS subjects has suggested the possibility that mitochodropathies may be present. However, no clear evidence for this generalization has emerged. Case reports of Kearns-Sayer syndrome and CVS have been reported, but a common and consistent identification of mitochondrial disease is lacking.[154] Yet, mitochondrial dysfunction may still be a risk factor among others. The search for unique subgroups within the larger cohorts of CVS children has suggested the possible validity of "cyclic vomiting plus and cyclic vomiting minus" categories. The "plus" group includes those with cognitive, neuromuscular, epileptic, and cranial nerve disturbances, and those subjects without them, the "minus" group.[155] Careful analysis of over sixty-seven subjects who could be subgrouped failed to discern a genetically distinct primary genetic or mitochondrial DNA sequence-mediated factor. However, the child with clinical features characterizing the cyclic vomiting plus group is a child likely to have a younger age of vomiting episodes and suffer additional neuromuscular-cognitive, dysautonomic, and constitutional ailments.[155] Therapeutic interventions with both antimigraine and pro-mitochondrial approaches may be suggested.

The association of CVS with migraine was postulated over 100 years ago by Langmead.[156] This stems logically from the foregoing discussion in that although headache is not a prominent feature of the syndrome in childhood, by adolescence this ultimately evolves. Family history data from 214 subjects with CVS revealed that 82% of these subjects had a positive family history for migraine or developed migraine attacks at later ages.[152] When this migraine subgroup was compared to the non-migraine subgroup, the migraine subset had milder episodes (20.7 $\pm$ 27.3 SD vs. 39.5 $\pm$ 66.5 emeses/episode, $p = 0.006$); more symptoms of abdominal pain (83% vs. 66%), headache (41% vs. 24%), social withdrawal (40% vs. 22%), photophobia (36% vs. 16%, all $p<0.05$); more frequent triggering events (70% vs. 49%, $p = 0.013$) including psychological stress (39% vs. 22%), physical exhaustion (23% vs. 3%), and motion sickness (10% vs. 0%); and a higher positive response rate to antimigraine therapy (79% vs. 36%, $p = 0.002$).[157] Although CVS can be identified utilizing the current diagnostic criteria, the exclusion of comorbid and contributing factors needs to be undertaken. In a study of 225 subjects referred for evaluation after at least three episodes of vomiting, 83% were ultimately diagnosed with idiopathic CVS after extensive investigations.[158] A full 41% had contributing comorbid causes to their vomiting additionally identified.[158] Nonetheless, there have been families with "pure" CVS, without comorbid symptomatology, migraine, or other gastroenterological or neurological disease.[154] These families have had mitochondrial disorders and oxidation defects excluded on the basis of laboratory testing.[159]

Interventions for CVS are both supportive and largely empiric but includes hydration, sedation, and antiemetics. These approaches have included anticonvulsants, antimigraine therapies, antidepressants, antacids, benzodiazepines, prokinetics, and non-steroidal anti-inflammatories.[160, 161] Abortive measures with analgesics and triptans have also been utilized in the prodromal phase.[160, 161] A typical approach will include pre-emesis prodromal phase of treatment with analgesics and triptans, followed by ondansetron and benzodiazepines with IV glucose fluid therapy as emesis ensues in the attack phase.[160, 161] Further sedation, antiemetics, and anticholinergic therapy with chlorpromazine, promethazine, metaclopramide, and diphenhydramine may be added to H_2-receptor antagonists.[160, 161] Newer approaches with alpha$_2$ receptor agonists, clonidine, and dexmedetomidine have received additional attention.[161] The reinstitution of oral intake in the postdrome phase after maintaining hydration and glucose supplementation throughout the attack should be gradual. Longer-term migraine prophylaxis with cyproheptadine, amitriptyline, topiramate, zonisamide, levetiracetam, a calcium channel blocker, or a beta-blocker is generally recommended.[160–166]

Abdominal Migraine Syndrome

Abdominal migraine syndrome (AMS) is less well described within the literature than are other periodic syndromes. It has been distinguished from cyclic vomiting syndrome as a distinct entity after many years of uncertain categorization (Table 8-10). AMS develops in school-aged children and presents as repetitive attacks of rather dull midline periumbilical pain lasting several hours with variable intensity (moderate to severe) but significant enough to interfere with function.[167–171] Repeated attacks can last on average a duration of up to 24–36 hours, with a frequency of —fifty to sixty times a year.[167] Reminiscent of migraine are the concomitant findings of pallor, dark circles under the eyes, anorexia, and nausea. Many children will experience motion sickness when riding in the car (50%).[167] Motion sickness has been identified as a common

Table 8-10 2004 International Classification of Headache Disorders Criteria for Abdominal Migraine1.3.2

Description

1. An idiopathic recurrent disorder seen mainly in children and characterized by episodic midline abdominal pain, manifesting in attacks lasting 1–72 hours, with normality between episodes
2. The pain is of moderate-to-severe intensity and associated with vasomotor symptoms, nausea, and vomiting

Diagnostic criteria:

(1) At least five attacks fulfilling criteria 2–4
(2) Attacks of abdominal pain lasting 1–72 hours
(3) Abdominal pain has all of the following characteristics:
    (a) Midline location, periumbilical or poorly localized
    (b) Dull or "just sore" quality
    (c) Moderate-or-severe intensity
(4) During abdominal pain, at least two of the following:
    (a) Anorexia
    (b) Nausea
    (c) Vomiting
    (d) Pallor
(5) Not attributed to another disorder; history and physical examination do not show signs of gastrointestinal or renal disease, or such disease has been ruled out by appropriate investigations

Source: Modified from Reference.[8]

feature of childhood migraine even in the absence of AMS.[4,171] Some children will develop prominent vasomotor instability during their attacks, characterized by periodic flushing.[167,172] Vomiting and vertigo can also occur but are not generally prominent features of the attacks. The estimated prevalence of AMS with and without headache was identified as 0.7% and 1.7%, respectively, from one population sample using a structured interview method and up to as high as 4.1%–6% in two other population-based cross-sectional samples.[168,170,173] The highest prevalence rates of 8.7%–18.5% have been noted in headache-referred migraneur cohorts.[67,170] Most children with abdominal migraine (70%) will develop clinical migraine headaches at some point in life.[170] Children with AMS are 2.6 times more likely to have a maternal history of migraine than the general population.[168] By the same token, children with migraine headaches were twice as likely to have had abdominal migraine and children with abdominal migraine were twice as likely to have had migraine headaches as the general population.[173]

As a matter of assessment, there are no clear biologic markers or diagnostic tests to identify AMS as one specific cause of chronic abdominal pain in children. A technical report from the American Academy of Pediatrics Subcommittee and the North American Society for Pediatric Gastroenterology, Hepatology, and Nutrition Committee on Chronic Abdominal Pain identified that the presence of alarm symptoms or signs was associated with a higher prevalence of organic disease.[174] These symptoms included weight loss, gastrointestinal bleeding, persistent fever, persistent right upper or lower quadrant pain, chronic severe diarrhea, family history of inflammatory bowel disease, and significant vomiting, all of which justify the performance of diagnostic tests.[175]

In a study of ten adult migraineurs compared to controls who underwent gastric scintigraphy to determine gastric motility, the time to half empting was delayed during the migraine ictus in 78% and interictally in 80% of migraineurs compared to none of the controls.[175] This omnipresent and significant delay in gastric emptying in migraineurs compared to controls suggests that there may be a baseline underlying gastric autonomic dysregulation in migraineurs.[175]

Previous studies identifying higher rates of specific genetic polymorphisms in the serotonin transporter genes (5-HTTLPR and STin2) have been equivocal in adult migraneur populations.[120–122] Genotyping and allele distribution in a Hungarian pediatric migraine cohort ($n = 38$ with aura, $n = 49$ without aura) compared to controls ($n = 464$) also found no differences in allele distributions among groups.[176] This suggests that it is not associated with a predisposition to the disease. However, subgroup analyses demonstrated an association between STin2 (12,12 homozygote genotype) polymorphism and migraine with aura.[176] Furthermore, this genotype was associated with migraine characterized by excessive vomiting and severe abdominal pain.[176] Whether genotypes such as this will have relevance in AMS diagnosis in the future awaits further clarification; however, treatment for AMS with a 5-HT2A receptor antagonist, such as pizotifen (not approved for use in the United States), has shown benefit.[177]

Treatment for children with AMS has been suggested to follow several logical steps.[167] Explain and reassure parents and child that there is no serious abdominal pathology. Attempt to identify and avoid trigger mechanisms when present. Triggers can vary with each child and with each attack, but many children will identify specific instances with high likelihood of attack precipitation. These include stress from school and family dynamics, whether this be anxiety or anticipatory excitement; travel in a car or bus; prolonged fasting; sleep deprivation or excessive sleep times, particularly when there are erratic patterns; flickering or glaring lights and, in some instances, exercise.[167] Specific food avoidance, particularly those with high dietary amines, such as aged cheese, chocolate, preserved and processed meats, and caffeine, among others could be considered. Drug therapies are somewhat empiric with the exception of pizotifen, which showed benefit in a placebo-controlled crossover trial.[177] Retrospective analyses have identified both propranolol and cyproheptadine as beneficial, with fair to excellent response in 75%–83%.[178] Other agents such as triptans, alpha$_2$ receptor blockers, and valproate have also been tried.[167] Recent trials of flunarazine, a calcium channel blocker (not approved for use in the United States), was found to improve gastric emptying times, abdominal pain, headache, and vomiting.[179] In a report of two children who had suffered recurrent abdominal migraine attacks, one had attacks associated with aggressive behavior, confusion, and self-mutilation, and the second with associated biting, self-induced vomiting, and auditory hallucinations.[180] Each was treated with intravenous valproic acid with benefit in terms of both the abdominal pain and the ensuing behavioral changes.[180] These two case descriptions offer the opportunity to appreciate the spectrum of migraine symptoms associated with the periodic syndromes. These two subjects manifest symptomatology of both abdominal migraine and confusional migraine. Thus, the alteration in mental status displayed by some migraineurs with AMS may have genesis in the concept of an overlap migraine syndrome.

Benign Paroxysmal Vertigo

Benign paroxysmal vertigo (BPV) is a migraine variant seen in toddler-age children, with an average age of onset at 2–3 years with a range between 14 months and 10 years (Table 8-11).[181–184] Characteristically, these attacks of vertigo without headache are abrupt in onset and associated with sudden fear, apprehension, nausea, and pallid color. There is no loss of awareness and the child typically seeks out a parent or nearby stanchion for stability. The child will cling to the parent, unable to stand or walk steadily, and appear somewhat limp. Older children may describe acroparesthesiae and transient visual disturbances. If observed carefully, there may be jerk nystagmus of the eyes and a compensatory thrusting of the head. These attacks typically last 20–30 seconds to at most few minutes and may occur as frequently as several times

Table 8-11 2004 International Classification of Headache Disorders Criteria for Benign Paroxysmal Vertigo of Childhood 1.3.3

Description

This probably heterogeneous disorder is characterized by recurrent brief episodic attacks of vertigo occurring without warning and resolving spontaneously in otherwise healthy children.

Diagnostic Criteria:

- At least five attacks fulfilling criterion B
- Multiple episodes of severe vertigo (often associated with nystagmus or vomiting; unilateral throbbing headache may occur in some attacks), occurring without warning and resolving spontaneously after minutes to hours
- Normal neurological examination, and audiometric and vestibular functions between attacks
- Normal electroencephalogram

Source: Modified from Reference.[8]

per week but average about monthly. The individual attacks are self-limited and suddenly resolve without intervention. The attacks may be recurrent for several months to years but will usually spontaneously remit within 1–3 years. After early childhood, children with BPV will often evolve and begin to experience more readily identifiable migraine. Over 50%–70% of these children will have immediate family members who also experience migraine headache or recurrent vertigo.[181–184]

The BPV syndrome was first described in 1964 by Basser, who originally ascribed the phenomenon to vestibular neuritis.[181] Later authors began to associate the familial pattern and prevalence of symptoms typically associated with migraine headache.[182, 183] Early descriptions of BPV include reference to the paroxysmal dysequilibrium syndrome.[184] The prevalence of BPV is not well known. The estimated prevalence of BPV was identified as 0.6% (7/4237) in a compilation of EEG telemetry cohort samples, 2.4% (9/380) of a population referred for evaluation of non-epileptic phenomenon, and up to as high as 38% (41/108) in a general child neurology headache-referred migraneur cohort (see Chapter 1, Table 1-6).[68] The prevalence increases further when the population under study is drawn from smaller otorhinolaryngological specialty clinics, where among evaluations of vertiginous children, 19%–65% of children have migraine or BPV-induced vertiginous attacks.[184–190]

The underlying pathogenesis of the syndrome is not better understood than the association to mechanisms that produce migraine. Early studies of vestibular function utilizing the Hallpike method of cold water caloric testing and Barany chair postrotational nystagmus evaluation disclosed abnormal vestibular responses in all seventeen children (3–7 years old).[183]

Data from one general otolaryngology clinic revealed that from 24,580 referred patients with vertigo, pediatric subjects numbered only 98 (0.39%).[190]

Migraine, BPV, or benign paroxysmal torticollis (BPT) was the etiology in 34.7% (34/98) of all pediatric subjects. This later smaller cohort of thirty-four subjects was further studied. Migraine was diagnosed in 52.9% (18/34 subjects), BPV in 44.1% (15/34 subjects), and there was one case of BPT. Subsequent evaluations comparing these groups included audiology tests, electronystagmography studies (rotatory and caloric stimulation), dynamic posturography, CT, and MRI examination.[190] Neuroimaging studies were normal in all subjects. Hearing was impaired in seven subjects with concurrent otitis media and effusion.[190] The vertigo was rotatory in most subjects of all groups (66.6%); comparisons of the electronystagmography results between groups showed no differences.[190] The results prompted the authors to suggest that the etiology was of central origin and not a peripheral process.[190] Furthermore, the vertigo and torticollis may be generated from stimulation (ischemia) to the inferior vestibular nucleus that is prominent in young children, whereas nystagmus may be a symptom arising from stimulation to the more superior portions of the nucleus.[190]

In a more recent study, twenty children with BPV underwent caloric and vestibular-evoked myogenic potential (VEMP) tests to evaluate whether subjects with BPV demonstrate similar vestibular abnormalities as subjects with basilar artery migraine.[191] The VEMP reflects the sacculo-collic reflex, originating in the saccule and transmitted through the inferior vestibular nerve to the lateral vestibular nucleus via the medial vestibulospinal tract to the sternocleidomastoid muscle. Twenty BPV subjects and twenty controls underwent audiometry, caloric, and VEMP tests.[191] All subjects had normal hearing. Caloric testing revealed abnormal responses in 7/20 (35%) of BPV subjects, and VEMP testing was abnormal in 10/20 (50%) of BPV subjects.[191] Combined testing revealed that 70% of the studied children with BPV had abnormalities similar to and as frequent as the 75% frequency of abnormal testing noted in subjects with basilar-type migraine.[191] These two tests selectively evaluate the integrity of brainstem pathways extending from the inferior pons to the midbrain level. Disturbances in their reflex responses again suggest brainstem-initiated disturbances, not peripheral sensitivity as suggested earlier.[191]

Data from a prospective study of twenty-two children (seventeen girls) with BPV demonstrated some intriguing results.[192] The twenty-two subjects were followed clinically and with serial serum CPK-MB measurements over an average of 2.8 years after onset of symptoms at mean age of 17 months. The CPK measures were persistently elevated in all children (mean, 6.0 μg/L, normal <3 μg/L).[192] The elevation was not related to duration of symptoms, frequency of attacks, or time since last attack. Concurrent elevation of aspartate aminotransferase in 14/22 (64%) and normal cardiac troponin-I in 16/16 (100%) were obtained.[192] The measures normalized in 7/22 (32%) subjects, whose BPV spontaneously remitted during the study period.[192] The authors suggested a possible muscular involvement in BPV, however the reason or mechanism is not known.

ALTERNATING HEMIPLEGIA OF CHILDHOOD

Alternating hemiplegia of childhood (AHC) is a rare and dramatic non-epileptic syndrome of children that causes recurrent attacks of hemiplegia and progressive neurological deficits.[193,194] Since the first description in 1971 by Verret and Steele, diagnostic criteria have been proposed and considerable research has been undertaken to uncover the pathophysiologic mechanism(s).[195] In their original report of the syndrome, eight children as young as 3 months old were described as having intermittent abrupt onset alternating hemiplegic events lasting several hours to days and up to 3 weeks in duration.[195] All eight of the children had a parent with migraine of whom four had hemiplegic migraines.[195] Common features of their attacks included abdominal pain and vomiting; however, only four ever had concurrent headache. These acephalgic events persisted despite repeated attacks of hemiplegia with intermittent paroxysmal dystonic and tonic spells. Four children also experienced "minor" attacks consisting of choreo-athetosis.[195] Because during attacks all children had normal EEG, or only slowing contralateral to the hemiplegia on repeated recordings, with no abnormalities identified on cerebral arteriogram or CFS examinations, a vascular ischemic mechanism was postulated.[195] Remarkable to the authors was the poor outcome attained with an eventual development of cognitive impairment, movement disorders, and epileptic seizures identified in 50% of the children.[195]

The diagnostic criteria for this syndrome have evolved over the decades since Verret and Steele initially called attention to AHC. With the recognition of additional children who displayed "complicated migraine syndromes," and poor cognitive outcomes, combined with the observation of complex ocular nystagmus and dystonic posturing in conjunction with hemiplegic events, Krageloh and Aicardi proposed that AHC was an entity distinct from hemiplegic migraine, specifically characterized by the affected child's poor neurological and cognitive outcomes.[196–198] These criteria were again updated at an international symposium in 1991, after worldwide clinical experience with the disorder had broadened.[194] The underlying pathophysiology and other hypothetical etiopathological considerations were further critically debated in a subsequent international conference in 1997.[199] High priority was given to the identification of candidate genes associated with the disorder as it was likely a result of contributions from both genetic and environmental influences.[199] A consideration was asserted that AHC may represent a type of mitochondropathy, cerebrovascular disorder, or channelopathy, potentially exploitable by modern neuroimaging and genetic analysis, and additional future investigational directions (see discussion below).[199] The possibility that AHC is not a single disorder but mechanistically heterogeneous remains a viable hypothesis.

The most recent iteration of current diagnostic criteria can be found within the ICHD-II (Table 8-12). Despite a rather profound clinical presentation, very little pathophysiologic abnormality is identified on both routine

Table 8-12 2004 International Classification of Headache Disorders Criteria Alternating Hemiplegia of Childhood. A1.3.4

Description

Infantile attacks of hemiplegia involving each side alternately, associated with a progressive encephalopathy, other paroxysmal phenomena, and mental impairment.

Diagnostic Criteria:

- Recurrent attacks of hemiplegia alternating between the two sides of the body.
- Onset before the age of 18 months.
- At least one other paroxysmal phenomenon is associated with the bouts of hemiplegia or occurs independently, such as tonic spells, dystonic posturing, choreoathetoid movements, nystagmus or other ocular motor abnormalities, or autonomic disturbances.
- Evidence of mental and/or neurological deficit(s).
- Not attributed to another disorder.

Source: Modified from Reference[8] Appendix.

and more sophisticated laboratory, neurophysiological, and neuroradiological examination.[199] Clinical attacks may begin in infancy (<3 months) but always before the age of 18 months. The recognition of these early symptoms may be overlooked if brief or ascribed to intercurrent illness, especially when this manifestation takes on a tonic or dystonic posture.[193, 194, 200] Writhing movements associated with crying have been described, but individual children will vary in their unique attack presentation. An important characteristic of the attacks in most affected children is the beneficial response to the induction of sleep.[193, 194] Although sleep will induce remission from an attack, there is often resumption into one upon awakening 20–30 minutes later.

Hallmark paroxysmal features of attacks are provided in Tables 8-13 and 8-14. The paroxysmal features of an infantile attack are more usually manifest by a tonic or dystonic spell.[193, 194, 200] This can be brief or more prolonged and heralded by a scream and crying. Other paroxysmal features can also be observed during the same episode, particularly nystagmus, which often leads to the incorrect inference that this is epileptic in origin. These more complex events will later evolve into hemiplegic events either prior to or immediately after the paroxysmal features surface.[193, 194, 200] It is uncommon for hemiplegia to be the initial or sole manifestation and persist unaccompanied by other features after the disorder establishes recurrence. The sequence of hypotonia-nystagmus-hemiplegia usually gives way to hemiplegic attacks alone. The hemiplegia has been observed for short and prolonged intervals. When there are prolonged events (several hours to days), shifting hemiplegia is usually observed, involving bilateral sides and affecting bulbar function.[193, 194, 200] Prominent drooling and difficulty in swallowing are experienced. The hemiplegia has been observed to affect the upper extremity to a greater degree than the lower and can be quite flaccid in tone. Despite this degree of weakness,

Table 8-13 Alternating Hemiplegia: Paroxysmal Clinical Characteristics – A

Hemiplegic Attacks (100%):

Onset: <18 months old

Prodrome: moodiness, autonomic changes with flushing, pallor, sweating, nausea and vomiting

Provocation: cold, excitement, fatigue, bathing, light, minor intercurrent illness, minor head trauma

Frequency: variable with infrequent attacks at onset and gradual escalation to biweekly and up to 20 times/month

Duration: from 20 minutes to 21 days (the duration is individually consistent for subsequent attacks)

Topography: predominantly unilateral, but may shift side-to-side or display bilateral plegia during individual attacks.

- Unilateral:
  Head and eye deviation toward the paretic side
  Complex gaze dysfunction (monocular nystagmus with impaired gaze)
- Shifting:
  Expressionless, fluctuating severity w/o ocular signs
- Bilateral (90%):
  Neck hypotonia evolves to complete paralysis, expressionless facies, drooling, irregular breathing, blinking and normal ocular movement. There may be fluctuating severity with tonic/dystonic posturing.

Source: Modified from References.[110, 191–196, 198]

children attempt to function and may be observed to have dystonic tremor affecting the hemiplegic limbs. An outstanding feature of AHC is the ocular motor manifestations. The unusual and complex combinations of nystagmus can be quite remarkable, with some children displaying a continually changing pattern of nystagmoid activity during a single observation period. Monocular horizontal coarse jerk nystagmus would appear to be the most prominent; however, all descriptions appear possible either in isolation or in a constant metamorphosis state.[193, 194] Prominent vasomotor instability and respiratory distress and irregularity can be at times compromising and force invasive supportive interventions.[193, 194, 200] Compounding these already complex symptoms is the additional possible occurrence of epileptic seizures in about half of affected children.[193, 194, 200] The hemiplegic attacks escalate in frequency over the first 5–10 years, then plateau but rarely remit completely. In addition, children with AHC will be burdened with other nonparoxysmal symptoms (Table 8-15). These are comprised by significant degrees of hypotonia, ataxia, and involuntary movements.[193, 194, 200] These will surface over the early period of 3–5 years after onset. Developmental and cognitive delays evolve over time until it becomes apparent that a progressive neurocognitive decline has occurred, with an eventual plateau.[193, 194, 200] The hemiplegic attacks

Table 8-14 Alternating Hemiplegia: Paroxysmal Clinical Characteristics – B

Paroxysmal Nystagmus (>90%):

- Horizontal plane more often than vertical, but both may occur within the same attack.
- Large amplitude more often than fine amplitude, but both may occur within the same attack.
- Monocular more often than binocular and associated with strabismus, both may occur within the same attack or in different attacks. The nystagmus, whether monocular or binocular, has a fast component that beats toward the hemiplegic or tonic side.
- Rotatory component can be observed as the attack evolves.
- Gaze disturbances can be appreciated, with relative paresis or deviation of up-gaze, down-gaze, and horizontal-gaze, with frequently observed dysconjugate gaze.

Paroxysmal Autonomic Phenomenon (>70%):

- Dyspnea and hyperpnea.
- Vasomotor blanching or flushing of the face or one limb, unilateral segment or trunk involved in the attack (60%).
- Clammy or cold skin associated with the vasomotor instability.
- Profuse diaphoresis.
- Mydriasis to a much greater frequency than miosis.
- Diarrhea and or abdominal distension.

Tonic or Dystonic Attacks (90%):

- Usually begin early (<4 months old).
- Tonic contractions, with vibratory tremor of one limb or side and ipsilateral head turning.
- Often accompanied by a scream or crying.

Source: Modified from References.[110, 191, 196, 198]

Table 8-15 Alternating Hemiplegia: Non-Paroxysmal Clinical Characteristics – C

Non-Paroxysmal Features:

- Hypotonia (20%–60%)
- Choreo-athetosis (45%–60%)
- Ataxia and truncal instability (11%–22%)
- Delayed global developmental milestones (45%–80%)
- Delayed cognitive development and mental retardation (85%–95%)
- Epileptic seizures (45%–60%)

Source: Modified from References.[110, 191, 196, 198]

are commonly identified by parents as having been provoked by emotional stress and excitement (55%–61%), fatigue (45%), minor trauma, particularly head bumps (38%), bathing or high activity levels (32%), cold weather (29%), and illness (13%), among others.[194, 200] The profound neurological deficits especially those of complex nystagmus, autonomic disturbances and alterations of tone and posture suggest preferential pathophysiological effects within the anatomic region of Mollarette's triangle (cerebello-rubro-olivary tract) circuitry.

Cerebral ischemia attributed to complicated migraine was the mechanism initially postulated for AHC.[195] Numerous case studies utilizing both standard (brain MRI, CT, angiography) and advanced (SPECT, PET) neuroimaging techniques, however, have failed to strongly support this mechanism or conclusively advance underlying cerebrovascular dysfunction.[195, 199] Other investigated mechanisms involving concurrent investigations of intermediate metabolism, evoked potentials, brain, and muscle MRI spectroscopy (MRS) studies have revealed essentially normal or transiently abnormal results during ictal hemiplegia. Similarly, although EEG recordings have demonstrated only hemispheric slowing or normal findings ictally, an epileptic mechanism is not operative. SPECT scans have shown somewhat contradictory results, rarely demonstrating increased flow, or more often decreased flow in the hemisphere contralateral to the hemiplegia, with other reports showing no change at all.[194, 201–204] PET scans have only been obtained in few patients. FDG (2-deoxy-2[^{18}F]-fluoro-D-glucose) PET studies have shown single or multiple areas of relative hypometabolism.[194, 199] Studies with [^{11}C]-flumazenil PET for benzodiazepine receptor binding in one patient showed increased binding in the hemisphere contralateral to the hemiplegia. Increased serotonin synthesis in the frontal and mediolateral temporal cortices of the striatum and thalamus was shown in two other children studied with [^{11}C]-α-methyltryptophan PET for regional serotonin synthesis.[199] Data from six additional patients with AHC studied in the ictal or pos-tictal state using alpha[^{11}C]methyl-L-tryptophan PET showed increased serotonin synthesis capacity in the frontal-parietal cortex, lateral, and medial temporal structures, striatum, and thalamus when compared to controls and subjects studied interictally.[205] Increased whole-brain serotonin synthesis capacity (reported in migraine subjects without aura) was not found in these children with AHC. What these data imply in total from a pathophysiologic perspective is that the existence of a neuronal and cellular disturbance is primary. Furthermore, there may be important differences in results stemming from the timing of these studies relative to the age of onset of the attacks. This needs to be taken into consideration interpretively. Progressive neuronal dysfunction and functional decline may be reflected in abnormal functional imaging studies, such as these, only in children with a more advanced disease process. More sensitive or even different evaluative measures altogether may be needed to identify neuronal dysfunction in real time during an ictal attack of AHC.

Phosphorous MRS of muscle has been performed on nine AHC subjects.[206,207] Abnormally high-resonance intensities from inorganic phosphate and low phosphocreatine coupled with low calculated cytosolic phosphorylation potentials and low-resonance intensities from phosphocreatine coupled with an abnormally high calculated cytosolic-free adenosine diphosphate concentrations have been found.[206] Using ^{31}P MRS, five subjects with AHC, aged 8–30 years old (mean age 18 years), compared to matched controls, were studied at rest, during incremental aerobic exercise, and at recovery.[207] There were no significant differences in resting muscle between subjects and controls.[207] However, exercise performance was reduced in AHC subjects to only 30% of normal duration.[207] During recovery, both the initial rate of phosphocreatine resynthesis and calculated mitochondrial capacity were reduced by about 35%, which implied a mitochondrial cause of the exercise deficiency.[207] How these findings in muscle relate to the CNS neurological manifestations require extrapolation and further study. There is a single report of a brain MRS study in another subject with AHC during an attack, which revealed elevated brain lactate concentration.[208] Nezu et al. reported on a subject with AHC who was followed for over 23 years and studied at age 24 years.[209] Brain proton MR spectroscopy interictally was normal, with no abnormal lactate peak despite significant neurological impairments. There was diffuse hypoperfusion identified on ^{123}I-IMP SPECT with normal MRI and MR angiography.[209] Brain MRS of selected grey and white matter regions ipsilateral and contralateral to the hemiplegia in addition to SPECT scanning in one additional patient with AHC were both normal during an attack (DiMario FJ, unpublished data). These combined studies suggest that there may be a component of mitochondrial dysfunction, possibly primary but more likely secondary, although the evidence is scant.

Biopsy findings of skin and muscle vascular smooth muscle cells studied from four AHC subjects have shown intracytoplasmic vacuoles, osmiophilic deposits, and apoptotic nuclei of undetermined significance.[210] A neurovascular mechanism similar to cerebral autosomal-dominant arteriopathy with subcortical infarcts and leukoencephalopathy (CADASIL) was proposed to explain the ultrastructural findings, but these would have to be confirmed in brain as well.[211] The reported findings may, however, serve as a possible biomarker for AHC if confirmed. More subtle regional disturbances in neurophysiologic function may be evident even in the absence of structural disease. Support for this comes from recent studies of six children with AHC who underwent neurophysiologic testing with evoked potentials.[212] These measures identified no abnormalities in somatosensory or motor-evoked potentials; however, the blink reflex recording demonstrated significantly longer ($p < 0.01$) latencies of both the ipsilateral (iR2) and contralateral (cR2) R2 components during the interictal phase compared to normal controls.[212] Furthermore, during the ictal phase, after stimulation of the hemiplegic side, the ipsilateral R2 latency was significantly decreased compared with the results obtained during the interictal phase ($p < 0.05$).[212] These resultant abnormalities suggest baseline and transiently augmented disturbances in brainstem function. Thus far, however, neuropathology has been limited and etiologically unrevealing.[213] Muscle studies examining mitochondria and respiratory chain enzymes have also been normal.[214]

The rationale for a probable genetic cause has been suggested by sibships and identical twins concordant for AHC, autosomal dominant transmission, and affected half-siblings.[213-216] Genetic evaluations have identified a single family with a balanced translocation [46XY, t(3;9)(p26;q34)] in the affected child.[215] Because of the obvious clinical similarities between AHC and familial hemiplegic migraine and episodic ataxia syndromes, the *CACNA1A* gene has been investigated and found to be normal.[204] The *ATP1A2* has been investigated and mutations identified in the α-2 subunit in several kindreds with AHC, migraine, and seizures are now published.[130,204,217,218] A recently described subject with severe neurological deficits and a presentation consistent with AHC, but described as FHM, has been identified with a mutation in the SLC1A3 gene.[141] This encodes for the excitatory amino acid transporter 1 (EAAT1), which is critical for the clearance of glutamate from the synaptic clefts.[141] This proposed disturbance in glutamate clearance might serve as an additional mechanism for consideration in the pathophysiology of AHC. A benign variety has also recently been described (see Chapter 7).[219]

The long-term outcomes of affected children with AHC have generally been poor. The progressive decline across all neurocognitive function domains is insidious and manifest early. In combining and summarizing the outcomes of sixty-four subjects reported with the age of onset <18 months, follow-up over 3–29 years, in three outcome studies, the following can be stated: (1) 20/64 (31%) developed epilepsy; (2) 59/64 (92%) had abnormal neurological examinations demonstrating hypotonia, choreo-athetosis, dystonia, predominantly with lesser degrees of ataxia, and hemiparesis; (3) 29/64 (45%) were judged to have mild cognitive impairment; and (4) 35/64 (55%) had moderate-to-severe cognitive impairments.[193,200,220] The only consistently reported beneficial treatment has been with flunarazine (5–20 mg/day), a calcium channel blocker (unapproved by the FDA for use in the United States).[200,220,221] These results are not from randomized clinical trials, however, but are from unblinded parental assessments. This agent does not prevent attacks but rather has been able to reduce the severity and duration of attacks in 50% and decrease the frequency of attacks in 25%.[200,220-222] A few patients have responded to amantadine (4–8 mg/kg/day).[223] Numerous other agents, particularly antiepileptic drugs, have been tried with little clear success on ameliorating the hemiplegic attacks.[222] The author has utilized trihexaphenidyl (6–30 mg/day) with some benefit in two children.

Important considerations for the care of children affected with AHC involves the attention to avoidance of identified triggers, the early induction of sleep when attacks develop, targeted treatment for coexistent epilepsy,

and possible use of calcium channel-blockers, particularly flunarizine.[222] AHC
may have heterogeneous mechanisms, however; the current evidence suggests
a channelopathy as a probable mechanism with mitochondrial and vascular
mechanisms as possible contributors.[194,199,206,210,215]

Benign Paroxysmal Torticollis of Infancy

Benign paroxysmal torticollis (BPT) is defined as self-limited, recurrent,
stereotyped episodes of torticollis without lateral predilection, often associated with pallor, hypotonia, vomiting, and apathy (Table 8-16). A number
of clinical series have been published over time discerning clinical characteristics of this rather infrequent periodic syndrome of childhood.[67,224-233] The
prevalence of BPT is not well known. The estimated prevalence of BPT was as
high as 10.1% (11/108) from one general child neurology headache-referred
migraneur cohort of periodic syndromes.[67]

There is no loss of awareness when a typical attack of torticollis occurs, but
an unsteady gait and trunkal instability with resistance to head straightening
are notable. The child will generally turn to either side randomly upon subsequent events and only up to about 20%–25% of infants will preferentially be
noted to assume torticollis to one side over the other.[224-233] Some infants will
assume incurved truncal positions reminiscent of dystonia or tonic seizures.

**Table 8-16 2004 International Classification of Headache Disorders Criteria for
Benign Paroxysmal Torticollis of Childhood A1.3.5**

Description
Recurrent episodes of head tilt to one side, perhaps with slight rotation, which remit
spontaneously. The condition occurs in infants and small children, with onset in the first
year. It may evolve into 1.3.3 benign paroxysmal vertigo of childhood or 1.2 migraine with
aura, or cease without further symptoms.

Diagnostic criteria:
1. Episodic attacks, in a young child, with all of the following characteristics, and
   fulfilling criterion 2:
   a. tilting of the head to one side (not always the same side), with or without
      slight rotation
   b. lasting minutes to days
   c. remitting spontaneously, and tending to recur monthly
2. During attacks, symptoms and/or signs of one or more of the following:

   a. pallor
   b. irritability
   c. malaise
   d. vomiting
   e. ataxia*
3. Normal neurological examination between attacks
4. Not attributed to another disorder

Source: Modified from Reference[8] Appendix.
* Ataxia is more likely in older children within the affected age group.

Concurrent awkward trunk and pelvic postures with frank ataxia while the toddler attempts to walk have been described as the primary manifestations after several episodes of more limited torticollis have occurred.[225] There is no associated pain or clear discomfort associated with most of the events, which may help to distinguish them from posturing, associated with posterior fossa structural causes. However, young children may appear ill with pallid color, sweating, and vomiting, whereas in the older child, an unsteady gait and fearful appearance may predominate. More rarely, hypotonia and gaze deviations may be noted. More typical features associated with migraine, such as photophobia, phonophobia, and lethargy are much less usual but occasionally present.[232]

Parents identify trigger mechanisms in up to a third of the subjects reported.[232] The episodes may last from minutes to several hours, but as long as 3–4 days (60%) and, less usually, 1–2 weeks (<40%), with recurrences one to three times per month common.[224–228, 232, 233] Sleep can often help terminate the event. Most children (>50%) who develop BPT do so within the first 3 months of life, but onset before age 3 years is expected.[224–227, 232, 233]

In combining several smaller series, girls appear to be more often affected than boys in a ratio of 3:2. In most children there is either ultimate resolution (60%–70%) or evolution into paroxysmal vertigo or more typical migraine headaches after age 5 years (30%–40%).[224–233] This is in keeping with the fact that there is often a family history of similar events (<5%) or family members having migraine headaches (40%), which implies a possible genetic link.[225, 228, 231–233]

A surface EMG study of one child during an episode disclosed continuous electrical discharges within the contracted ipsilateral sternocleidomastoid and contralateral trapezius muscles, which suggests that the torticollis is indeed dystonic in origin.[234] It should be remembered that dystonia can be an atypical motor aura prior to migraine. The relationship to vestibular dysfunction remains a possibility as suggested by previous abnormalities in auditory and vestibular function testing.[224, 225]

Reports of several children are now available with family histories of hemiplegic migraine with ataxia.[235] In these subjects the propensity for atypical auras is usual and important in that calcium channel dysfunction has been suggested to contribute to its development. *CACN1A* gene mutations on chromosome 19 have been found in more than half of the families with hemiplegic migraine and episodic ataxia syndromes.[235] These syndromes have both shared symptoms and calcium channel dysfunction with the potential involvement of the cerebellum in common. This structure has been postulated to serve as the genesis of the dystonia associated with BPT. Now two children with BPT, within a family whose members had migraine with ataxia and hemiplegia and migraine without aura, have been found to harbor the *CACNA1A* mutation.[236] How this genetic mutation is related to BPT remains speculative. The author suggests a link to cerebellar dysfunction as seen in experimental models.[236] Also plausible may be the relationship of these channel disturbances with the genesis of migraine aura during cortical spreading depression and possible effects upon subcortical motor systems and the basal ganglia in particular.

Neuroimaging, CSF analysis, and neurotransmitter measurement as well as EEG recordings are generally normal and are not routinely required in an otherwise normal child with typical features. When the onset is in the neonatal age range or additional clinical findings are present, laboratory and neuroradiological evaluation may be needed. No specific treatment is of proven benefit; however, prophylaxis with antimigraine therapies has been commonly utilized.

Other Considerations

Migraine and its variants together with the well-defined periodic syndromes of childhood make up a vast proportion of the clinical problems encountered by general pediatric practitioners and specialists alike. In this closing section, a brief mention will be made of several additional periodic phenomena not as often encountered but nonetheless important to identify.

Paroxysmal headache and transient neurological deficits are the sine quo non of migraine with aura and other "complex migraine" entities. Migraine can be precipitated by a number factors that result in prodromes associated with (1) psychological symptoms (e.g.), mood depression, mood elevation, hyperactivity, irritability, drowsiness, restlessness, and others; (2) neurological symptoms (e.g.), inattention, dysphasia, heightened sense of smell, taste, and sound; and (3) systemic symptoms (e.g., meningismus, anorexia, hunger, intestinal upset, diarrhea/constipation, thermal sensitivity, thirst, urination, fluid retention, and lethargy. These prodromal symptoms are then often followed by the aura with altered visual perception, scotoma, general sensory disturbances, olfactory hallucinations, motor impairments (weakness, ataxia, posturing), language dysfunction, psychic phenomena, and impaired consciousness and memory. These symptoms ultimately evolve prior to headache, and in the case of children, the headache is often inconsequential or nonexistent. Hence the "migraine equivalents" become an important category of neurological dysfunction appreciated in children, especially the youngest of them. Equally important and often the most difficult to categorize are the myriad of autonomic symptoms that often accompany these equivalents or present as isolated paroxysmal symptoms.

As children age this phenomenon of associated paroxysmal symptoms remains evident but transformed such that in adults the most commonly associated manifestation of autonomic dysfunction with migraine is syncope. The only population-based study to date to address this coexistence is from the Netherlands, the CAMERA study (Cerebral Abnormalities in Migraine, an Epidemiologic Risk Analysis study).[237] Results from 6491 adults have demonstrated an elevated lifetime prevalence of both syncope and orthostatic intolerance among migraineurs, even in the presence of normal interictal autonomic function, compared to controls that did not have migraine.[237] Syncope was noted in up to 45% of women and 41% of all migraneurs compared to 31% controls ($p = 0.001$), and orthostatic intolerance was identified in 32% of migraineurs compared to only 12% controls ($p<0.001$).[237] These results suggest that migraine sufferers have an intrinsic propensity to dysautonomic symptomatology over and above the neurological disturbances associated with the migraine itself.

Episodic Spontaneous Recurrent Hypothermia is an infrequently encountered and rarely reported periodic syndrome of childhood. This syndrome may be recognized as Shapiro's syndrome, after the author who, in 1969, called attention to the phenomenon in association with agenesis of the corpus callosum and surgical sectioning of the callosum in the absence of hypothalamic dysfunction.[238] There has been reference to this syndrome as a diencephalic seizure, but epileptic discharges have not been demonstrated in conjunction with symptoms. Since its initial descriptions, variations on the components have been described. For the purposes of this discussion, the periodic syndrome of spontaneous recurrent hypothermia is without midline brain lesion or associated endocrinopathy as noted in children and adults.[239, 240]

Thus, as the name implies, these are children (and adults) who experience spontaneous episodes of hypothermia, with body temperatures ≤34°C–35°C, generally associated with hyperhydrosis, and less consistently with the additional symptoms of bradycardia, pallor, hypertension, somnolence, abdominal pain, and headache. The events are first manifest between the ages of 2 and 5 years, but children as young as 2 months and as old as 12 years have been reported.[239, 241–243] These are recurrent events with a periodicity as often as 2–4 times per month, lasting from 1 hour to 4–5 days. Most reported children experience less than 12–24 hours of symptoms, with many manifesting symptoms for only 1–4 hours. There has been little physiological study applied to unraveling the genesis of this syndrome, but importantly, normal neuroimaging studies have been obtained, thus excluding midline structural CNS lesions as prerequisites.[241, 243] Although it may be associated with more diffuse encephalopathy as seen in cerebral palsy with heterogeneous etiologies, the periodic syndrome can be identified in otherwise normal children without any neurodevelopmental disorder or disease.

One important observation made during the onset of hypothermic episodes is the fact that sweating and not shivering is present despite the degree of lowered body temperature experienced.[242] Shivering may be noted later in the course of the event. This infers that a dysregulation in the normal physiologic thermoregulatory response and maintenance of core temperature is operative. The observed sweating during the initial period of hypothermia has been explained as contributing to the cooling of core temperature. This sequence is opposite of that observed in infectious processes, where shivering serves to escalate core body temperature and sweating counteracts this.[244] A dysfunction in serotonergic regulation has been suggested as an explanation, as it is a primary neurotransmitter involved in the regulation of body temperature, serotonergic syndromes incorporate similar symptomatology, and cyproheptadine (antiserotonergic properties) has been used as a successful treatment.[239]

A clear understanding of the pathophysiologic mechanism of episodic spontaneous recurrent hypothermia awaits further study and identification. No definitive treatment is suggested. Combinations of centrally acting sympathetolytic, antidopaminergic (clonidine, gabapentin, chlorpromazine, and levodopa-carbidopa), and antiserotonergic (cyproheptadine) compounds deserve trials.[244–246]

Sympathetic storms are a related phenomenon consisting of sympathetic hyperactivity manifest by periodic hypertension, tachycardia, hyperpnea, hyperhydrosis, agitation with less evident tremor or posturing, bruxism, vasomotor instability, lacrimation, mydriasis/miosis, and nystagmus.[247–253] Although paroxysmal sympathetic hyperactivity predominate the clinical picture, bradycardia and hypothermia (similar to or confused with Shapiro's syndrome) may emerge. Penfield had also referred to these episodes as diencephalic seizures initially, in 1929, although an epileptic mechanism is not evident.[248]

Common to all reported cases is the presence of hydrocephalus, diencephalic tumor, or lesion secondary to trauma or surgery.[247–255] Activation or disinhibition of central sympathetic pathways would seem the likely mechanism, especially with evident diencephalic lesions of various types.[251,254] A review of seven such cases by Goh et al., with the addition of a 7- and a 21-year-old (four cases between 1 and 21 years old), failed to show epileptiogenic activity during storming episodes.[247,249,254] Similar dysautonomic symptoms are regularly observed after diffuse axonal injury, compounded by hypoxic ischemic encephalopathy during rehabilitative hospitalization stays.[254,255] In this context, one study compiled outcomes of subjects with traumatic brain injury with diffuse axonal injury and hypoxic ischemic encephalopathy, and compared those subjects with sympathetic storms to a matched comparator control group without them.[255] Analysis revealed significantly longer rehabilitation hospital stays, and longer periods of both posttraumatic amnesia and chronic amnesia.[255] Furthermore, the group with dysautonomia had poorer Glasgow outcome scores and lesser improvements in functional independence measures at time of discharge.[255] The course of the dysautonomia appears to take on a predictable timetable when it develops after traumatic brain injury.[255] Phase 1 presymptomatic phase ends when sedation and paralytic agents are stopped. Phase 2 evolves from that point and incorporate the set of symptoms described previously. This phase may endure over a range of weeks (mean 74 days, range 15–204 days); its termination is marked by the termination of hyperhydrotic periods.[255] One additional report noted the paroxysms to continue for over 1 year.[254]

The paroxysmal dysautonomic storms represent disruption of the integrated central autonomic system within the diencephalon and brainstem. Specific disinhibitory impact centering around the sympathetoexcitatory regions including the paraventricular hypothalamic nucleus, lateral periaqueductal grey matter, lateral parabrachial nucleus, and rostral ventrolateral medulla are likely responsible.[251,254] These effects can be intermittently exaggerated with increases in intracranial pressure.[251]

Treatment is aimed at reducing the potentially injurious effects of a hypersympathetic state, particularly hyperthermia. Centrally acting sympathetolytic, dopaminergic, and antiserotonergic compounds may again be useful but are empiric. Commonly utilized substances include benzodiazepines, bromocriptine, and morphine; carbidopa-levodopa, alpha2 adrenergic receptor antagonists; nonselective beta-adrenergic antagonists; and selective alpha1-, beta1-, and beta2-adrenergic receptor blockers.[251,255–257] A recent trial of gabapentin therapy coupled with intrathecal baclofen has also been successful.[256]

Stroke-Like Migraine Attacks after Radiation Therapy (SMART syndrome) is a recognizable clinical syndrome that occurs typically several years after the completion of cranial irradiation.[258–263] This is a unique sequela apparent mainly in children, but also in adults, after treatment with high-dose cranial irradiation ($\geq$5000 cGy) for intracranial neoplasm. Symptoms are similar to migraine with visual aura with additional complicating neurological deficits. These deficits include expressive aphasia, confusion, homonymous hemianopsia, hemiparesis, hemisensory disturbances, dysesthesias, clumsiness, and lateralized headache. The symptoms gradually resolve often over a period of hours to —days, but have been present for as long as 3 weeks.[261] The syndrome appears to result uniquely after treatment to those malignancies confined to the posterior fossa and pineal region. These were initially referred to as a "complicated migraine-like episodes," but with recognition of the symptoms and recent examination with modern neuroimaging techniques, ongoing damage to the posterior circulation and brainstem has been suggested.[258,262,263]

Symptoms have been reported to develop as early as 14 months after cranial irradiation to as long as 21 years later.[262,263] Although the majority of reports describe children who had undergone treatment for the neoplasm and subsequently developed symptoms, there has been only one subject who was 23 years old when the cranial irradiation was first given.[262] This raises speculation as to whether there may be some vulnerability for children and protection for adults undergoing similar posterior fossa treatment.

Extensive evaluations to identify recurrent tumor, stroke, concurrent seizure, and vasculopathy have been unrewarding. Diagnostic considerations of carcinomatous meningitis, tumor recurrence, vasculitis, subarachnoid hemorrhage, venous thrombosis, cerebral ischemia, seizures, and encephalitis are often contemplated. EEG recording has demonstrated attenuation over the hemisphere corresponding to the symptoms but without epileptiform activity.[262] MRI utilizing fluid-attenuated inversion recovery (FLAIR), T_2, and diffusion-weighted sequences usually reflect no changes from the subject's baseline findings. However, gyral thickening and cortical enhancement have been evident during attacks, with resolution of these MRI findings at follow-up in several subjects.[259–263] Use of [^{18}F]-fluoro-D-glucose (FDG) PET studies in two subjects during an attack revealed intense cortical hyperactivity corresponding to gyral hyperintensity identified on MRI.[263] Each abnormality resolved in a short interval at follow-up when the subject was back to baseline.

The underlying mechanism of this syndrome is not known. Whether there is an underlying accumulated vascular endothelial injury, triggering effect upon the trigeminovascular system, alteration to mitochondria or membrane ion channels is speculative. The identification of CNS angiomas, siderosis, and hearing loss in a subject as a result of cranial irradiation may serve as marker for increased risk of the syndrome.[263] Treatment has been empiric, with steroids given most commonly and short-term anticonvulsants offered without clear indication.

Trauma-Induced Migraine

Minor head trauma, such as that acquired in sporting events and not resulting in concussion (immediate loss of consciousness or amnesia), may trigger migraine with aura several minutes afterward.[264–266] These migraine attacks have been sometimes referred to as "footballer's migraine," after the trauma experienced with "heading" a soccer ball.[266–269] The precipitated events classically develop after a symptom-free interval and begin with typical visual aura symptoms and or motor weakness, sensory disturbances with or without brainstem signs of diplopia, vertigo, or facial paresthesias. The aura can take on more profound symptoms of basilar artery migraine syndrome with associated nausea, vomiting, confusion, ataxia, limb paresthesias, myoclonus, somnolence, and headache.[270] Rarely cortical blindness with preserved pupillary light responses have been reported.[271,272] This evolution of symptoms is often erroneously attributed to an epileptic seizure, concussion, or intracranial hemorrhage. An arterial dissection is always a consideration with acute neurological deficits in the young. It is important, however, to differentiate short duration neurologic deficits (<24 hours) from more prolonged deficits.[272] In the later scenario, intracranial contusion is a more common explanation.[272]

Minor trauma-induced migraine is well documented in children and has been less frequently identified in adults.[263–266] The aura symptoms evolve over 30–40 minutes, with subsequent headache persisting for up to 24 hours and spontaneous resolution. There is a high propensity for repeated migraine events upon subsequent minor head trauma as well as spontaneous migraines without trauma in a minority.[264,265] Cerebrovasospasm triggering the cortical spreading depression phenomenon has been suggested as a mechanism, but recent evidence for trigeminovascular activation and reactive hyperemia without cerebral edema may also be operative.[273,274] Head collisions is not a prerequisite, as symptoms of basilar artery migraine and confusional migraine syndromes can also develop after whiplash-type injuries.[275,276] Hemiplegic migraines have also been associated with coughing paroxysms in cystic fibrosis.[277] The hemiplegic migraine precipitated by minor trauma should also provoke consideration of possible sporadic hemiplegic migraine syndrome with *CACNA1A* gene mutations and alternating hemiplegia syndrome if it occurs in toddlers (see above).[140,200]

Treatment Approaches for Migraine

The treatment of migraine in children follows parallel approaches as for adults. A number of evidence-based reviews are available on this topic, including guidance from the American Academy of Neurology Quality Standards Subcommittee and the Practice Committee of the Child Neurology Society. Principles of migraine management are offered in succeeding sections. A summary of commonly prescribed nonpharmacologic, acute, and preventative pharmacologic therapies is provided in the accompanying tables (Tables 8-17, 8-18, and 8-19). It is important to note, however, that despite the number of treatment options available, there is a paucity of well-designed,

Table 8-17 Non-Pharmacologic Migraine Therapy

Identification and Elimination of Migraine Triggers
Regular exercise
Regular and adequate sleep schedule

Dietary Interventions
Avoidance of fasting
Limitation of stimulants (caffeine, etc.)
Avoidance of food sensitivities (aged cheese, chocolate, processed meats, strong smells)
Herbal interventions (feverfew, ginkgo balboa)
Vitamin and minerals (riboflavin, magnesium)

Biofeedback Training
Thermal

Relaxation Techniques
Meditation
Self-hypnosis

Stress Management
Yoga
Guided imagery
Massage therapy

Acupuncture
Aromatherapy

Source: Modified from References.[278,279]

Table 8-18 Acute Pharmacologic Migraine Therapy Studied in Randomized Placebo-Controlled or Open Trials

Drug	Onset of Action	Dosage	Efficacy (Approximate)	Ages Studied (RPCT or OT)
Acetaminophen	PO: 30 min to 1 hr	10–15 mg/kg	PO: 54%	4–16 years old
Ibuprofen	PO: 30 min to 1hr	7.5–10 mg/kg	PO: 68%–76%	4–16 years old
Dihydroergotamine	PO: 2 hrs	PO: 20–40 mcg/kg	PO: 58%	5–15 years old
Sumatriptan	PO: 1–3 hrs	PO: 50–100 mg	PO: 30% @ 2 hrs	8–16 years old
	SQ: 15 min to 1 hr	SQ: 3–6 mg	SQ: 64%–78% @ 2 hrs	6–18 years old
	IN: 15–60 min	IN: 5–20 mg	IN: 64%–85% @ 2hrs	6–17 years old
Zolmitriptan	PO: 1–3 hrs	PO: 2.5–5 mg	PO: 28%–85% @ 2 hrs	6–18 years old
Almotriptan	PO: 1–3 hrs	PO: 6.25–12.5 mg	PO: 86% @ 4 hrs	11–17 years old
Rizatriptan	PO: 1–2 hrs	PO: 5 mg	PO: 56%–70% @ 1 hr	12–17 years old

278–282,284 Notes:RPCT = randomized placebo-controlled trials, OT = open trials, PO = per oral, SQ = subcutaneous, IN = intranasal, min = minutes, hr(s) = hour(s)
mg = milligrams, kg = kilograms, mcg = micrograms.
Source: Modified from References.276–281

Table 8-19 Chronic Preventative Migraine Therapy Studied in Randomized Placebo-Controlled or Open Trials

Drug	Dosage	Efficacy (approximate)	Ages Studied (RPCT or OT)
Serotonergic			
Cyproheptadine	2–8 mg/d	83%	3–12 years old
Pizotifen	1–1.5 mg/d	NS	7–14 years old
Antihypertensives			
Propranolol	1–4 mg/kg/d–120 mg/d	82%	6–16 years old
Clonidine	0.07–0.1 mcg/kg/d	NS	7–15 years old
Anticonvulsants			
Divalproex sodium	15–45 mg/kg/d 500–1000 mg/d	76%	7–17 years old
Topiramate	0.7–2.1 mg/kg/d	75%	8–15 years old
Levetiracetam	250–1500 mg/d	>placebo	3–17 years old
Gabapentin	15 mg/kg	80%	6–17 years old
Zonisamide	5.8 mg/kg/d	66%	10–17 years old
Antidepressants			
Amitriptyline	1 mg/kg/d–10 mg/d	80%–89%	3–15 years old
Trazadone	1 mg/kg	NS	7–18 years old
Calcium channel blockers			
Flunarazine	5 mg/d	66%	5–13 years old
Nimodipine	10–20 mg/d	NS	7–18 years old

Notes: RPCT = randomized placebo-controlled trials, OT = open trials, PO = per oral, SQ = subcutaneous, IN = intranasal, min = minutes, hr(s) = hour(s) mg = milligrams, kg = kilograms, mcg = micrograms, NS = nonsignificance compared to placebo.
Source: Modified from References.[278–284]

sufficiently powered, randomized, controlled, clinical trials data from which to guide most therapeutic decision making. The accompanying tables include those drugs that have had some study with randomized placebo-controlled trial or open-label trial data available. These tables are not all-inclusive; additional treatment options exist with less well-documented evidenced-based data. Within the previous sections, specific treatment approaches were enumerated for specific migraine syndromes; many of these recommendations are based on series, anecdotal evidence, and expert opinion pertaining to these specific syndromes. The additional tables here are provided as an overview to migraine therapy in children.

There is consensus that paramount to any intervention for childhood migraine the establishment of a clear diagnosis is needed. This may require more than one interview and supplementation of the history with a detailed diary calendar and symptom catalogue made by the patient or family. Defining exactly what the symptoms refer to and their meaning in the context of diagnosis will be necessary to further educate the child and family on what is important to observe and how to best intervene. An assessment of the impact the headache syndrome has upon the daily function of the child is also needed. This impact can be defined in terms of not just hours present but what changes in usual activity or routine are required as a direct result of the migraine itself. The identification of avoidable triggers is advisable but often not easily accomplished. Advising the family and patient on the general physiologic mechanisms of the migraine event may help to dispel undoubted pent-up anxiety with regard to the severity and consequences of each occurrence. Headache hygiene in terms of preventative measures and the development of a better tolerance to the migraine attacks when they surface is essential. Stressing the importance of regular exercise and sleep, good nutrition, and regular eating schedules, with an avoidance of trigger foods and excessive caffeine will be an important first step in prevention. Realistic expectations surrounding any treatment plan will have to be discussed explicitly. Overall management plans implementing nonpharmacologic and pharmacologic interventions need to be clear and initiated in a timely manner so as to avoid unnecessary prolongation of symptoms and increased disability. The consideration of using oral versus non-oral drug administration routes, antiemetics, and self-administered abortive and rescue medications when needed should be included in the plan. Attempts to limit the overuse of acute therapies should be encouraged so as to avert the development of rebound and overuse headache syndromes. Chronic preventative therapies would be advisable if the need to enlist acute therapies regularly approaches a weekly or more frequency.

REFERENCES

1. King NJ, Sharpley CF. Headache activity in children and adolescents. J Paediatr Child Health 1990; 26; 500–554.
2. Scheller JM. The history, epidemiology, and classification of headaches in childhood. Semin Pediatr Neurol 1995; 2(2); 102–108.
3. Vahlquist B. Migraine in children. Int Arch Allergy 1955; 7; 348–352.
4. Bille B. Migraine in school children. Acta Paediatr Scand 1962; 51(Suppl 136); 1–151.
5. Prensky AL, Sommer D. Diagnosis and treatment of migraine in children. Neurology 1979; 29; 506–510.
6. Headache Classification Committee of the International Headache Society. Classification and diagnostic criteria for headache disorders, cranial neuralgias and facial pain. Cephalalgia 1988; 8(Suppl 7); 1–96.
7. Winner P, Martinez W, Mante L, et al. Classification of pediatric migraine; proposed revisions to the IHS criteria. Headache 1995; 35; 407–410.
8. Oleson J. The Headache Classification Subcommittee of the International Headache Society. The International Classification of Headache Disorders. Cephalalgia 2004; 24(Suppl 1); 1–160.
9. Lewis DW. Migraine and Migraine Variants in Childhood and Adolescence. Semin Pediatr Neurol 1995; 2(2); 127–143.
10. Sillanpaa M. Prevalence of migraine and other headache in Finnish children starting school. Headache 1976; 15; 288–290.

11. Linet MS, Stewart WF, Celentano DD, et al. An epidemiologic study of headache among adolescents and young adults. JAMA 1989; 261; 2211–2216.
12. Sillanpaa M. Changes in the prevalence of migraine and other headaches during the first seven school years. Headache 1983; 23; 15–19.
13. Sillanpaa M, Piekkala P, Kero P. Prevalence of headache at preschool age in an unselected child population. Cephalalgia 1991; 11; 239–242.
14. Mortimer MJ, Kay J, Jaron A. Epidemiology of headache and childhood migraine in an urban general practice ad hoc, Vahlquist and IHS criteria. Dev Med Child Neurol 1992; 34; 1095–1101.
15. Abu-Arafeh I, Russel G. Prevalence of headache and migraine in schoolchildren. BMJ 1994; 309; 765–769.
16. Raieli V, Raimondo D, Cammalleri R, et al. Migraine headache in adolescents: a student population-based study in Monreal. Cephalalgia 1995; 15; 5–12.
17. Lu SR, Fuh JL, Juang KD, et al. Migraine prevalence in adolescents aged 13–15: a student population-based study in Taiwan. Cephalalgia 2000; 20(5); 479–485.
18. Al Jumah M, Awada A, Al Azzam S. Headache syndromes amongst schoolchildren in Riyadh, Saudi Arabia. Headache 2002; 42(4); 281–286.
19. Zwart JA, Dyb G, Holmen TL, et al. The prevalence of migraine and tension-type headaches among adolescents in Norway. The Nord-Trondelag Health Study (Head-HUNT-Youth), a large population-based epidemiological study. Cephalalgia 2004; 24(5); 373–379.
20. Split W, Neuman W. Epidemiology of migraine among students from randomly selected secondary schools in Lodz. Headache 1999; 39; 494–501.
21. Karli N, Akis N, Zarifoglu M, et al. Headache prevalence in adolescents aged 12 to 17: a student-based epidemiological study in Bursa. Headache 2006; 46(4); 649–655.
22. Lima MM, Padula NA, Santos LC. Critical analysis of the international classification of headache disorders diagnostic criteria (ICHD I-1988) and (ICHD II-2004). Cephalalgia 2005; 255(11); 1042–1047.
23. Hershey AD, Winner P, Kabbouche MA, et al. Use of the ICHD-II criteria in the diagnosis of pediatric migraine. Headache 2005; 45(10); 1288–1297.
24. Bille B. A forty-year follow-up of school children with migraine. Cephalalgia 1997; 17; 488–491.
25. Hockaday JM. Definitions, clinical features and diagnosis of childhood migraine. In *Migraine in Children*. Ed: Hockaday JM. London, England, Butterworth, 1988; 5–24.
26. Congdon PJ, Forsythe WI. Migraine in childhood: a study of 300 children. Dev Med Child Neurol 1979; 21; 209–216.
27. Goadsby PJ. Migraine pathophysiology. Headache 2005; 45(Suppl 1); S14–S24.
28. Russell MB. Genetic epidemiology of migraine and cluster headache. Cephalalgia 1997; 17; 683–701.
29. Ulrich V, Gervil M, Kyvik KO, et al. Evidence of a genetic factor in migraine with aura in a population-based Danish twin study. Ann Neurol 1999; 45; 242–246.
30. Carrera P, Stenirri S, Ferrari M, et al. Familial hemiplegic migraine: an ion channel disorder. Brain Res Bull 2001; 56; 239–241.
31. Ducros A, Denier C, Joutel A, et al. The clinical spectrum of familial hemiplegic migraine associated with mutations in a neuronal calcium channel. N Engl J Med 2001; 345; 17–24.

32. Haan J, Terwindt GM, Ferrari MD. Genetics of migraine. Neurol Clin 1997; 15; 43–60.

33. Kors EE, Terwindt GM, Vermeulen FL, et al. Delayed cerebral edema and fatal coma after minor head trauma: role of the CACNA1A calcium channel subunit gene and relationship with familial hemiplegic migraine. Ann Neurol 2001; 49; 753–760.

34. De Fusco M, Marconi R, Silvestri L, et al. Haploinsufficiency of ATP1A2 encoding the Na/K pump a2 subunit associated with familial hemiplegic migraine type 2. Nat Genet 2003; 33(2); 192–196.

35. Riant F, De Fusco M, Aridon P, et al. ATP1A2 mutations in 11 families with familial hemiplegic migraine. Hum Mutat 2005; 26(3); 281.

36. Dichgans M, Freilinger T, Eckstein G, et al. Mutation in the neuronal voltage-gated sodium channel SCN1A in familial hemiplegic migraine. Lancet 2005; 366; 371–377.

37. Bernard G, Shevell MI. Channelopathies: a review. J Child Neurol 2008; 38; 73–85.

38. Ducros A, Tournier-Lasserve E, Bousser MG. The genetics of migraine. Lancet Neurol 2002; 1(5); 285–293.

39. Blau JN. Migraine prodromes separated from the aura: complete migraine. BMJ 1980; 281; 658–660.

40. Cady RK, The convergence hypothesis. Headache 2007; 47(Suppl 1); S44–S51.

41. Dodick D, Silberstein S. Central sensitization theory of migraine: clinical implications. Headache 2006; 46(Suppl 4); S182–S191.

42. Sanchez-del-Rio M, Uwe R, Moskowitz MA. New insights into migraine. Curr Opin Neurol 2006; 19(3); 294–298.

43. Shields KG, Goadsby PJ. Serotonin receptors modulate trigeminovascular responses in ventroposteromedial nucleus of thalamus: a migraine target? Neurobiol Dis 2006; 23; 491–501.

44. Potrebic S, Ahn AH, Skinner K, et al. Peptidergic nociceptors of both trigeminal and dorsal root ganglia express serotonin 1D receptors: implications for the selective antimigraine action of triptans. J Neurosci 2003; 23(34); 10988–10997.

45. Leao AAP. Spreading depression of activity in the cerebral cortex. J Neurophysiol 1944; 7; 359–390.

46. Teive HAG, Kowacs PA, Filho M, et al. Leao's cortical spreading depression: from experimental "artifact" to physiological principle. Neurology 2005; 65; 1455–1459.

47. Ayata C, Jin H, Kudo C, et al. Suppression of cortical spreading depression in migraine prophylaxsis. Ann Neurol 2006; 59; 652–661.

48. Levy D, Burnstein R, Strassman AM. Mast cell involvement in the pathophysiology of migraine headache: a hypothesis. Headache 2006; 46(Suppl 1); S13–S18.

49. Dalkara T, Zervas NT, Moskowitz MA. From spreading depression to the trigeminovascular system. Neurol Sci 2006; 27; S86–S90.

50. Malick A, Burstein R. Peripheral and central sensitization during migraine. Funct Neurol 2000; 15(Suppl 3); 28–35.

51. Strassman AM, Levy D. Response properties of dural nociceptors in relation to headache. J Neurophysiol 2006; 95; 1298–1306.

52. Borsook D, Burstein R, Moulton E, et al. Functional imaging of the trigeminal system: applications to migraine pathophysiology. Headache 2006; 46(Suppl 1); S32–S38.

53. Bartolini M, Baruffaldi R, Paolino I, et al. Cerebral blood flow changes in the different phases of migraine. Funct Neurol 2005; 20(4); 209–211.

54. Cutrer FM, Black DF. Imaging findings of migraine. Headache 2006; 46; 1095–1107.

55. Weiller C, May A, Limmroth V. Brainstem activation in spontaneous human migraine attacks. Nat Med 1995; 1; 658–660.

56. Afridi SK, Giffin NJ, Kaube H, et al. A positron emission tomographic study in spontaneous migraine. Arch Neurol 2005; 62(8); 1270–1275.

57. Matharu MS, Cohen AS, McGonigle DJ, et al. Posterior hypothalamic and brainstem activation in hemicrania continua. Headache 2004; 44(8); 747–761.

58. Airy GB. On hemiopsy. The London, Edinburgh, and Dublin Philos Mag J Sci. 1865; 30; 19–21.

59. Airy H. On a distinct form of transient hemiopsia. Philos Trans R Soc 1870; 160; 247–264.

60. Lashley KS. Patterns of cerebral integration indicated by the scotomas of migraine. Arch Neurol Psychiatry 1941; 46; 331–339.

61. Schott GD. Exploring the visual hallucinations of migraine aura: the tacit contribution of illustration. Brain 2007; 130; 1690–1703.

62. Murray TJ. The neurology of Alice in Wonderland. Can J Neurol Sci 1982; 9(4); 453–457.

63. Golden GS. The Alice in Wonderland syndrome in juvenile migraine. Pediatrics 1979; 63(4); 517–519.

64. Evans RW, Rolak LA. The Alice in Wonderland syndrome. Headache 2004; 44(6); 624–625.

65. Hachinski VC, Porchawka J, Steele JC. Visual symptoms in the migraine syndrome. Neurology 1973; 23; 570–589.

66. Kirchmann M, Thomsen LL, Olesen J. Basilar-type migraine. Clinical, epidemiologic, and genetic features. Neurology 2006; 66; 880–886.

67. Al-Twaijiri WA, Shevell MI. Pediatric migraine equivalents: occurrence and clinical features in practice. Pediatr Neurol 2002; 26; 365–368.

68. Lai C-W, Ziegler DK, Lansky LL, et al. Hemiplegic migraine in childhood: diagnostic and therapeutic aspects. J Pediatr 1982; 101(5); 696–699.

69. Gascon G, Barlow CF. Juvenile migraine presenting as acute confusional states. Pediatrics 1970; 45; 628–635.

70. Jensen TS. Transient global amnesia in childhood. Dev Med Child Neurol 1980; 22; 654–667.

71. Bigal ME, Lipton RB, Cohen J, et al. Epilepsy and migraine. Epilepsy Behav 2003; 4; S13–S24.

72. Andermann F, Zifkin B. The benign occipital epilepsies of childhood: an overview of the idiopathic syndromes and of the relationship to migraine. Epilepsia 1998; 39; 9–23.

73. Andermann F. Migraine and the benign partial epilepsies of childhood: evidence for an association. Epileptic Disord 2000; 2; S37–S39.

74. Deprez L, Peeters K, Van Paesschen W, et al. Familial occipitotemporal lobe epilepsy and migraine with visual aura. Linkage to chromosome 9q. Neurology 2007; 68; 1995–2002.

75. Ludvigsson P, Hesdorffer D, Olafsson E, et al. Migraine with aura is a risk factor for unprovoked seizures in children. Ann Neurol 2006; 59; 210–213.

76. Kuo Y-T, Chiu N-C, Shen E-Y, et al. Cerebral perfusion in children with Alice in Wonderland syndrome. Pediatr Neurol 1998; 19; 105–108.

77. Parain D, Guegan-Massardier E, Lebas A, et al. Migraine aura lasting 1–24 hours in children: a sequence of EEG slow-wave abnormalities vs. vascular events. Cephalalgia 2007; 27; 1043–1049.
78. Lewis DW, Dorbad D. The utility of neuroimaging in the evaluation of children with migraine or chronic daily headache who have normal neurological examinations. Headache 2000; 40; 629–632.
79. Lewis DW, Ashwal S, Dahl G, et al. Practice parameter: evaluation of children and adolescents with recurrent headaches. Reprt of the Quality Standards Subcommittee of the American Academy of Neurology and the Practice Committee of the Child Neurology Society. Neurology 2002; 59; 490–498.
80. Knezevic-Pogancev M. Specific features of migraine syndrome in children. J Headache Pain 2006; 7; 206–210.
81. Russell MB, Iselius L, Olesen J. Migraine without aura and migraine with aura are inherited disorders. Cephalalgia 1996; 16; 305–309.
82. Svensson DA, Larsson B, Bille B, et al. Genetic and environmental influences on recurrent headaches in eight to nine year old twins. Cephalalgia 1999; 19(10); 866–872.
83. Gardner KL. Genetics of migraine: an update. Headache 2006; 46(Suppl 1); S19–S24.
84. Stewart WF, Bigal ME, Kolodner K, et al. Familial risk of migraine. Variation by proband age at onset and headache severity. Neurology 2006; 66; 344–348.
85. Russell MB, Olesen J. Increased familial risk and evidence of genetic factors in migraine. Br Med J 1995; 31; 541–544.
86. Winner P, Rothner AD, Putnam DG, et al. Demographic and migraine characteristics of adolescents with migraine: Glaxo Wellcome clinical trials' database. Headache 2003; 43; 451–457.
87. Guidetti V, Galli F. Evolution of headache in childhood and adolescence: an 8-year follow-up. Cephalalgia 1998; 18(7); 449–454.
88. Monastero R, Camarda C, Pipia C, et al. Prognosis of migraine headaches in adolescents. A 10-year follow-up study. Neurology 2006; 67; 1353–1356.
89. Wang SJ, Fuh JL, Juang KD, et al. Evolution of migraine diagnoses in adolescents: a 3-year annual survey. Cephalalgia 2005; 25; 333–338.
90. Mazzotta G, Carboni F, Guidetti V, et al. Outcome of juvenile headache in outpatients attending 23 Italian headache clinics. Italian Collaborative Study Group on Juvenile Headache (Societa Italiana Neuropsichiatria Infantile [SINPI]). Headache 1999; 39; 737–746.
91. Zebenholzer K, Wober C, Kienbacher C, et al. Migrainous disorder and headache of the tension-type not fulfilling the criteria: a follow-up study in children and adolescents. Cephalalgia 2000; 20; 611–616.
92. Lance JW, Anthony M. Some clinical aspects of migraine. Arch Neurol 1966; 15; 356–361.
93. Gascon G, Barlow C. Juvenile migraine presenting as an acute confusional state. Pediatrics 1970; 45; 628–635.
94. Emery ES. Acute confusional state in children with migraine. Pediatrics 1977; 60; 110–114.
95. Ehyai A, Fenichel GM. The natural history of acute confusional migraine. Arch Neurol 1978; 35; 368–369.
96. Brott T, Leviton A. Headache rounds: "violence". Headache 1976; 16; 203–209.
97. Jensen TS. Transient global amnesia in childhood. Dev Med Child Neurol 1980; 22; 654–667.

98. Haas DC, Pineda GS, Lourie H. Juvenile head trauma syndromes and their relationship to migraine. Arch Neurol 1975; 32; 727–730.

99. Evans RW, Gladstein J. Confusional Migraine or Photoepilepsy? Case History and Follow-up. Headache 2003; 43; 506–508.

100. Podoll K. Migraine art – the migraine experience from within. Cephalalgia 1998; 18; 376.

101. Willkinson M, Robinson D. Migraine art. Cephalalgia 1985; 5; 151–157.

102. Podoll K, Robinson D. Out-of-body experiences and related phenomena in migraine art. Cephalalgia 1999; 19; 886–896.

103. Lippman CW. Hallucinations of physical duality in migraine. J Nerv Ment Dis 1952; 117; 345–350.

104. Lippman CW. Certain hallucinations peculiar to migraine. J Nerv Ment Dis 1953; 116; 346–351.

105. Bickerstaff ER, Birm MD. Basilar artery migraine. Lancet 1961; 1; 15–17.

106. Kirchmann M. Migraine with aura: new understanding from clinical epidemiologic studies. Cur Opin Neurol 2006; 19; 286–293.

107. Cutrer FM, Baloh RA. Migraine-associated dizziness. Headache 1992; 32; 300–304.

108. Sturzenegger MH, Meinenberg O. Basilar artery migraine: a follow-up study of 82 cases. Headache 1985; 25; 408–415.

109. Neuhauser H, Leopold M, von Brevern M, et al. The interrelations of migraine, vertigo, and migrainous vertigo. Neurology 2001; 56; 436–441.

110. Golden GS, French JH. Basilar artery migraine in young children. Pediatrics 1975; 56; 722–726.

111. Liao LJ, Young YH. Vestibular evoked myogenic potentials in basilar artery migraine. Laryngoscope 2004; 114(7); 1305–1309.

112. Maytal J, Libman RB, Lustrin ES. Basilar artery migraine and reversible imaging abnormalities. Am J Neuroradiol 1998; 19; 1116–1119.

113. Ambrosetto P, Bacci A. Basilar artery migraine and reversible imaging abnormalities. Am J Neuroradiol 2000; 21; 234–235.

114. Ramelli GP, Sturzenegger M, Donati F, et al. EEG findings during basilar migraine attacks in children. Electroencephal & Clin Neurophysiol 1998; 107(5); 374–378.

115. De Romanis F, Buzzi MG, Assenza S, et al. Basilar migraine with electroencephalographic findings of occipital spike-wave complexes: a long-term study in seven children. Cephalalgia 1993; 13(3); 192–196.

116. Kinast M, Leuders H, Rothner AD, et al. Benign focal epileptiform discharges in childhood migraine (BFEDC). Neurology 1982; 32; 1309–1311.

117. Sand T. Electroencephalography in migraine: a review with focus on quantitative electroencephalography and the migraine vs. epilepsy relationship. [erratum appears in Cephalalgia. 2003 July; 23(6); 483]. Cephalalgia 2003; 23 (Suppl 1); 5–11.

118. Ambrosini A, D'Onofrio M, Grieco GS, et al. Familial basilar migraine associated with a new mutation in the *ATP1A2* gene. Neurology 2005; 65; 1826–1828.

119. Eriksen MK, Thomsen LL, Andersen I, et al. Clinical characteristics of 362 patients with familial migraine with aura. Cephalalgia 2004; 24; 564–575.

120. Marziniak M, Mossner R, Schmitt A, et al. A functional serotonin transporter gene polymorphism is associated with migraine with aura. Neurology 2005; 64; 157–159.

121. Borroni B, Brambilla C, Liberini P, et al. Functional serotonin 5-HTTLPR poly-morphism is a risk factor for migraine with aura. J Headache Pain 2005; 6; 182–184.

122. Todt U, Freudenberg J, Goebel I, et al Variation of the serotonin transporter gene SLC6A4 in the susceptibility to migraine with aura. Neurology 2006; 67; 1707–1709.

123. Loder E, Harrington MG, Cutrer M, et al. Selected confirmed, probable, and exploratory migraine biomarkers. Headache 2006; 46; 1108–1127.

124. Black DF. Sporadic and familial hemiplegic migraine: diagnosis and treatment. Semin Neurol 2006; 26(2); 208–216.

125. Thomsen LL. Familial hemiplegic migraine: update. Cephalalgia 2008; 28; 415–470.

126. Dodick D, Roarke M. Familial hemiplegic migraine: permanent attack-related neurologic deficits. Headache 2007; 47(8); 1210–1212.

127. Masuzaki M, Utsunomiya H, Yasumoto S, et al. A case of hemiplegic migraine in childhood: transient unilateral hyperperfusion revealed by perfusion MR imaging and MR angiography. Am J Neuroradiol 2001; 22; 1795–1797.

128. Gutschalk A, Kollmar R, Mohr A, et al. Multimodal functional imaging of prolonged neurological deficits in a patient suffering from familial hemiplegic migraine. Neurosci Lett 2002; 332; 115–118.

129. Jen JC, Bolthauser E, Cartwright MS, et al. Prolonged hemiplegic episodes in children due to mutations in ATP1A2. J Neurol Neurosurg Psychiatr 2007; 78; 523–526.

130. Vanmolkot KRJ, Stroink H, Koenderink JB, et al. Severe episodic neurological deficits and permanent mental retardation in a child with a novel FHM2 ATP1A2 mutation. Ann Neurol 2006; 59; 310–314.

131. Le Fort D, Safran AB, Picard F, et al. Elicited repetitive daily blindness: a new famil-ial disorder related to migraine and epilepsy. Neurology 2004; 63(2); 348–350.

132. Dichgans M, Herzog J, Freilinger T, et al. ^{1}H-MRS alterations in the cerebellum of patients with familial hemiplegic migraine type 1. Neurology 2005; 64; 608–613.

133. Kors EE, et al. Delayed cerebral edema and fatal coma after minor head trauma: role of the CACNA1A calcium channel subunit gene and relationship with familial hemiplegic migraine. Ann Neurol 2001; 49; 753–760.

134. Takahashi T, Arai N, Shimamura M, et al. Autopsy of acute encephalopathy linked to familial hemiplegic migraine with cerebellar atrophy and mental retardation. Neuropathology 2005; 25(3); 228–234.

135. Thomsen LL, Olesen J. Sporadic hemiplegic migraine. Cephalalgia 2004; 24(12); 1016–1023.

136. Thomsen LL, Ostergaard E, Romer SF, et al. Sporadic hemiplegic migraine is an aetiologically heterogeneous disorder. Cephalalgia 2003; 23; 921–928.

137. Terwindt G, Kors E, Haan J, et al. The International Hemiplegic Migraine Group. Mutation analysis of the CACNA1A calcium channel subunit gene in 27 patients with sporadic hemiplegic migraine. Arch Neurol 2002; 59; 1016–1018.

138. Vahedi, K, Denier C, Ducros A, et al. CACNA1A gene de novo mutation caus-ing hemiplegic migraine, coma, and cerebellar atrophy. Neurology 2000; 55(7); 1040–1042.

139. Ducros A, Denier C, Joutel A, et al. Recurrence of the T666M calcium chan-nel CACNA1A gene mutation in familial hemiplegic migraine with progressive cerebellar ataxia. Am J Hum Genet 1999; 64(1); 89–98.

140. Curtain RP, Smith RL, Ovcaric M, et al. Minor head trauma induced sporadic hemiplegic migraine coma. Pediatr Neurol 2006; 34; 329–332.

141. Jen JC, Wan J, Palos TP, et al. Mutation in the glutamate transporter EAAT1 causes episodic ataxia, hemiplegia, and seizures. Neurology 2005; 65; 529–534.

142. Wang H-S, Kuo MF, Chou ML, et al. Transcranial ultrasound diagnosis of intracranial lesions in children with headaches. Pediatr Neurol 2002; 26; 43–46.

143. Gee S. On fitful or recurrent vomiting. St. Bartholomew's Hosp Report. 1882; 18; 1–6.

144. Fleicher DR, Matar M. The cyclic vomiting syndrome: a report of 71 cases and literature review. J Pediatr Gastroenterol Nutr 1993; 17; 361–369.

145. Abu-Arafeh I, Russell G. Cyclical vomiting syndrome in children: a population-based study. J Pediatr Gastroenterol Nutr 1995; 21; 454–458.

146. Cullen K, MacDonald WB. The periodic syndrome. Its nature and prevalence. Med J Aust 1963; 2; 167–172.

147. Li BU. Cyclic vomiting: the pattern and syndrome paradigm. J Pediatr Gastroenterol Nutr 1995; 21(Suppl 1); S6–S10.

148. To J, Issenman RM, Kamath MV. Evaluation of neurocardiac signals in pediatric patients with cyclic vomiting syndrome through power spectral analysis of heart rate variability. J Pediatr 1999; 135(3); 363–366.

149. Rashed H, Abell TL, Familoni BO, et al. Autonomic function in cyclic vomiting syndrome and classic migraine. Digest Dis Sci 1999; 44(8 Suppl); 74S–78S.

150. Chelimsky TC, Chelimsky GG. Autonomic abnormalities in cyclic vomiting syndrome. J Pediatr Gastroenterol Nutr 2007; 44(3); 326–330.

151. Sato T, Igarashi N, Minami S, et al. Recurrent attacks of vomiting hypertension and psychotic depression: a syndrome of periodic catecholamine and prostaglandin discharge. Acta Endocrinol (Copenhagen) 1988; 117; 189–197.

152. Tache Y. Cyclic vomiting syndrome: the corticotrophin-releasing factor hypothesis. Dig Dis Sci 1999; 44(Suppl); 79S–86S.

153. Li BU, Balint J. Cyclic vomiting syndrome: evolution in our understanding of a braingut disorder. Adv Pediatr 2000; 47; 117–160.

154. Boles RG, Baldwin EE, Prezant TR. Combined cyclic vomiting and Kearns-Sayre syndromes. Pediatr Neurol 2007; 36; 135–136.

155. Boles RG, Powers LR, Adams K. Cyclic vomiting syndrome plus. J Child Neurol 2006; 21; 182–188.

156. Langmead F. On recurrent vomiting of childhood (cyclical vomiting), with the reports of two cases. BMJ 1905; 1; 350–352.

157. Li BU, Murray RD, Heitlinger LA, et al. Heterogeneity of diagnosis presenting as cyclic vomiting. Pediatrics 1998; 102; 583–587.

158. Li BU, Murray RD, Heitlinger LA, et al. Is cyclic vomiting syndrome related to migraine? J Pediatr 1999; 134(5); 567–572.

159. Haan J, Kors EE, Ferrari MD. Familial cyclic vomiting syndrome. Cephalalgia 2002; 22(7); 552–554.

160. Fleicher DR. Management of cyclic vomiting syndrome. J Pediatr Gastroenterol Nutr 1995; 21(Suppl 1); S52–S56.

161. Khasawinah TA, Ramirez A, Berkenbosch JW, et al. Preliminary experience with dexmedetomidine in the treatment of cyclic vomiting syndrome. Am J Therap 2003; 10; 303–307.

162. Andersen JM, Sugerman KS, Lockhart JR, et al. Effective prophylactic therapy for cyclic vomiting syndrome in children using amitriptyline or cyproheptadine. Pediatrics 1997; 100; 977–981.

163. Li BU. Cyclic vomiting: new understanding of an old disorder. Contemp Pediatr 1996; 13; 48–62.

164. Olmez A, Kose G, Turanli G. Cyclic vomiting with generalized epileptiform discharges responsive to topiramate therapy. Pediatr Neurol 2006; 35(5); 348–351.

165. Clouse RE, Sayuk GS, Lustman PJ, et al. Zonisamide or levetiracetam for adults with cyclic vomiting syndrome: a case series. Clin Gastroenterol Hepatol 2007; 5(1); 44–48.

166. Chepyala P, Svoboda RP, Olden KW. Treatment of cyclic vomiting syndrome. Curr Treat Options Gastroenterol 2007; 10(4); 273–282.

167. Russell G, Abu-Arafeh I, Symon DNK. Abdominal migraine: evidence for existence and treatment options. Paediatr Drugs 2002; 4(1); 1–8.

168. Mortimer MJ, Kay J, Jaron A. Clinical epidemiology of childhood abdominal migraine in an urban general practice. Dev Med Child Neurol 1993; 35; 243–248.

169. Catto-Smith AG, Ranuh R. Abdominal migraine and cyclical vomiting. Semin Ped Surg 2003; 12(4); 254–258.

170. Dignan F, Abu-Arafeh I, Russell G. The prognosis of childhood abdominal migraine. Arch Dis Child 2001; 84; 415–418.

171. Barabas G, Schempp Mathews W, et al. Childhood migraine and motion sickness. Pediatrics 1983; 72; 188–190.

172. Lee K. Abdominal migraine in childhood. Cephalalgia 2007; 27(C016); 633.

173. Abu-Arafeh I, Russell G. Prevalence and clinical features of abdominal migraine compared with those of migraine headache. Arch Dis Child 1995; 72; 413–417.

174. A technical report from the American Academy of Pediatrics Subcommittee and the North American Society for Pediatric Gastroenterology, Hepatology, and Nutrition Committee on Chronic Abdominal Pain. J Pediatr Gastroenterol Nutr 2005; 40; 249–261.

175. Aurora SK, Kori SH, Barrodale P, et al. Gastric stasis in migraine: more than just a paroxysmal abnormality during a migraine attack. Headache 2006; 46; 57–63.

176. Szilagyi A, Boor K, Orosz I, et al Contribution of serotonin transporter gene polymorphysims to pediatric migraine. Headache 2006; 46; 478–485.

177. Symon DN, Russell G. Double blind placebo controlled trial of pizotifen syrup in the treatment of abdominal migraine. Arch Dis Child 1995; 72; 48–50.

178. Worawatttanakul M, Rhoads JM, Lichtman SN, et al. Abdominal migraine prophylactic treatment and follow-up. J Pediatr Gastroenterol Nutr 1999; 28(1); 37–40.

179. Boccia G, Del Giudice E, Crisanti AF, et al. Functional gastrointestinal disorders in migrainous children: efficacy of flunarizine. Cephalalgia 2006; 26; 1214–1219.

180. Tan V, Sahami AR, Peebles R, et al. Abdominal migraine and treatment with intravenous valproic acid. Psychosom 2006; 47(4); 353–355.

181. Basser LS. Benign paroxysmal vertigo of childhood. Brain 1964; 87; 141–152.

182. Fenichel GM. Migraine as a cause of benign paroxysmal vertigo. J Pediatr 1967; 71; 114–115.

183. Koenigsberger MR, Chutorian AM, Gold AP, et al. Benign paroxysmal vertigo of childhood. Neurology 1970; 20; 1108–1113.

184. Watson P, Steele JC. Paroxysmal disequilibrium in the migraine syndrome of childhood. Arch Otolaryngol 1974; 99; 177–179.

185. Choung Y-H, Park K, Moon S-K, et al. Various causes and clinical characteristics in vertigo in children with normal eardrums. Int J Pediatr Otorhinolaringol 2003; 67(8); 889–894.
186. Erbek SH, Erbek SS, Yilmaz I, et al. Vertigo in childhood: a clinical experience. Int J Pediatr Otorhinolaringol 2006; 70(9); 1547–1554.
187. Balatsouras DG, Kaberos A, Assimakopoulos D, et al. Etiology of vertigo in children. Int J Pediatr Otorhinolaringol 2007; 71(3); 487–494.
188. Niemensivu R, Ilmari P, Kentala E. Vertigo and imbalance in children. Arch Otolaryngol Head Neck Surg 2005; 131; 996–1000.
189. Russell G, Abu-Arafeh I. Paroxysmal vertigo in children-an epidemiological study. Int J Pediatr Otorhinolaringol 1999; 49(Suppl 1); S105–S107.
190. Herraiz C, Calvin FJ, Tapia MC, et al. The migraine: benign paroxysmal vertigo of childhood complex. Int Tinnitus J 1999; 5(1); 50–52.
191. Chang C-H, Young Y-H. Caloric and vestibular evoked myogenic potential tests in evaluating children with benign paroxysmal vertigo. Int J Pediatr Otorhinolaringol 2007; 71; 495–499.
192. Rodoo P, Hellberg D. Creatinine kinase MB (CK-MB) in benign paroxysmal vertigo of childhood: a new diagnostic marker. J Pediatr 2005; 146; 548–551.
193. Bourgeois M, Aicardi J, Goutieres F. Alternating hemiplegia of childhood. J Pediatr 1993; 122; 673–679.
194. Aicardi J, Bourgeois M, Goutieres F. Alternating hemiplegia of childhood: clinical findings and diagnostic criteria. In *Alternating Hemiplegia of Childhood*. Eds: Andermann F, Aicardi J, Vigevano F. New York, Raven Press, 1995; 3–18.
195. Verret S, Steele JC. Alternating hemiplegia in childhood: a report of eight patients with complicated migraine beginning in infancy. Pediatrics 1971; 47; 675–680.
196. Hosking GP, Cavanaugh NPC, Wilson J. Alternating hemiplegia of childhood: complicated migraine of infancy. Arch Dis Child. 1978; 53; 656–659.
197. Dittrich J, Havlova M, Nevsimova S. Paroxysmal hemipareses of childhood of childhood. Dev Med Child Neurol 1979; 21; 800–807.
198. Krageloh I, Aicardi J. Alternating hemiplegia in infants: report of five cases. Dev Med Child Neurol 1980; 22; 784–791.
199. Rho JM, Chugani HT. Alternating hemiplegia of childhood: insights into its pathophysiology. J Child Neurol 1998; 13; 39–45.
200. Mikati M, Kramer U, Zupanc ML, et al. Alternating hemiplegia of childhood: clinical manifestations and long-term outcome. Pediatr Neurol 2000; 23(1); 134–141.
201. Zupanc ML, Dobkin JA, Perlman SB. ^{123}I-iodamphetamine SPECT brain imaging in alternating hemiplegia. Pediatr Neurol 1991; 7; 35–38.
202. Aminian A, Strashun A, Rose A. Alternating hemiplegia of childhood: studies of regional cerebral blood flow using ^{99m}Tc-hexamethylpropylene amine oxime single-photon emission computed tomography. Ann Neurol 1993; 33; 43–47.
203. Siemes H, Cordes M. Single-photon emission computed tomography investigations of alternating hemiplegia. Dev Med Child Neurol 1993; 35; 346–358.
204. Wong-Kisiel LC, Renaud DL, Collins DA. Single-photon emission computed tomography in a child with recurrent alternating hemiplegia and quadriplegia. Pediatr Neurol 2008; 38(3); 221–222.
205. Pfund Z, Chugani DC, Muzik O, et al. Alpha[11C] methyl-L-typtophan positron emission tomography in patients with alternating hemiplegia of childhood. J Child Neurol 2002; 17(4); 253–260.

206. Arnold DL, Silver K, Andermann F. Evidence for mitochondrial dysfunction in patients with alternating hemiplegia of childhood. Ann Neurol 1993; 33; 604–607.

207. Kemp GJ, Taylor DJ, Barnes PR, et al. Skeletal muscle mitochondrial dysfunction in alternating hemiplegia of childhood. Ann Neurol 1995; 38(4); 681–684.

208. Rust RS, Thomas A, Zupanc ML. 1H volume localized in vivo magnetic resonance spectroscopy and single-photon emission computed tomography in alternating hemiplegia. Ann Neurol 1992; 32; 452.

209. Nezu A, Kimura S, Ohtsuki N, et al. Alternating hemiplegia of childhood: report of a case having a long history. Brain & Dev 1997; 19; 217–221.

210. Auvin S, Joriot-Chekaf S, Cuvellier JC, et al. Small vessel abnormalities in alternating hemiplegia of childhood. Neurology 2006; 66; 499–504.

211. Ruchoux MM, Maurage CA. CADASIL: cerebral autosomal dominant arteriopathy with subcortical infarcts and leukoencephalopathy. J Neuropathol Exp Neurol 1997; 56; 947–964.

212. Rinalduzzi S, Valeriani M, Vigevano F. Brainstem dysfunction in alternating hemiplegia of childhood: a neurophysiological study. Cephalalgia 2006; 26(5); 511–519.

213. Becker L. Alternating hemiplegia of childhood: a neuropathologic review. In: *Alternating Hemiplegia of Childhood*. Eds: Andermann F, Aicardi J, Vigevano F. New York, Raven Press, 1995; 57–65.

214. Kramer U, Nevo Y, Margalit D, et al. Alternating hemiplegia of childhood in half-sisters. J Child Neurol 2000; 15(2); 128–130.

215. Mikati M, Maguire H, Barlow CF, et al. A syndrome of autosomal dominant alternating Hemiplegia: clinical presentation mimicking intractable epilepsy; chromosomal studies; physiologic investigations. Neurology 1992; 42; 2251–2257.

216. Kanavakis E, Xaidara A, Papathanasiou-Klontza D, et al. Alternating hemiplegia of childhood: a syndrome inherited with an autosomal dominant trait [erratum appears in Dev Med Child Neurol. 2004 April; 46(4); 288] Dev Med Child Neurol 2003; 45(12); 833–836.

217. Swoboda KJ, Kanavakis E, Xaidara A, et al. Alternating Hemiplegia of Childhood or Familial Hemiplegic Migraine?: a novel ATP1A2 Mutation. Ann Neurol 2004: 55; 884–887.

218. Bassi MT, Bresolin N, Tonelli A, et al. A novel mutation in the ATP1A2 gene causes alternating hemiplegia of childhood. J Med Genet 2004; 41; 621–628.

219. Chaves-Vischer V, Picard F, Andermann E, et al. Benign nocturnal alternating hemiplegia of childhood: six patients and long-term follow-up. Neurology 2001; 57(2); 1491–1493.

220. Silver K, Andermann F. Alternating hemiplegia of childhood: a study of 10 patients and results of flunarizine treatment. Neurology 1993; 43; 36–41.

221. Sasaki M, Sakuragawa N, Osawa M. Long-term effect of flunarizine on patients with alternating hemiplegia of childhood in Japan. Brain & Devel 2001; 23; 303–305.

222. Neville BGR, Ninan M. The treatment of alternating hemiplegia of childhood. Dev Med Child Neurol 2007; 49; 777–780.

223. Sone K, Oguni H, Katsumori H, et al. Successful trial of amantadine hydrochloride for two patients with alternating hemiplegia of childhood. Neuropediatr 2000; 31; 307–309.

224. Snyder CH. Benign paroxysmal torticollis in infancy. A possible form of labyrynthitis. Am J Dis Child 1969; 117; 458–460.
225. Deonna T, Martin D. Benign paroxysmal torticollis in infancy. Arch Dis Child 1981; 56; 956–958.
226. Hanukoglu A, Somekh E, Fried D. Benign paroxysmal torticollis of infancy. Clin Pediatr 1984; 23; 272–274.
227. Cataltepe SU, Barron TF. Benign paroxysmal torticollis presenting as "seizures" in infancy. Clin Pediatr 1993; 32; 564–565.
228. Roulet E, Deonna T. Benign paroxysmal torticollis in infancy. Dev Med Child Neurol 1988; 30; 409–410.
229. Andermann F, Ohtahara S, Andermann E, et al. Infantile hypotonia and paroxysmal dystonia – a variant of alternating hemiplegia of childhood. Mov Disord 1994; 9; 227–229.
230. Dunn DW, Snyder CH. Benign paroxysmal vertigo of childhood. Am J Dis Child 1976; 130; 1099–1100.
231. Sanner G, Bergstrom B. Benign paroxysmal torticollis in infancy. Acta Paediatr Scan 1979; 68; 219–223.
232. Drigo P, Carli G, Laverda A M. Benign paroxysmal torticollis of infancy. Brain & Devel 2000; 22(3); 169–172.
233. Cohen HA, Nussinovitch M, Ashkenasi A, et al. Benign paroxysmal torticollis in infancy. Pediatr Neurol 1993; 9; 488–490.
234. Kimura S, Nezu A. Electromyographic study in an infant with benign paroxysmal torticollis. Pediatr Neurol 1998; 19; 236–238.
235. Ducros A, Denier C, Joutel A, et al. The clinical spectrum of familial hemiplegic migraine associated with mutations in a neuronal calcium channel. N Engl J Med 2001; 345; 17–24.
236. Giffin NJ, Benton S, Goadsby PJ. Benign paroxysmal torticollis of infancy: four new cases and linkage to CACN1A mutation. Dev Med Child Neurol 2002; 44; 490–493.
237. Thijs RD, Kruit MC, van Buchem MA, et al. Syncope in migraine. The population-based CAMERA study. Neurology 2006; 66; 1034–1037.
238. Shapiro WR, Williams GH, Plum F. Spontaneous recurrent hypothermia accompanying agenesis of the corpus callosum. Brain 1969; 92; 423–436.
239. Arroyo HA, DiBlasi M, Grinszpan G. A syndrome of hyperhydrosis, hypothermia, and bradycardia possibly due to central monoamine dysfunction. Neurology 1990; 40; 556–557.
240. Arroyo HA, DiBlasi M, Fejerman N. Episodic spontaneous hypothermia with hyperhydrosis. Pediatr Neurol 1994; 11; 266.
241. Arroyo HA, DiBlasi M, Fejerman N. Episodic hypothermia with sweating and bradycardia without habeas callosum agenesis: a new syndrome? Brain Dev (abstract) 1991; 12; 625.
242. Sheth RD, Barron TF, Harlage PL. Episodic spontaneous hypothermia with hyperhydrosis: implications for pathogenesis. Pediatr Neurol 1994; 10; 58–60.
243. Ruiz C, Gener B, Garaizar C, et al. Episodic spontaneous hypothermia: a periodic childhood syndrome. Pediatr Neurol 2003; 28; 304–306.
244. Klingler ET, Meyer K. Shapiro's Syndrome: a Renewed Appreciation for Vital Signs. Clin Infect Dis 2004; 38; e107–e108.

245. Kloos RT. Spontaneous periodic hypothermia. Medicine (Baltimore) 1995; 74; 268–280.
246. Walker BR. Anderson JA, Edwards CR. Clonidine therapy for Shapiro's syndrome. Q J Med 1992; 82; 235–245.
247. Goh KYC, Conway EJ, DaRosso RC, et al. Sympathetic storms in a child with a midbrain glioma: a variant of diencephalic seizures. Pediatr Neurol 1999; 21; 742–744.
248. Penfield W. Diencephalic autonomic epilepsy. Arch Neurol Psychiatry 1929; 22; 358–374.
249. Solomon GE. Diencephalic autonomic epilepsy caused by a neoplasm. J Pediatr 1973; 83; 277–280.
250. Talman WT, Florek G, Bullard DE. A hyperthermic syndrome in two subjects with acute hydrocephalus. Arch Neurol 1988; 45; 1037–1040.
251. Bullard DE. Diencephalic seizures: responsiveness to bromocriptine and morphine. Ann Neurol 1987; 21; 609–611.
252. McClean AJ. Autonomic epilepsy: report of a case with observation at necroscopy. Arch Neurol Psychiatry 1934; 32; 189.
253. Engle GL, Aring CD. Hypothalamic attacks with thalamic lesion. I. Physiologic and psychologic considerations. II. Anatomic considerations. Arch Neurol Psychiatry 1945; 54; 37–44.
254. Boeve BF, Wijdicks EFM, Benarroch EE, et al. Paroxysmal sympathetic storms (diencephalic seizures) after severe diffuse axonal head injury. Mayo Clin 1998; 73; 148–152.
255. Baguley IJ, Nicholls JL, Felmingham KL, et al. Dysautonomia after traumatic brain injury: a forgotten syndrome? J Neurol Neurosurg Psychiatr 1999; 67(1); 39–43.
256. Baguley IJ, Heriseanu RE, Gurka JA, et al.. Gabapentin in the management of dysautonomia following severe traumatic brain injury: a case series. J Neurol Neurosurg Psychiatr 2007; 78(5); 539–541.
257. Do D, Sheen VL, Bromfield E. Treatment of paroxysmal sympathetic storm with labetalol. J Neurol Neurosurg Psychiatr 2000; 69(6); 832–833.
258. Shuper A, Packer RJ, Vezina LG, et al. "Complicated migraine-like episodes" in children following cranial irradiation and chemotherapy. Neurology 1995; 45; 1837–1840.
259. Murthy SN, Cohen ME. Pseudomigraine with prolonged aphasia in a child with cranial irradiation for medulloblastoma. J Child Neurol 2002; 17; 134–138.
260. Bartleson JD, Krecke KN, O'Neill BP, et al. Reversible, strokelike migraine attacks in patients with previous radiation therapy. Neuro-oncol 2003; 5; 121–127.
261. Lachance DH, Black DF, Bartleson JD. SMART: stroke-like migraine attacks after radiation therapy. Neurology 2005; 64(Suppl 1); A220.
262. Partap S, Walker M, LongstrethWT, et al. Prolonged but reversible migraine-like episodes long after cranial irradiation. Neurology 2006; 66; 1105–1107.
263. Pruitt A, Dalmau J, Detre J, et al. Episodic neurologic dysfunction with migraine and reversible imaging findings after radiation RRH. Neurology 2006; 67; 676–678.
264. Solomon S. John Graham Senior Clinicians Award Lecture. Posttraumatic migraine. Headache 1998; 38(10); 772–778.
265. Bennett DR, Fuenning SI, Sullivan G, et al. Migraine precipitated by head trauma in athletes. Am J Sports Med 1980; 8(3); 202–205.

266. Ashworth B. Migraine, head trauma and sport. Scot Med J 1985; 30(4); 240–242.
267. Espir ML, Hodge IL. Matthews PH. Footballer's migraine. BMJ 1972; 3(5822); 352.
268. Matthews WB. Footballer's migraine. Am Heart J 1973; 85(2); 279–280.
269. Lucas RN. Footballer's migraine. BMJ 1972; 2(5812); 526.
270. Neinstein L, Milgrom E. Trauma-triggered migraine and acute confusional migraine. J Adolesc Health 2000; 27(2); 119–124.
271. Harrison DW. Walls RM. Blindness following minor head trauma in children: a report of two cases with a review of the literature. J Emerg Med 1990; 8(1); 21–24.
272. Kaye EM, Herskowitz J. Transient post-traumatic cortical blindness: brief versus prolonged syndromes in childhood. J Child Neurol 1986; 1(3); 206–210.
273. Sakas DE, Whittaker KW, Whitwell HL, et al. Syndromes of posttraumatic neurological deterioration in children with no focal lesions revealed by cerebral imaging: evidence for a trigeminovascular pathophysiology. Neurosurgery 1997; 41(3); 661–667.
274. Packard RC, Ham LP. Pathogenesis of posttraumatic headache and migraine: a common headache pathway? Headache 1997; 37(3); 142–152.
275. McBeath JG, Nanda A. Roller coaster migraine: an underreported injury? Headache 2000; 40(9):745–747.
276. Jacome DE. Basilar artery migraine after uncomplicated whiplash injuries. Headache 1986; 26; 515–516.
277. Rao DS, Infeld MD, Stern RC, et al. Cough-induced hemiplegic migraine with impaired consciousness in cystic fibrosis. Pediatr Pulmonol 2006; 41; 171–176.
278. Pakalnis A. Current therapies in childhood and adolescent migraine. J Child Neurol 2007; 22(11); 1288–1292.
279. Balottin U, Termine C. Recommendations for the management of migraine in paediatric patients. Expert Opin Pharmacother 2007; 8(6); 731–744.
280. Hamalainen ML. Migraine in children and adolescents. A guide to drug therapy. CNS Drugs 2006; 20(10); 813–820.
281. Mathew NT, Kailasam J, Meadors L. Early treatment with rizatriptan: a placebo controlled study. Headache 2004; 44; 669–673.
282. Lewis D, Ashwal S, Hershey A, et al. Silberstein S. Practice parameter: pharmacological treatment of migraine headache in children and adolescents. Report of the American Academy of Neurology Quality Standards Subcommittee and the Practice Committee of the Child Neurology Society. Neurology 2004; 63; 2215–2224.
283. Lewis D. Toward the definition of childhood migraine. Curr Opin Pediatr 2004; 16; 628–636.
284. Damen L, Jacques KJ, Bruijn JKJ, et al. Symptomatic Treatment of Migraine in Children: a Systematic Review of Medication Trials. Pediatrics 2005; 116; e295–e302.

9

Further Considerations

INTRODUCTION

In the previous chapters an organization and description of the clinical conditions and epidemiology of non-epileptic paroxysmal childhood disorders was presented. These entities individually and as a group can in many instances be mistakenly considered diagnostically for epileptic seizures.[1–6] An emphasis has been placed upon phenomenon that display variations in normal childhood behavior and physiologic functioning with special consideration to other pathological conditions that require additional identification, further investigation, and treatment. Although many events have a distinctive clinical character (e.g., severe breath-holding spells), there are many others that require prior clinical experience beyond a detailed description (e.g., alternating hemiplegia of childhood) and some that necessitate selected laboratory evaluation to clarify their exact nature (e.g., opsoclonus-myoclonus-ataxia syndrome).

OVERVIEW

Although there is neither an absolute nor a foolproof approach to arriving at the correct non-epileptic diagnosis, there are logical means to do so. There is no substitution for the direct observation of the clinical event by the clinician. However, in the absence of such direct observation, substitute methods with home video or, at the very least, careful detailed parental observations will assist immeasurably. A simple stratification into those elements of the history which suggest that the child experiences an alteration in consciousness or that the events happen during sleep versus those events where neither of these elements are present will help to direct a reasonable thought process.[1,3] Further clinical distinctions can be made by the subsequent identification of other specific critical signposts or "nodal points" (Table 9-1). Implicit in all diagnostic endeavors is the continual follow-up of the patient to assure that the expected natural course of disease is evolving. Deviations from an expected clinical course for a given diagnostic entity should prompt rethinking of the problem and reconsideration of other diagnostic possibilities.

The clinician must always be mindful of the patient who may have multiple diagnoses that are not always mutually exclusive. This point is generally emphasized with respect to the concurrence of epileptic seizures and psychogenic non-epileptic seizures. Although this emphasis is deserved, there are

Table 9-1 Clinical Nodal Points

Elements

- Specific provocatives
- Autonomic symptoms
- Color changes
- Alterations in respiratory pattern (apnea, hyperventilation, breath holding, etc.)
- Enuresis
- Emesis
- Eye deviations
- Vertigo
- Abrupt changes in mood and behavior
- Involuntary movements
- Alteration in posture and/or muscle tone
- Event recollection
- Exclusive observers

other equally compelling concurrences: epileptic seizures and breath-holding spells, syncope and non-epileptic seizures, and sleep disorders with an involuntary movement disorder, among others. By the same token, the presence of a somatoform disorder may develop from or occur concurrently with an organically definable entity. The fact that many children develop this de novo does not exclude a child with a readily explicable non-epileptic disorder to additionally develop a conversion disorder at a later time. Often the most problematic and certainly most critical entity to identify is the factitious disorder, especially when it concerns childhood Munchausen by proxy abuse. The evanescent nature of the complaints together with the often perplexing and dramatic symptomatology without identifiable cause should always arouse suspicion.

The concepts of symptom evolution and contextual age deserve emphasis here as well. Certain symptoms may well define a specific entity in younger ages, whereas other symptomatology defines the same entity at older ages. Conversely, the same diagnostic symptomatology at one age may be more specific of another diagnostic entity when present at another age. These are best evidenced by the many types of migraine manifestations encountered in childhood. In infants, paroxysmal torticollis may evolve into paroxysmal vertigo as a migraine variant when a child reaches the toddler age. The same symptoms of paroxysmal torticollis or vertigo in adolescents may signal the onset of an involuntary movement disorder or of peripheral vestibular disease, respectively, rather than that of migraine in view of this age context.

The contribution of a detailed family history can be immensely contributory when other family members are encountered with similar phenomena as presented by the child under evaluation. This contribution is apparent for clear genetic entities, such as some of the various movement disorders (e.g., the paroxysmal dyskinesias) but also in those disorders with a "familial" component, such as chronic tic disorder, several sleep disorders, and migraines.

Perhaps less familiar examples of this contribution but equally as relevant are the familial patterns noted with the development of syncope and breath-holding spells, somatization disorder, and Munchausen by proxy abuse in children of affected parents. Many other clinical entities described in prior chapters of the book refer to the currently known inheritance patterns. As more children are precisely identified with specific non-epileptic disorders, the relationship to genetic contribution and familial occurrence will become clearer.

It must be reemphasized that despite our best efforts at syndrome delineation and differentiation of and from epilepsy, there exists a significant fraction of children for whom a definitive diagnosis cannot be identified. This uncertain diagnosis does not include the even more important proportion of children for whom an incorrect diagnosis of epilepsy has been given. A misdiagnosis of epilepsy in children with non-epileptic events can be as high as 39%.[7–11] The identification of an inappropriate diagnosis may ultimately be arrived at only after repeated evaluations or in view of serendipitous findings.[7–11] Thus, the concept of a "suspected" diagnosis or comfort with the idea of an "uncertain" or "unclassified paroxysmal event" diagnosis should be accepted.[12]

FINAL CONSIDERATIONS

Episodic Behavioral Syndromes

A number of behavioral events can be confused as epileptic. Young children are generally easily recognized when temper tantrums occur. These are usually situation specific, gradual in escalation, and goal directed. The child may follow the parent or guardian to another location if they remove themselves from the child's presence. There is no loss of consciousness and/or deliberate self-injury. Older children and adolescents, however, may escalate the behavior beyond simple interventions. The potential for self-injury, injury to others, or destruction of property is much greater because of the size of the child and the nature of the attacks. Previously described as rage attacks or episodic dyscontrol, these attacks are more appropriately diagnosed as part of **Intermittent Explosive Disorder** (IED), now defined in the DSM-IV-TR (Table 9-2).[13,14] These episodes are discrete and extreme, often preceded by a sense of tension or arousal. The child fails to resist their innate aggressive impulses, which results in serious assaults (physical or verbal) to others and destruction of valued property. There must be a degree of aggression that is clearly far out of proportion to the initial stress or trigger. Later, the individual may feel upset, remorseful, regretful, or embarrassed about the aggressive behavior. A diagnosis of IED can only be made after the exclusion of other causative mental disorders, effects of a substance, or another general medical condition. They are suddenly provoked, behaviorally extreme to the point of verbal and physical violence, and directed toward a specific individual. There is a degree of

Table 9-2 Intermittent Explosive Disorder

Diagnostic Criteria for Intermittent Explosive Disorder (312.34)

1. Several discrete episodes of failure to resist aggressive impulses that result in serious assaultive acts or destruction of property.
2. The degree of aggressiveness expressed during the episodes is grossly out of proportion to any precipitating psychosocial stressors.
3. The aggressive episodes are not better accounted for by another mental disorder (e.g., antisocial personality disorder, borderline personality disorder, a psychotic disorder, a manic episode, conduct disorder, or attention deficit/hyperactivity disorder) and are not due to the direct physiological effects of a substance (e.g., a drug of abuse, a medication) or a general medical condition (e.g., head trauma, Alzheimer's disease).

Source: Modified from Reference.[13]

irrationality, and the individual often reports only a vague recollection of their actions afterwards.[13, 14] Data suggest that mood disorders, anxiety disorders, eating disorders, substance use disorders, and other impulse-control disorders may be associated with IED.[13, 15] Children may have experienced prior severe temper tantrums, impaired attention, hyperactivity, and other behavioral difficulties, such as stealing and fire setting. An association with chronic tic disorders has also been noted. There is a lifetime prevalence estimate of 5.4%–7.3% in persons 18 years of age and older, and a mean age of onset of 14 years old.[15]

Other Ocular Phenomenon

Camfield and colleagues have described nineteen children with idiopathic generalized epilepsy and photosensitivity who also exhibited **non-epileptic paroxysmal eyelid fluttering**.[16] Each child had paroxysmal attacks of eyelid movement that differed from absence seizures. The observed eyelid fluttering attacks were characterized by initial slow eyelid closure, rapid eyelid flutter, and strong upward eye deviation, without loss of consciousness or epileptiform EEG correlation.[16] The attacks could be initiated voluntarily or precipitated by stress. The attacks are slow, and halting with complete (or nearly complete) eyelid closure. The eyelids flutter at 8–10 Hz, with contracted facial muscles (upper and lower), raised eyebrows, and no automatisms.[16] Fine "twitchy" movements around the lips were observed in a single patient. Most importantly, there is complete preservation of consciousness. The children could speak and respond to questioning and commands without hesitation. The mothers of 5/19 children were also observed to display similar eyelid fluttering without evidence of epilepsy. In seven other cases, there was a history of similar eye movements in second-degree relatives.

A less well described phenomenon identified in late adolescence and young adulthood is that of transient benign unilateral pupillary dilation.[17–19] This can mimic the initial ictal changes of partial seizures or potentially a post-ictal finding. The pupillary asymmetry has been measured to be as much as

4–5 mm with preserved reactivity and consensual response, with an otherwise completely normal neurological examination.[17–19] The pupillary dilatation has lasted up to 24–48 hours. Precipitants have been identified as sleep deprivation, caffeine consumption, and later development of migraine headache, but no homogeneous etiologic cause has been clearly identified.[17–19] A number of other specific causes of mydriasis must be considered as exclusionary in order to be confident of the benign nature of the phenomenon in each individual patient.

In Closing

As more careful observation and clinical characterization of additional childhood paroxysmal phenomenon are reported, it is apparent that we will all benefit from a broader understanding and deeper appreciation for the many non-epileptic childhood paroxysmal events that befall our children.

REFERENCES

1. DiMario FJ. Paroxysmal non-epileptic events of childhood. Semin Pediatr Neurol 2006; 13; 208–221.
2. Fenichel GM. Paroxysmal disorders, In *Clinical Pediatric Neurology, A Signs and Symptoms Approach*, 5th edition. Philadelphia, PA, W.B. Saunders Co., 2005; 1–45.
3. DiMario FJ. The nervous system. In Rudolph's *Fundamentals of Pediatrics*. Eds: AM Rudolph, RK Kamei, KJ Overby. 3rd edition. New York, Mcgraw Hill, 2002; 796–846.
4. Kotagal P, Costa M, Wyllie E, et al. Paroxysmal nonepileptic events in children and adolescents. Pediatrics 2002, 110:e46.
5. Chaves-Carballo E. Syncope and paroxysmal disorders other than epilepsy. In *Pediatric Neurology: Principles & Practice*. Eds: Swaiman KF, Ashwal S, Ferriero DM. 4th edition. Philadelphia, PA, Mosby-Elsevier, 2006; 1209–1223.
6. Paolicchi JM. The spectrum of non-epileptic events in children. Epilepsia 2002; 43(Suppl 3); 60–64.
7. Scheepers B, Clough P, Pickles C. The misdiagnosis of epilepsy: findings of a population study. Seizure 1998; 7; 403–406.
8. Stroink H, van Donselaar CA, Geerts AT, et al. The accuracy of the diagnosis of paroxysmal events in children. Neurology 2003; 60; 979–982.
9. Leach JP, Lauder R, Nicolson A, et al. Epilepsy in the UK: Misdiagnosis, mistreatment, and undertreatment? The Wrexham area epilepsy project. Seizure 2005; 14; 514–520.
10. Somoza MJ, Forienza RH, Brussino M, et al. Epidemiological survey of epilepsy in the primary school population in Buenos Aires. Neuroepidemiology 2005; 25; 62–68.
11. Uldall P, Alving J, Hansen LK, et al. The misdiagnosis of epilepsy in children admitted to a tertiary epilepsy centre with paroxysmal events. Arch Dis Child 2006; 91; 219–221.
12. Beach R, Reading R. The importance of acknowledging clinical uncertainty in the diagnosis of epilepsy and non-epileptic events. Arch Dis Child 2005; 90; 1219–1222.

13. *Diagnostic and Statistical Manual of Mental Disorders (DSM-IV-TR)*, 4th edition, text revision, Arlington, VA: American Psychological Association, 2000.
14. Elliott FA. The episodic dyscontrol syndrome and aggression. Neurol Clin 1984; 2; 13–20.
15. Kessler RC, Coccaro EF, Fava M, et al. The prevalence and correlates of DSM-IV intermittent explosive disorder in the National Comorbidity Survey replication. Arch Gen Psychiatr 2006; 63; 669–678.
16. Camfield CS, Camfield PR, Sadler M, et al. Paroxysmal eyelid movements. A confusing feature of generalized photosensitive epilepsy. Neurology 2004; 63; 40–42.
17. Edelson RN, Levy DE. Transient benign unilateral pupillary dilation in young adults. Arch Neurol 1974; 31; 12–14.
18. Hallett M, Cogan DG. Episodic unilateral mydriasis in otherwise normal patients. Arch Ophthalmol 1970; 84; 130–136.
19. Walsh FB, Hoyt WF. *Clinical Neuro-Ophthalmology* 3rd edition. Baltimore, MD: Williams & Wilkins Co., 1969, 523.

Index

Note: In this index, tables are indicated by "t", figures by "f"

A

abdominal migraine syndrome, 321–323,
   321t
abdominal pain, in conversion disorder, 184
abuse, illness falsification disorder by proxy,
   179
acetazolamide, for infant apnea, 121
acetylcholine
   projections of, 237t
   in sleep, 111t
actigraph, 103
active standing test (AST), in syncope
   evaluation, 50
adenoidectomy, for OSA, 124
adenosine, in sleep, 111t
adenotonsillar hypertrophy, OSA due to,
   122–123
adolescent(s)
   movement disorders in, 256–261
      BHDS, 259–260
      EPT, 260–261
      head tremor, 258–259
      non-epileptic head drops, 258
      transient tics, 256–258, 257t
   non-epileptic childhood paroxysmal
      disorders in
      autonomic and sensory phenomena as
        presenting features in, 34t, 35–36
      ocular movements/deviations, 33t
      paroxysmal paralysis or collapse as
        presenting feature in, 29t
      paroxysmal posturing, shaking, jerking,
        or twitching as presenting feature of,
        31t
adult-onset breath-holding spells, 179
adult somatization disorder, development of,
   181–182

age
   as factor in conversion disorder, 182
   as factor in habit movements, 250t
   as factor in migraine, 299–300
   in interpretation of normal sleep behavior
      and sleep architecture, 106–108
AHC. *see* alternating hemiplegia of childhood
   (AHC)
akathasia, 220t
algorithmic approach, in non-epileptic
   childhood paroxysmal disorders, 25–26
"Alice in Wonderland" syndrome, 311
ALTE. *see* apparent life threatening events
   (ALTE)
alternating hemiplegia
   of childhood, in non-epileptic childhood
      paroxysmal disorders, 29–30
   non-paroxysmal clinical characteristics of,
      329t
   paroxysmal clinical characteristics of,
      328t–329t
alternating hemiplegia of childhood (AHC),
   326–333, 327t–329t
Ambulatory Sentinel Practice Network
   (ASPN), in somatoform disorder, 181
American Academy of Neurology, Quality
   Standards Subcommittee of, 306
American Academy of Pediatrics
   OSA treatment guidelines of, 124
   on snoring studies, 124
American Professional Society on the Abuse of
   Children (APSAC), 205
   gamma-aminobutyric acid (GABA)
      for cyanotic breath holders, 60
      projections of, 237t
      in sleep, 111t
anemia, BHS and, 57–58
anhidrosis (HSAN type IV), 72–73